Clinics in Developmental Medicine No. 143/144

NEUROPHYSIOLOGY AND NEUROPSYCHOLOGY
OF MOTOR DEVELOPMENT

© 1997 Mac Keith Press
High Holborn House, 52–54 High Holborn, London WC1V 6RL

Senior Editor: Martin C.O. Bax
Editor: Pamela A. Davies
Managing Editor: Michael Pountney
Sub Editor: Pat Chappelle

Set in Times and Avant Garde on QuarkXPress

The views and opinions expressed herein are those of the authors and do not necessarily represent those of the publisher

First published in this edition 1997

British Library Cataloguing-in-Publication data:
A catalogue record for this book is available from the British Library

ISSN: 0069 4835
ISBN: 1 898683 10 7

Printed by The Lavenham Press Ltd, Water Street, Lavenham, Suffolk
Mac Keith Press is supported by **Scope** (formerly The Spastics Society)

Clinics in Developmental Medicine No. 143/144

Neurophysiology & Neuropsychology of Motor Development

Edited by

KEVIN J. CONNOLLY
University of Sheffield
Sheffield, England

HANS FORSSBERG
Karolinska Institute
Stockholm, Sweden

1997
Mac Keith Press

Distributed by 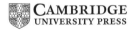 **CAMBRIDGE**
UNIVERSITY PRESS

CONTENTS

CONTRIBUTORS

J. Armand

CNRS, Laboratoires de Neuroscience Cognitives, 31 Chemin Joseph Aiguier, 13402 Marseille Cédex 20, France

P. Ashby

Toronto Hospital, Western Division, Playfair Neuroscience Unit, MTP 13-319, 399 Easthurst Street, Toronto, Ontario M5T 2S8, Canada

J. Keith Brown

Edinburgh Sick Children's NHS Trust, Royal Hospital for Sick Children, Sciennes Road, Edinburgh EH9 1LF, Scotland

E. Cafarelli

Toronto Hospital, Western Division, Playfair Neuroscience Unit, MTP 13-319, 399 Easthurst Street, Toronto, Ontario M5T 2S8, Canada

L.J. Carr

Wolfson Centre, Institute of Child Health, Mecklenburgh Square, London WC1N 2AP, England

Kevin J. Connolly

Department of Psychology, University of Sheffield, Western Bank, Sheffield S10 2TP, England

Ester Cotton

19 Lambole Road, London NW3 4HS, England

Volke Dietz

Schweizerisches Paraplegikerzentrum, Universitätsklinik Balgrist, Frochstrasse 340, 8008 Zürich, Switzerland

S.A. Edgley

Department of Anatomy, University of Cambridge, Downing Street, Cambridge CB2 3DY, England

Andrew Lloyd Evans

Department of Child Health, Royal Free Hospital, Pond Street, London NW3 2QG, England

Hans Forssberg

Motor Control Laboratory, Department of Pediatrics, St Görans Hospital, 11281 Stockholm, Sweden

A.M. Gordon

Department of Movement Science, Box 119, Teachers College, Columbia University, 525 West 120th Street, New York, NY 10027, USA

David N. Lee

Perception in Action Laboratories, Department of Psychology, University of Edinburgh, 7 George Square, Edinburgh EH8 9JZ, Scotland

R.N. Lemon

Sobell Department of Neurophysiology, National Hospital for Neurology and Neurosurgery, Queen Square, London WC1N 3BG, England

J-P. Lin

Guy's Hospital, St Thomas' Street, London SE1 9RT, England

Edison deJ. Manoel

Departamento de Pedagogica do Movimento do Corpo Humano, Escola de Educação Física, Universidade de São Paulo, Av Prof Mello Morais, 65 - Butanta, São Paulo - SP, CEP: 05508-900, Brazil

Dafne Matiello

Department of Exercise and Movement Science, College of Arts and Sciences, Eugene, OR 97403-1240, USA

P. Vernon McDonald

Krug Life Sciences, 1290 Hercules Drive, Suite 120, Houston, TX 77058, USA

M.D. Neilson

Cerebral Palsy Research Unit, The Prince Henry Hospital, Little Bay, NSW 2036, Australia

P.D. Neilson

Cerebral Palsy Research Unit, The Prince Henry Hospital, Little Bay, NSW 2036, Australia

Karl M. Newell

Department of Kinesiology, Pennsylvania State University, 109 White Building, University Park, PA 16802, USA

N.J. O'Dwyer

Cerebral Palsy Research Unit, The Prince Henry Hospital, Little Bay, NSW 2036, Australia

E. Olivier

Sobell Department of Neurophysiology, National Hospital for Neurology and Neuro-surgery, Queen Square, London WC1N 3BG, England

Tarek Omar

Edinburgh Sick Children's NHS Trust, Royal Hospital for Sick Children, Sciennes Road, Edinburgh EH9 1LF, Scotland

Mary O'Regan

Edinburgh Sick Children's NHS Trust, Royal Hospital for Sick Children, Sciennes Road, Edinburgh EH9 1LF, Scotland

E. Palmer

Toronto Hospital, Western Division, Playfair Neuroscience Unit, MTP 13-319, 399 East-hurst Street, Toronto, Ontario M5T 2S8, Canada

Heinz F.R. Prechtl

Department of Physiology, University of Graz, Harrachgasse 21/5, A-8010 Graz, Austria

Peter L. Rosenbaum

Department of Pediatrics, McMaster University Medical Centre, 1200 Main Street West, Hamilton, Ontario L8N 3ZS, Canada

David Scrutton

Wolfson Centre, Institute of Child Health, Meck-lenburgh Square, London WC1N 2AP, England

J.A. Stephens

Department of Physiology, University College London, Gower Street, London WC1E 6BT, England

Beverly D. Ulrich

Motor Development Laboratory, Kinesiology Department, Indiana University, Bloom-ington, IN 47405, USA

Claes von Hofsten

Department of Psychology, Umea University, S-90187 Umea, Sweden

Marjorie Woollacott   Department of Exercise and Movement
                             Science, College of Arts and Sciences,
                             Eugene, OR 97403-1240, USA

FOREWORD

This book brings together insights from clinical and basic sciences to normal and pathological motor development. The developmental perspective on any neurological function is inevitably more difficult than study of the mature (adult) situation. Developmental neuroscience requires age-appropriate assessment tools and a dialogue between those with technological skills, developmental neurobiologists and clinicians. The importance of input from pathological conditions to the study of normal development is in the natural experiments that occur. This field sets rigorous standards for clinical case and problem definition which is only recently becoming possible in the central motor disorders of early onset: the cerebral palsies. This group of conditions is clinically unsatisfactory because of an arbitrary focus upon motor aspects of an impairment complex that may include epilepsy, and cognitive, special and general sensory and psychiatric disorders. It is also biologically flawed because of the wide range of pathologies from periventricular leucomalacia to cortical dysplasias that are included within a single phenotype, *e.g.* congenital hemiplegia. Notwithstanding the eventual need for pathogenetically based separation of syndromes for scientific study, the editors' view that research into motor function had something important to say now about this difficult group of disorders is, I think, justified by the high quality of the chapters. Nevertheless, the gap between good science and effective treatment remains wide. We should expect an attempt to close this gap by those working in the field and, increasingly, we should expect more sophisticated case definition than 'the child with diplegia' or even 'the cerebral palsied child'.

The opening chapter is a comprehensive review of the embryological and behavioural aspects of human motor development. It is paired with a helpful review of the seminal work of the Groningen group on fetal movements by Heinz Prechtl—that such studies have been taken up so slowly outside Holland is surprising.

The chapter by Forssberg and Dietz on normal and impaired locomotor development is an excellent review of neurophysiological research which has produced a clear outline of levels of motor control and how these should be measured in normal and pathological situations. It is followed by a most helpful and original description of locomotor development in children with cerebral palsy by Scrutton and Rosenbaum. It contains critical reviews of problematic issues such as 'quality of movement'. It also brings the now widely used Gross Motor Function Measure into a dialogue with those concerned with pathological and therapeutic sequences of development. A number of neurophysiologically oriented chapters explore maturational issues in both normal and pathological conditions/circumstances; convincing evidence for reorganization in the nervous system at spinal cord level in early unilateral cerebral cortical damage is provided by Carr and Stephens. The account of the development of skilled action and the corticospinal tract by Lemon, Armand, Olivier and Edgley is masterly. One of the high points of the book is a series of three chapters focused on 'grasping' which will inform those wishing to perform research in this area.

There is in this book one most extraordinary and original chapter on 'Perception in action approach to cerebral palsy', taking the form of a dialogue, which rewards close study. It is followed by a helpful synthesis of work on the development of skilled action by Manoel and Connolly and contributions on current research into integrated models for motor actions from a developmental perspective.

This book is a very high quality review of the state of motor research in the context of pathology in the developing human nervous system. The writers are leaders in their field and are to be congratulated in putting so much of their time and energy at the service of disabled people, their professional advisers and investigators in the field. It is an essential book for those researching in the area of motor development and developmental disorders of action for whom it may provide anything from the methodology for solving a problem to the conclusion that the research is ill advised.

One hopes that this group will keep in contact and assist the development of the cross-disciplinary research for which this book provides the groundwork.

BRIAN NEVILLE, FRCP
Professor of Paediatric Neurology,
Institute of Child Health (UCL) and
Great Ormond Street Hospital for
Children NHS Trust, London

PREFACE

Much of the important work on child development during the first half of the 20th century was concerned with motor development. The appearance and mastery of static and dynamic balance, crawling, locomotion, reaching, grasping, etc., were all described and the pattern and timing of their appearance carefully charted. When this was accomplished concern shifted to other aspects of development. However, as is the way in science, attention has switched back again to the development of skilled action and the control of movements with the appearance of new techniques and concepts. Over the past decade there have been important advances in our understanding of the mechanisms underlying behaviour and we are on the threshold of many more.

This book is based on the first Mac Keith Meeting held at the Royal Society of Medicine in London in 1994. The participants in the meeting and the contributors to this volume are drawn from a wide range of disciplines and specialities and from several countries. One of the ideas which lay behind the planning of the meeting was the desirability of making connections across what is now a large and complex interplay of ideas and approaches: connections between levels of explanation, normal and pathological processes, basic and clinical research, and so forth. Underlying themes, therefore, are: linking neurophysiological and psychological explanations, pre- and postnatal behaviour, input and output processes; ballistic and graded movements; stability and variability; and so on. We hope that the range and juxtaposition of ideas presented will tempt specialists in one area to acquaint themselves with the ideas and approaches developed by those in others, and thus lay sound foundations for an applied science of movement.

Research on motor development is important for a number of reasons, not least because of the many individuals who suffer from movement disorders. Most of the therapeutic programmes for children with movement disorders lack an adequate scientific base which is necessary for testing treatment strategies and essential for formulating new approaches. If this book contributes to linking clinical and scientific effort it will serve a good purpose.

KEVIN CONNOLLY
HANS FORSSBERG

1
BRAIN DEVELOPMENT AND THE DEVELOPMENT OF TONE AND MOVEMENT

J. Keith Brown, Tarek Omar, Mary O'Regan

In examining the adult nervous system we are dealing with either a relatively static system or one which is in decline. The neurological examination is similarly static, but the paediatric neurologist in contrast must learn not only to examine the various components of the nervous system but also when developmental landmarks occur and the distribution of their timing in a population. For example, in Edinburgh 50% of infants can take five steps by their first birthday whereas only 20% of preterm infants can take five steps unaided one year from their expected date of delivery. Does this constitute a developmental disorder or a neurological abnormality? Some families, particularly of shufflers, have children who do not walk until about 20 months. Should this slow and different pattern of development be regarded as abnormal, or is it a normal variant? A further important point for the neurologist is that many of the abnormalities seen in clinical practice such as spinal flexor tone, decerebration, decortication and ataxia can also be explained in developmental terms. When the child first walks the gait is broad based, the arms are held out to the side and foot strike is flat. The gait is in fact classically ataxic and has been called physiological ataxia. In this chapter we shall restrict our consideration to development from 12 weeks of gestation to 12 months of postnatal age. Knowledge of development *in utero* has been advanced by the availability of ultrasonography and magnetic resonance imaging (MRI), and development after birth can now be studied from gestations as low as 23 weeks as increasing numbers of these extremely immature infants survive.

The brain is a developing organ

The development of the brain can be considered in a series of phases (Table 1.1). The process is epigenetic in character and not predetermined, genetic information interacting with non-genetic (environmental) factors in the creation of the system. The role of the extrinsic factors is complicated. The ectodermal cells which transform into the neural plate do so because of induction through contact with chordomesoderm tissues; without such induction they develop into skin. Neural development is not a simple linear progressive increase in the numbers of cells and their connections, it also includes remodelling processes by pruning connections and removing excess cells.

The ectoderm itself has the ability to differentiate along many different lines, for example into skin, spinal cord, thyroid, melanocytes and sympathetic ganglia. This is called prospective potency. The prospective potency of the neuroectoderm gradually undergoes

TABLE 1.1
Phases of brain development

1. Cell division and specification in subependymal germinal matrix
2. Cell migration along the Bergmann glial fibres
3. Cell differentiation
4. Cell long process, axon, formation
5. Myelination
    Rapid phase—long association fibres
    Slow phase—short association fibres
6. Dendritic maturation, Nissl substance formation, synaptogenesis
7. Cell death and dissolution, terminal axon pruning, synaptic stabilization
8. Dominance
9. Psychogenesis
10. Full brain maturity
11. Senescence

restriction until it will differentiate only as a neural tissue when translocated to another site in the embryo or when isolated in *in vitro* culture. This restriction, known as determination, occurs in two overlapping phases. First, activation of the ectoderm by the underlying chordomesoderm determines the size and form of the neural plate and also results in the development of forebrain structures. Second, transformation of the already activated neuro-ectoderm is brought about by interaction with mesoderm and results in the development of more caudal structures of the nervous system. Various inducer substances are involved in brain development. Which part of the brain differentiates depends not only on the specific inducer substance but also on its concentration and the timing of exposure (Sharpe *et al.* 1987, Dixon and Kintner 1989).

By the fifth week after conception the spinal cord is closed and three primitive vesicles (prosencephalon, mesencephalon and rhombencephalon) are already well demarcated, with the rostral flexures and the primitive cerebral hemispheres and cerebellar placode easily visible.

The telencephalon and the diencephalon develop from the anterior of the three cerebral vesicles, the prosencephalon. The eyes, thalami, globus pallidus and hypothalamus develop from the diencephalon, therefore when development fails, *i.e.* anencephaly occurs, the eyes and thalami are usually well formed. The two telencephalic vesicles are joined at the lamina terminalis, and as they grow the lamina does not become more infolded to the anterior end of the third ventricle. If this fails then a single holosphere, *i.e.* holoprosencephaly, results.

The thin walled primitive telencephalic vesicle is most marked in the occipital pole by day 40 and in the temporal pole by day 50, even though the temporal archicortex is phylogenetically older than the neocortex over the surface of the hemispheres.

Histogenesis (cell division)
The neurons and glia of the cerebral cortex are formed in the subependymal germinal layer, a stratified neuroepithelium which surrounds the lateral ventricle including the temporal lobe. It regresses after 28 weeks gestation when it is the site of subependymal haemorrhage.

It regresses last of all in the region of the head of the caudate nucleus. The cells are pre-programmed in all mammals for a set number of divisions and for a predetermined destination. The stem cells themselves change shape from elongated to round and move towards the ependyma; they then divide into two by mitosis, one daughter cell migrating to the cortical plate along a glial fibre and the other moving back higher into the ventricular zone ready to undergo the next of its programmed number of divisions. This up and down movement of the stem cells is called interkinetic nuclear migration. Most neurons destined for the human neocortex are produced between eight and 20 weeks of gestation (Casaer 1993). The second DNA increase between 20 and 40 weeks of gestation is the result of glial cell proliferation. The number of divisions each cell undergoes is genetically determined and is similar in other mammals (Brodal 1992). The neuroectodermal cells reach their maximum volume in the ventricular or germinal zone around the 26th gestational week.

Migration

A basic feature of central nervous system (CNS) development is that most cells are generated in sites different from those at which they will reside in the mature organ. This principle of migration is particularly clear in the case of cerebral cortex formation. The cells find their way to the distant cortex using the Bergmann glial fibres as guides. The radially oriented glial cells themselves ultimately disappear, many transforming into astrocytes (Sidman and Rakic 1974, Casaer 1993). Radial migration seems to be more important than tangential migration in the human cerebral cortex, although tangential migration occurs in the formation of the external granular layer of the cerebellum.

These glial 'guide wires' are attached at both ventricular/ependymal and cortical surfaces. The outer pial membrane, also formed by the foot processes of the radial glial cells, offers a barrier to the distance travelled by the cells unless it is breached as in some cortical dysplasias. The primitive cells are obligatory anaerobes and are not killed by cyanide or glutamate agonists. There are very few capillaries and so the cells derive their nutrition from glycogen which is abundant in the glial fibres. This substrate store is obtained at pial and ventricular surfaces where there is a blood supply. The primitive cells swarm up the fibres by amoeboid movement at a rate of about 1 mm per day (Fig. 1.1). Genetically determined diseases such as neurofibromatosis, tuberous sclerosis and Zellweger syndrome interfere with the programmed migration, while toxins such as cocaine and alcohol also affect cells during their migration (Marret *et al.* 1995).

The last cells to leave the germinal matrix travel the furthest to the outermost parts of the cortex; known as the 'inside out' rule, this enables the gyral pattern to form. The first migration forms the deepest cortical layer, the next population of neurons moves through the deepest cortical layer to form the second layer, and so on until the six cortical layers are formed. The final position of the migrating cells is dictated by their interaction with processes of other cells, a positioning mechanism which is extrinsic to the cell itself and independent of the migration mechanism (Sidman and Rakic 1974). Chemotropism is important in guidance and regulation of migration, *e.g.* fibronectin and laminin are thought to be associated with the glial fibres and cerebroglycan and astrotactin with the migrating cells. It is believed that the layer of the cerebral cortex to which the cell migrates is predetermined

3

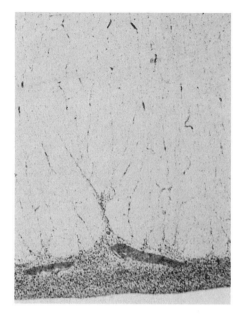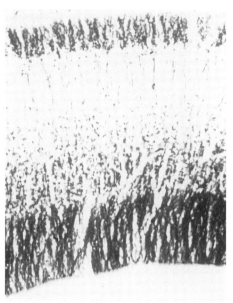

Fig. 1.1. *(Left)* The germinal layer, showing faint lines of the glial fibres along which the primitive neuroblasts swarm to form the cerebral cortex. *(Right)* The very vascular subependymal layer with cells migrating upwards in columns.

at the time of mitosis in the germinal matrix, and if transferred to another embryo the cell will continue to form neurons in the same predetermined layer of cortex.

Each 'guide wire' in all mammalian species allows 130 cells to move into vertical arrays in the future cortex. The Bergmann glial fibres themselves comprise bundles of about eight fibres which fan out as they reach the cortical plate, permitting about 1000 cells to form a unit in the cerebral cortex which may be the embryological basis of the learning modules described later. The cerebral cortex can therefore be regarded like a computer as made up of millions of individual learning units or modules, *i.e.* similar to electronic chips.

Differentiation and maturation
Four fundamental embryonic zones can be distinguished at different depths in the developing telencephalon. From the external surface to the ventricle, they are as follows.
• *The marginal zone.* This, the outermost zone, initially contains only the cytoplasmic processes of cells whose nuclei are at deeper levels. Later it becomes sparsely populated by neurons that form layer I of the cerebral cortex, which is the first cortical layer to develop. By 12 weeks of gestation there is an external granular layer in the cerebral cortex similar to that in the cerebellum, but it is not thought that tangential migration of cells moving inwards from this layer is important compared to radial migration from the ventricular zone outwards.
• *The intermediate zone.* This develops as a result of the ingrowth of afferent axons and

4

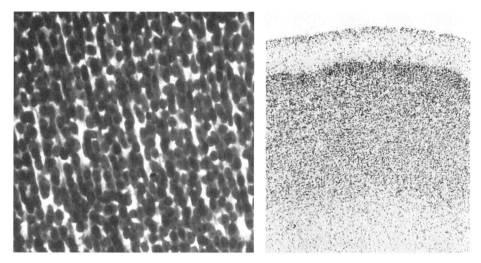

Fig. 1.2. *(Left)* High magnification view of the cerebral cortex at 14 weeks gestation showing the columns of primitive neuroblasts. *(Right)* Low magnification view of a non-stratified cerebral cortex.

the migration of cells to form the cortical plate. As the cells and fibres continue to invade this zone, the cortical plate undergoes progressive differentiation to form the definitive layers of the cerebral cortex.

• *The subventricular zone.* This zone, also known as the subependymal zone, contains proliferating cells that mainly give rise to macroglia (astrocytes and oligodendrocytes). The zone persists after birth. While its role in gliogenesis during the early postnatal period is well established, its only role in adult life may be to replace glial cells. The subventricular cells have been considered a potential source of gliomas and it is one of the commonest sites for brain tumours induced by chemical carcinogens. The incidence of glial tumours in different species is directly related to the size of the residual subventricular zone in the adult brain of that species.

• *The ventricular zone.* This contains the ventricular germinal cells. It is the first zone to develop, giving rise to the other zones and disappearing at an early stage of development.

The migrated primitive cells are arranged first, up to the 16th gestational week, in vertical columns of deeply staining cells looking like a neuroblastoma (Fig. 1.2). The neuroblasts differentiate into neurons with the axon pointing in the correct direction. Dendrites form and arborize, synapses form, excess dendrites and synapses are pruned and Nissl substance and neurofibrils appear; the neuron has to develop an association with the astrocytes and their foot processes and becomes aerobic. There are hundreds or thousands of different cells in the CNS depending on how they are classified: size, shape, position, Nissl, dendritic pattern, axonal direction and arborization, etc.

Dendrites appear first in the brainstem and thalamus, and the resultant increase in synapses requiring ATP means that they become aerobic and thus susceptible to damage earlier. The Rohon–Beard cells and large pyramidal neurons migrate and differentiate first,

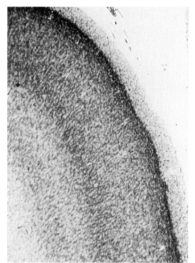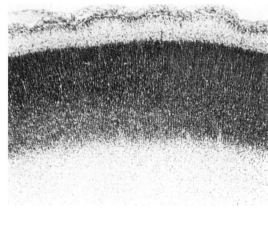

Fig. 1.3. *(Left)* The completely unstratified cortex with primitive darkly staining neuroblast cells. *(Right)* Development of stratification between 18 and 22 weeks gestation.

followed by small local intracortical circuit neurons and finally glia. Glial cells can divide once migrated, whereas neurons cannot. Microglia are not really glia because they do not arise from glioblasts but are mesodermal cells. The cells gradually become organized into the six layers of the cortex and spread out with a horizontal pattern replacing the primitive vertical stratification of the cell layers (Fig. 1.3). The oldest cells by the inside out rule are layer 6, and the youngest the subpial, so maturation occurs inside out, layers 6–1. The six layers of cerebral cortex develop from 16 weeks in an odd sequence of 5 – 6 – 3 (c, b then a) – 4 – 2 – 1. The granule cells of the fourth and second layers are particularly slow to differentiate, doing so around 38–40 weeks (Marin-Padilla 1988). This gives rise to the gradual increase in gyrification of the cortex.

In the precentral gyrus, area 4 of the motor cortex, the arrival of afferent fibres follows a regular sequence, occurring in each layer before and during the time of arrival of neurons in that layer. The first fibres arrive in layer I and are followed by the Cajal–Retzius cells, which are the first neurons to originate and to differentiate in the human motor cortex. Thereafter, the pyramidal cells of layers VI and V can be seen at 5 months gestation. These are followed by the interneurons of layer IV (cortical basket cells) around the seventh prenatal month, then the pyramidal cells of layer III, and finally those of layer II can be readily recognized at 7.5 months gestation (Jacobson 1978). The greatest disruption is seen in lissencephaly or pachygyrias. In polymicrogyria, layer 5 is absent. This is the first layer to become aerobic, and it can be disrupted by glutamate in the extremely immature infant at about 20–24 weeks, before the other layers have formed or become aerobic (Marret *et al.* 1995). Towards 30 weeks when more layers are aerobic, ulegyria is more common, and by term full cortical thickness neuronal necrosis occurs following hypoxic–ischaemic damage or experimental glutamate toxicity. In severe failure of the cortical plate one sees a radial microbrain in which only a very tiny brain (50 g) is seen at term. In true genetic primary microcephaly the cells of layer 2 are always absent.

Neuronal development

In general, large neurons are produced before the small ones in any part of the nervous system and those produced last are invariably local circuit neurons. In the retina, the ganglion cells are formed first; in the cerebellar cortex, the Purkinje cells; and in the cerebral cortex, the pyramidal cells. Furthermore, there is a tendency for motor nuclei to commence their histogenesis and complete their cell populations before the sensory nuclei at the same level of the neuraxis, and for the histogenesis of the motor system to have a shorter duration than that of the sensory system. Each distinct set of neurons originates in a fairly invariant timetable. Thus, in any one neuronal set (which may contain several neuronal types) the entire population of each type of neuron completes the final cell cycle and becomes permanently postmitotic within a relatively short period, and in each region they are always produced before their associated glial cells. Glial cells in any region withdraw from the mitotic cycle over a much longer time than the neurons in the same region. It has been concluded that neurons stimulate proliferation of glial cells, as evidenced by failure of production of glial cells after the death of the associated neurons.

The first sign of differentiation of the neuron is the obvious increase of the amount of rough endoplasmic reticulum as well as smooth cytoplasmic membranes. The final degree of development is related directly to the characteristic amount of Nissl substance finally attained by a particular type of cell. Nissl substance consists of cisternae of rough endoplasmic reticulum made of RNA. All these changes reflect the increase in protein synthesis associated with cellular growth and differentiation. Other aspects of cellular differentiation include an increase in the numbers of mitochondria, neurofilaments and neurotubules (Jacobson 1978).

The thickness of the cortex continues to increase, *e.g.* Broca's area grows rapidly in the first postpartum month although it does not reach adult thickness until 4 years. By 25 weeks gestation the pyramidal cells are differentiating but have no shape, no basal dendrites and a very tortuous apical dendrite with a prominent growth cone. By 3 years the pyramidal cell is morphologically complete; the discharge in the axon is a result of summation from the dendritic tree. The first synapses in the human cerebral cortex develop at about 23 weeks gestation (Molliver *et al.* 1973).

Lamination starts at 25 weeks and the dendritic explosion is at 32 weeks. Spines appear on the dendrites, the small pyramidal cells also mature in the last trimester, and dendritic trees increase ten fold in the first three months after birth. The gradual increase in area of the cerebral cortical mantle shows as increased surface infolding and gyral formation (Fig. 1.4). The corpus callosum, neurons from the thalamus and association areas all end as axo-dendritic synapses on dendritic spines which fatten and shorten when contact is made.

Development of glial cells

Neuroglial cells or macroglia include astrocytes and oligodendrocytes. Neurons are all

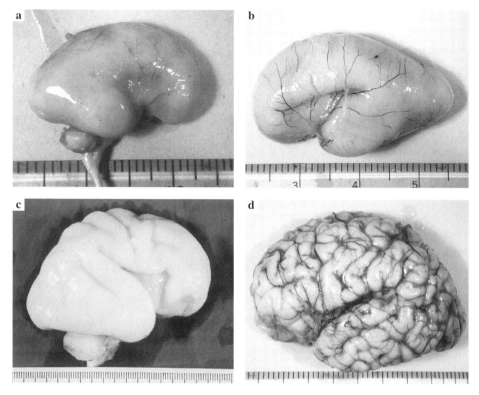

Fig. 1.4. Increasing gyral development between 16, 24, 32 weeks and term (a–d respectively).

formed in the germinal plate by 20 weeks of gestation, and it is from 20 to 28 weeks that the so-called second DNA spurt occurs with division and migration of the glioblast precursor of glial cells. These cells then migrate to organize themselves in the cerebral cortex in the case of astrocytes, and to align with axons in the case of oligodendroglia. Macroglia are ectodermal in origin, whereas microglia are of mesodermal origin. During the early stages of development their precursors, the Bergmann glial cells, function as guides to the migrating neurons, but later after neurogenesis has ceased they too are transformed into mature astrocytes in layers 3, 4 and 5, and oligodendrocytes.

Microglia, on the other hand, are true macrophages. They are mesodermal in origin, and remove the debris of cells that die (apoptosis) during normal development. They are especially numerous in those regions where massive cell death occurs during a short period of development, *e.g.* the subependymal germinal matrix.

The matured astrocytic cells organize themselves into the neuronal unit with some astrocyte foot processes attached to a blood vessel, the others attached to the neuron. This helps to form the blood–brain barrier, and the astrocyte acts as a 'mother cell' for the neuron. It also acts in a similar fashion to an hepatocyte, storing glycogen, detoxifying ammonia and maintaining the ionic concentration, *e.g.* of potassium in the extracellular fluid. The astrocyte is also mobilized after cell death, *i.e.* neuronal necrosis, from ischaemia or infection, to form the fibrillary glial scar of CNS healing.

The oligodendroglia are responsible for myelination, which occurs mainly postnatally in the human infant: they align themselves along the developed axon, wind cell membrane around up to 15 axons, and lay down myelin in the membrane.

Type 1 astrocytes develop earlier from a different glioblast precursor than oligodendroglia and type 2 astrocytes. The type 1 astrocyte is necessary to drive the other glial precursor through a set number of divisions. Two growth factors, platelet-derived growth factor (PDGF) and ciliary neurotrophic factor (CNTF), both of which are derived from type 1 astrocytes, are also necessary. If CNTF is high, a type 2 astrocyte is formed, and if PDGF is low an oligodendrocyte is formed. Glioblasts are very susceptible to chemical carcinogens, while neurons and their stem cells are greatly resistant to the same agents. Virtually all tumours induced by carcinogens are gliomas.

Growth of axons and establishment of specific connections

Neurites must grow from the pyramidal neurons as efferents and from the thalamus and midbrain tegmentum as afferents. Little is known about what guides the axons of, for instance, a Betz cell in the leg area towards the flexor hallucis longus, but it seems to be predetermined. A swelling develops at the end of the primitive axon forming an organelle or growth cone which contains mitochondria, microtubules and microfilaments. Continuous formation of membrane, microtubules and microfilaments is obviously necessary for continued growth in length. The membranous surface of the growth cone is covered with numerous different receptors, and the growth cone appears to release transmitter substances in its movements. The cone also puts out spikes or filopodia which are mobile and contain both muscle proteins, *i.e.* actin and myosin, and so can probe around. Laminar extensions issue transiently from the growth cone as the structure 'feels its way along' (Caviness 1989).

Axons grow best in groups on an adherent surface along a 'Laminin Lane', and are attracted by certain chemicals and repelled by other so-called guidance molecules (chemotropism). The neurite will actively withdraw in tissue culture from certain cells and be attracted to others. They are also affected by weak electrical fields. Substances such as lamellin and integrin are known to affect the neural filopodia in their search for target end organs. Semaphorins as their name suggests signal which way to go.

While growing, the axons must find their way and recognize the neurons with which they are going to establish synaptic contact. They may encounter many neurons without establishing synaptic contacts due to diffusable neuromodulators which repel them. After arriving in the target region, only some of the many neurons make synaptic contact with the ingrowing axons.

Many more contacts are made than will eventually be required, so dying back and synaptic stabilization will eventually prune an overexuberant system. Cells from the nasal part of the retina are destined to be connected topographically to a specific part of the superior colliculus; cells and membrane from the anterior tectum produce chemicals which attract neurites from one half of the retina and repel those from the other half. Moreover, axons have a tendency to grow along other axons, so that if a few pioneer axons have arrived safely, others may simply follow their course.

There are various molecules that have been identified by immunocytochemical techniques. Typically such molecules are expressed only during certain phases of development, *e.g.* during synapse formation. They then disappear. Nerve-cell adhesion molecules (N-CAMs) make the cells 'sticky', slowing down movement, and if they are present on the surface of certain neurons and not on others at a certain time, they may contribute to the establishment of selective contacts (Brodal 1992, Casaer 1993). Some guidance cues are expressed by cells along the paths of the axons and operate over a short range. In addition, there is evidence for the existence of longer-range guidance cues, *i.e.* diffusable chemo-attractants that emanate from the intermediate or final targets of the axons, and diffusable chemo-repellents that are secreted by cells in regions which the axons avoid.

Netrin-1 and netrin-2 function as chemo-attractants for developing spinal commissural axons *in vitro*. Netrin-1 is expressed by an intermediate target, the floor plate, a structure situated along the ventral midline of the neural tube, during the period when commissural axons grow along a ventral circumferential trajectory to the floor plate. Thus, netrin-1 secreted by floor plate cells probably plays a role in directing the circumferential migrations of commissural axons, attracting them to the ventral midline of the spinal cord. In the case of diffusable chemo-repellents, the semaphorin family of axon guidance cues includes two members, semaphorin-II and collapsin/semaphorin-III, which have been implicated as long-range inhibitory or repulsive cues (Colamarino and Tessier-Lavigne 1995). The growing neurite is therefore stationary, repelled or attracted. In addition to various matrix glycoproteins such as fibronectin, laminin and merosin there are substances such as PDGF, nerve growth factor (NGF) and ganglioside.

Cell process guidance is complicated and only just beginning to be understood. It is, however, extremely important since it is thought that in the adult CNS substances exist which inhibit cell division, migration and differentiation and so may prevent healing by regeneration in the nervous system. These substances may also prevent brain tumours.

Myelination

Structural lipid for membranes is important in all tissues from the red cell envelope, all cell membranes, organelle membranes and specialized membranes such as the myelination lamellae. In the mature nervous system, myelin is found as a multilamellar structure surrounding the nerve axon.

Myelination is not essential for the development and functioning of axons. Impulse conduction in axons starts before the formation of myelin sheaths, and the normal impulse traffic occurs in unmyelinated axons. However, myelination increases conduction velocity by some tenfold. The conduction velocity of the nerve impulse is directly proportional to the diameter of the nerve; for myelinated fibres, this ratio between conduction velocity and fibre diameter is 6:1. Even with the smallest nerve fibres (0.2 μm), conduction velocity is faster if they are myelinated. Because the propagation of the action potential in myelinated axons is saltatory, from node to node, the conduction velocity increases with maturation of the axon.

The amount of myelin from one node of Ranvier to the next is derived from one Schwann cell or oligodendrocyte (Davison 1974, Jacobson 1978).

STRUCTURE OF MYELIN

Myelin makes up one quarter of mature brain weight. It consists of a bimolecular layer of lipid/protein sandwich which is wrapped around the axon like a Swiss roll. There may be up to 100 whorls in a single myelin sheath. The membrane which forms the myelin is made from the oligodendrocyte cell membrane growing round and round as new membrane production causes the leading end to move under other outer layers. The axon does not move as was once thought.

The protein is myelin basic protein (now known to consist of seven proteins rich in lysine and arginine) in both central and peripheral myelin. Cerebroside and cerebroside sulfate (sulfatide) are the most prominent lipids in the myelin sheath. Cerebroside content is always higher in white matter, even unmyelinated, than in grey. There is a 400% increase in cerebroside between 34 weeks and term (Martinez 1989). The biochemical spurt at 32 weeks starts just before the histochemical spurt in myelination. Very rapid accumulation continues until 6 months and near adult values are found by 4 years.

The composition of myelin changes little during development (Martinez 1989). The first myelin sheaths are less tightly wound and have more water; only later in development do myelin lamellae appear. Myelin protein and proteolipid protein increase during maturation. Myelin is stable with a slow metabolic turnover, possibly greater than a year, so if different fatty acids are used in its composition, as from different infant feeds, slow replacement would be expected. Myelin continues to be formed while peripheral nerves elongate and increase in calibre during growth of the cell body. A single peripheral nerve axon may finally have up to 100 layers of myelin. The growth of the myelin sheath thus necessarily requires very considerable expansion and slippage of myelin lamellae over each other.

Unlike the Schwann cell, a single oligodendrocyte may myelinate more than one axon, and the glial cell body may not be adjacent to its myelin sheath. The main difference at the nodes of Ranvier is the presence of processes of Schwann cell cytoplasm covering the nodes in peripheral axons, whereas the central axons are exposed at the nodes. The point of exit of the cranial nerves and spinal roots is a boundary at which a transition zone between central and peripheral myelin occurs. The transition is not hard and fast.

Before the onset of myelination there is a period of intense proliferation of oligodendrocytes and Schwann cells, termed myelination gliosis (Fig. 1.5). It stops at the onset of myelination. Myelination in each region of the brain is always preceded by an increase in vascularization, followed by a period of greatly increased lipid synthesis in the Schwann cells and interfascicular oligodendrocytes. During this period, the increase in brain weight is largely due to the accumulation of myelin. Once compact myelin has been formed, its lipid constituents appear to be remarkably stable, with very slow turnover (Jacobson 1978).

MYELINATION OF THE PERIPHERAL NERVOUS SYSTEM

Schwann cells, which are solely responsible for the myelination of peripheral nerves, are derived from the neural crest and migrate out proximo-distally along the growing nerve

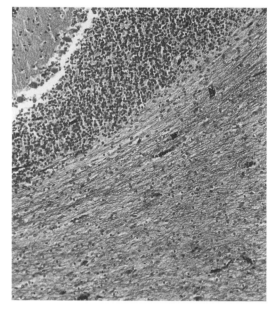

Fig. 1.5. Alignment of the oligodendroglia along the developing myelin.

fibres. The mechanism of their migration is poorly understood. Peripheral myelination begins before that at the centre, and the sciatic nerve is myelinated by 12 weeks gestation. Immediately before myelination begins in the CNS, there is proliferation of glial endoplasmic reticulum, and glycogen deposits and lipid droplets accumulate in Schwann cells and oligodendrocytes (Davison 1974). Myelination occurs in a proximo-distal direction, although sometimes a gap is left between two myelinated internodes, which becomes filled in later. Myelination starts near the nucleus of the Schwann cell and spreads from there in both directions. The myelin close to the nodes is most unstable, and breaks down under unfavourable conditions.

Schwann cells secrete a basal lamina that encloses the entire cell–axon complex. This acellular stocking is needed if Schwann cells are to myelinate their axons successfully (Sanes 1989) and it provides a persistent scaffolding after nerve degeneration to confine dividing Schwann cells and guide regrowing axons. Before myelination, all Schwann cells express N-CAMs, but after myelination N-CAM synthesis is downregulated leaving only the unmyelinating Schwann cells (Remak cells) with N-CAM on their surface membranes (Jessen *et al.* 1987).

The basic intercellular interactions which initiate and sustain myelination are not known. Whether the Schwann cell does or does not form a myelin sheath is determined by the type of axon with which it associates. The evidence indicates that the axon stimulates the Schwann cell to form the myelin. The formation of the myelin sheath is also affected by the diameter of the axon. In peripheral nerves, axons smaller than about 1 µm are unmyelinated, and in myelinated nerves, the number of lamellae of myelin is proportional to the diameter of the axon. Schwann cells continue dividing after migrating into dorsal roots and peripheral nerves. Most of the Schwann cells are formed by mitosis in the peripheral nerves rather than by migration of postmitotic cells from the neural crest. Schwann cells that have begun to form myelin no longer divide.

CENTRAL OLIGODENDROGLIAL MYELINATION

• *Oligodendroglial development.* Cell division in the germinal plate ceases at about 28 weeks, neuronal division is complete by 22 weeks, and glial division continues until term. Apoptosis with cell dissolution then removes the remaining precursor cells leaving unsupported thin walled capillaries. Blood flow to basal parts of the cerebral hemispheres from Heubner's artery diminishes, and the striate arteries are no longer as important. The developing cortex requires an increasing blood supply, and surface penetrating vessels become longer to supply the myelinating future white matter. The myelinating part of the brain was also shown in early autoradiographic studies to have an increased blood supply. Myelination is always preceded by increased vascularization; this comes from the developing long penetrating arteries and from the surface of the brain, as the basal circulation becomes less important following resolution of the germinal plate.

The second DNA spurt in the last trimester of pregnancy occurs when the oligodendrocytes are differentiating from the migrated satellite cells. Each oligodendrocyte myelinates between 15 and 50 axons, sending out amoeboid-type extensions of its plasma membrane. The oligodendrocytes, which are metabolically very active, take up fatty acids (33% polyunsaturated) and synthesize myelin and amino acids in order to construct the proteolipid membrane. If they are damaged during their differentiation at the time of the second DNA spurt then it may not be possible to replace them, so that myelination cannot proceed, *i.e.* there is a critical period for myelination. This may be why in encephalopathy of low birthweight infants and periventricular leukomalacia, thin or delayed myelination is seen on MRI scan.

• *The myelinogenetic cycle.* There is a definite order in which myelination takes place, the so-called myelinogenetic cycles of Yakovlev and Lecours (1967). The peripheral nerves, spinal cord, brainstem, cerebellum, basal ganglia and thalamus, and then the cortex, myelinate in a caudal to rostral order. The sciatic nerve is myelinated by 12 weeks gestation and the posterior columns begin to show myelin soon after. Short association pathways may not fully myelinate until the individual reaches the age of 16. Although the child develops in a cephalocaudal direction, the leg area and visual (optic nerve, optic tract and optic radiation to calcarine cortex) areas myelinate first in the cerebral cortex. This is in spite of leg area glia being late in migration. Myelin formation at term, and so metabolic activity and blood supply, is maximal in the leg area. At birth there is myelin in the superior cerebellar peduncle, the ventrolateral nucleus of the thalamus, the posterior limb internal capsule, the leg area of the cortex and the median longitudinal bundle in the brainstem. Myelination is subsequently very rapid from about 38 weeks gestation to six weeks after birth when the whole of the pons, middle cerebellar peduncle and cerebellar white matter, olives, brainstem, calcarine cortex and leg area myelinate over a very short time. By 3 months of life the cerebellum which was poorly myelinated at birth resembles that of the adult. However, cerebellar growth in terms of total size has still a long way to go. The corpus callosum starts to myelinate eight weeks after birth.

13

There is no definite correlation between myelination and the beginning of function. The leg area myelinates early yet walking is relatively late, and the leg area is also particularly vulnerable to damage. However, the onset of myelination in a system often mirrors function. There are regional differences and myelination occurs at specific times in various parts of the nervous system. Vestibular and spinal tracts, related to basic postural control, are myelinated at 40 weeks of gestation. Midbrain–cortical visual pathways are myelinated when the visual smile (smile in response to visual stimuli) emerges in infants at 2–3 months.

The extent of peripheral myelination can be measured as motor nerve conduction time. It increases by about 1 m/s per week between 20 and 30 weeks gestation from 20 to 30 m/s. In the adult it should be above 40 and usually about 60 m/s. The optic nerve can be examined by the visual evoked responses, and brainstem conduction time by brainstem evoked responses. It is claimed that corticospinal conduction times, and hence myelination, can be measured by cortical electromagnetic stimulation.

Elaboration of dendrites and synaptogenesis
The outgrowth of dendrites from the neuronal cell body always occurs after the outgrowth of axons. The young neuron has relatively short and thick dendritic processes which develop a complex system of branches. The branching leads to a great increase in the surface area of the dendrites, which form more than 90% of the postsynaptic surface of the neuron. The size, shape and pattern of dendritic branching is characteristic for each type of neuron. In any region of the brain, the dendrites of the neurons with short axons differentiate later than dendrites of principal neurons which have long axons. The spines show a dramatic increase from about 32 weeks gestation and are all formed by six months after birth. There are about 2000 spines per cortical neuron. Purpura *et al.* (1982) have suggested that failure of normal dendritic spine formation is the basis of learning disorders such as those associated with Down syndrome, hypothyroidism, ventilated preterm infants and West syndrome. Nissl substance and the soma may appear normal.

The maturation of dendrites tends to occur in a ventrodorsal or inside-out sequence: the dendrites of the cortex mature later than the dendrites of the central nuclei projecting to the cortex, and within the cortex, the dendrites of deeper layers tend to develop before those in more superficial layers. There also is a tendency for the dendrites of the motoneurons to develop before those of the sensory neurons in the same region of the brain. Within ascending sensory systems (auditory, somatosensory, visual and olfactory) the neurons mature in ascending order, beginning with those nearest the peripheral receptors (Jacobson 1978).

Synaptogenesis, the establishment of specific synaptic interactions between the neurons, is essential for functional neuronal activity. In the human brain, it starts during the second prenatal month in the cerebral cortex and is advanced by the time of birth (Molliver *et al.* 1973). Synaptogenesis and dendritic growth are independent processes. Both occur at the same time. Synaptogenesis starts before neurogenesis is completed, and the fact that synapses are commonly seen on dendrites as well as on axonal growth cones shows that neither need be completely mature to enable synaptogenesis to begin. Moreover, axodendritic synapses are formed over an extended period during the postnatal growth of dendrites. Development of synapses has been correlated with changes in the EEG and in evoked potentials.

14

Regressive events

Regressive events (cell death, axonal pruning and synaptic elimination) appear to be characteristic of many, perhaps all, regions of the CNS (Cowan *et al.* 1984). These events occur as final mechanisms of development and are generally delayed until projections approach their final configurations.

Many more neurons are formed in embryonic life than the number present in the mature nervous system. In fact, many are eliminated at the time their axons are establishing synaptic contacts. This is called the phase of selective cell death. As many as 50% of anterior horn cells and retinal ganglion cells may be eliminated by this naturally programmed cell death (Oppenheim and Chu-Wang 1983). About half of the neurons in a nucleus are also eliminated during this phase. The elimination is very rapid, apparently within days in some systems. Programmed cell death is genetically determined but may be influenced by functional changes such as motor activity or inactivity and by the size of the target group of neurons. If the target group is experimentally expanded, more of the neurons in a nucleus supplying it with axons survive. On the other hand, by reducing their number in the target nucleus, the elimination is increased. The most likely explanation is that they need some kind of trophic substance to survive. It is well known that the presence of NGF and brain-derived neurotrophic factor (BDNF) stimulates survival of the cells and axonal growth.

The extent of cell death for a given type of neuron is determined from estimates of their absolute number at a given site at different developmental stages. The number of neurons is found first to rise to a maximum as they proliferate and settle at their final destination, then to decline with the onset of cell death, finally to reach a plateau when the period of cell death has passed (Brown *et al.* 1991).

There are several different purposes or reasons for cell death, including the elimination of neurons whose axons fail to reach a target, scaling down neuron number to match the size of the target or the size of a presynaptic pool, and the elimination of connection errors. These purposes are not mutually exclusive and more than one may be served. Furthermore, a temporary excess of neurons might have a positive role to play in some circumstances. For example, the excess of motoneurons during development may be needed to ensure the production of enough muscle fibres because muscle fibre numbers are regulated by the number of innervating motoneurons.

Postnatal brain growth

There is a rapid phase of development in the first four years during which the brain increases in size greatly (Table 1.2).

The development of dendritic connections, synaptic stabilization, cellular apoptosis (for example, of the external granular layer of the cerebellum), myelination, formation of Nissl substance and maturation of association pathways occur postnatally and follow an orderly predetermined sequence (Conel 1939–1967, Yakovlev and Lecours 1967).

THE STRUCTURE OF THE CEREBRAL CORTEX

The gyral pattern of the cerebral cortex is most readily recognized in the preterm infant when the pre- and postcentral gyri, calcarine sulcus and primary areas are easily demarcated.

15

TABLE 1.2

TABLE 1.2
Average brain and body weight at various ages*

Age	Brain weight (g)	Body weight (kg)	Ratio %
Birth	350	3.5	10
1 year	1000	10.0	10
2 years	1200	20.0	6
Adult male	1400	70.0	2
Adult female	1250	60.0	2

*After Cockburn (1995).

As the cortex increases in area it needs to be infolded more and more, and the pattern becomes more complicated. This is seen on MRI at the time of the glial spurt as a thickening of the cortical grey matter. Primary and secondary, but not tertiary sulci are present at birth, and the frontal and temporal poles are not yet fully developed. There is a difference between the two sides of a single brain, and differences between brains are also evident, so the surface anatomy must not be regarded as sacrosanct. There is much more cortex in the insula and inferior frontal region as well as in the cingulate and medial surface than can be recognized simply from looking at the surface. It can be unfolded as in hydrocephalus when many more gyri, *i.e.* polymicrogyri, are seen, and yet intelligence can be quite normal even with the cortex unpacked and thinned.

There are three stages in the maturation of the cerebral cortex, as follows.
(1) The development of *primary areas* such as primary motor, (Brodman area 4), somatosensory (Brodman area 41) and Heschl's gyrus. These are areas of cerebral cortex which receive information from the environment via the senses. They have rich connections to the thalamus, with no long intracortical ones, or else have long efferent projections to the periphery, *i.e.* the muscle. Included with these early developing primary areas is the limbic system.
(2) The second areas to develop are the *association areas* which usually lie adjacent to the primary motor or sensory area. These secondary areas all have long intracortical association pathways and are connected via the corpus callosum to their equivalent region in the opposite hemisphere. The visual association area is adjacent to the primary visual calcarine area: the hearing association area is identical with the planum temporale (Wernicke's area) and is adjacent to the primary hearing area in Heschl's gyrus. The motor planning area for speech, Broca's area, is adjacent to the motor strip for lips, tongue and palate, and the graphomotor area for writing is adjacent to that for the hand. They are less dependent on hard wiring than the primary areas and can move from side to side.
(3) The third and final parts of the cerebral cortex to mature during childhood are called *terminal zones*. They represent the anterior pole of the frontal lobe and the angular gyrus and are areas which have no thalamic connections. Long association fibres, *e.g.* between frontal and occipital lobes, develop early, while short association fibres may only become operative in the second decade.

If there is any delay in brain maturation then parts of the brain important for motivation and cognitive function are the last to develop and consequently the most likely to be delayed.

Localization of function was first inferred from the clinical deficits associated with focal pathology, *e.g.* tumours, infarcts and gunshot wounds (see Luria 1966), and subsequently from the direct stimulation studies of Penfield and Roberts (1959). The notion of brain localization then became unfashionable, but studies of local blood flow, regional cerebral metabolism of glucose and oxygen and now functional MRI have changed this dramatically.

Broca (1861) showed that expressive speech came from the left hemisphere in an area adjacent to the motor strip for the lips, tongue and palate. Although 90% of people use their right hand to write, only 66% are strongly right handed for all tasks (Annett 1970). Lesions of the left hemisphere are 50 times more likely to produce dysphasia than lesions of the right hemisphere in right handed people. Among left handed people the left hemisphere still carries speech in 60% of individuals. Writing appears to be localized in the graphomotor area, again on the left and adjacent to the motor control of the right hand. Reading depends on the visual association area on the left but also requires the integration of the angular gyrus (a tertiary area). The right hemisphere controls musical tone recognition and tune memory, prosodic recognition in speech, facial expression and reception of nonverbal or emotional communication.

The planum temporale
The hard wiring of the auditory system extends from the cochlea via the eighth nerve to the cochlear nucleus, then decussates and passes via the lateral lemniscus to the inferior colliculus and then via the medial geniculate nucleus of the thalamus to Heschl's gyrus in the temporal lobe. Evidence to support this comes from electrocochleography, brainstem evoked responses and cortical auditory evoked responses. Behind Heschl's gyrus is the planum temporale which is the auditory association area. This, the most asymmetrical area of the brain, which differs markedly between man and the higher primates, is thought to be the anatomical basis of speech. It is larger and more cellular on the left (Geschwind and Levitsky 1968).

On the left hand side the occipital lobe is wider, the sylvian fissure longer and the angular gyrus more prominent. The crossed corticospinal tract is larger to the right hand, the direct corticospinal tract is also larger from the right hemisphere to the right hand

Dominance
It is believed that the young infant utilizes both sides of the brain in learning various skills with initially a mirroring of effect. Subsequently some skills, speech and facial recognition will become lateralized. To avoid interference there must be a suppression of one lateral pattern in favour of the other. This localization is effected by reciprocal cerebral inhibition through the corpus callosum. This is what is meant by the acquisition of dominance which tends to occur between 3 and 7 years, though some children do not achieve dominance until well into the school years and consequently may experience difficulties in school.

Development of the cerebellum
The cerebellum is also growing and developing in parallel with the cerebral cortex. The

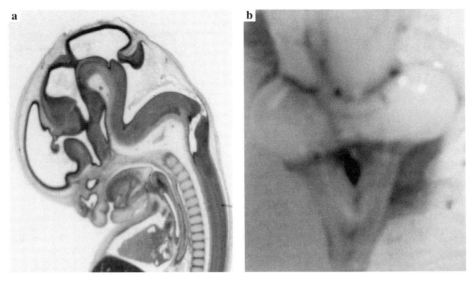

Fig. 1.6. *(a)* Primitive cerebellar placode budding from the hindbrain. *(b)* The two primitive cerebellar buds developing contact across the midline as the primitive vermis.

primitive cerebellar buds protrude on either side of the rhombencephalon by about 32 days gestation as shown in Figure 1.6a. These then fuse by 10 weeks as the primitive vermis (Fig. 1.6b). The germinal cells migrate from the rhomboid lip over the surface of the cerebellum to form the external granular layer (Fig. 1.7a). The cells then migrate inwards to form the Purkinje cells; this is the opposite of the outward migration observed in the cortex. The external granular layer persists until the end of the first year of life when apoptosis removes these millions of redundant cells. It is thought that medulloblastoma or primitive neuroectodermal tumours could arise from these remnants. The cerebellum differs from the cerebral cortex in that it has a uniform structure in archi-, paleo- and neocerebellum (Fig. 1.7b). The cerebellum has a greater sensory afferent input than the cerebral cortex. Myelination of the cerebellum is mainly a postnatal event occurring most rapidly in the first two postnatal months.

Posture and mobility
Motor behaviour can be divided broadly into two component classes, gross and fine motor. Gross motor behaviour involves the skilful use of the whole body and includes posture and mobility, whereas fine motor behaviour involves the use of individual body parts, particularly the hands, and other small muscle masses. Posture has two basic components, standing and balance. Standing requires constant antigravity muscle contraction to hold the body in an upright position while balance maintains the centre of gravity and prevents falling over.

Preyer (1885) was the first to note that fetal motility occurs several days before sensory stimuli become effective in evoking reflexes, an observation which implied that efferent (motor) systems begin to function before afferent (sensory) systems. He called these move-

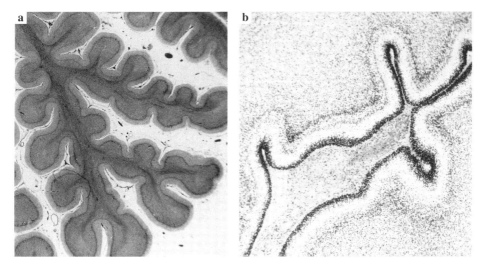

Fig. 1.7. *(a)* External granular layer of the cerebellum. *(b)* Homogenous structure of the cerebellum.

ments impulsive movements and claimed they were of central and not peripheral origin. These motility rhythms were described by Clarke and Clarke (1914) as being periodic, waxing and waning in a somewhat rhythmic fashion. Fetal breathing movements have also long been recognized (Ahlfeld 1888).

A number of early studies on fetal movement relied on maternal reports. However, the introduction of linear array real-time ultrasonography led to important new possibilities, and it is now known that both spontaneous and elicited movements can be detected at 7.5 weeks (de Vries *et al.* 1982).

Development of posture
Sustained contraction in antigravity muscles is obviously needed to keep the body upright, but normal pendular sway or movement means that constant adjustment of the position of different parts of the body, head or limbs is required to maintain the centre of gravity at the level of the symphysis pubis. This varying muscle contraction is what we mean by tone and as defined, it changes and is not constant.

In the mature nervous system muscle tone is fluid. The contraction of postural muscle is variable and is adjusted according to willed movements in addition to proprioceptive, visual and vestibular input. In subcortical states due to failure of maturation or damage there tends to be a constant pattern of either flexor or extensor dominant muscle contraction which resists attempts to reverse the pattern. This is what we mean by muscle tone. Muscle tone when present usually indicates a subcortical release mechanism of systems which in the mature state are kept inhibited but can be used as part of the motor repertoire. These primitive patterns must disappear before volitional cortical postures appear. No child can walk if extensor dystonia is present, and equally the child may lose walking and independent standing when these patterns return in disease. The presence of muscle tone is shown clinically by resistance to passive movement, the range of movement at joints, the tendency to adopt fixed postures and the presence of postural reflexes. The extensor reflexes, for example, appear when subcortical extensor dystonia fails to disappear, or when it reappears.

The remark by Sherrington (1947) that 'posture is the shadow of movements' is still apposite today. The capacity to link the motor system to the afferent sensory input is present from an early age *in utero*, but spontaneously generated and co-ordinated motor patterns of the fetus eventually become linked to specific stimulus conditions to which the infant is exposed after birth. The old idea that all development before birth is under genetic and not environmental control whereas after birth environmental control is predominant is plainly oversimplified and incorrect. For example, we now know that the fetus will respond to prosodic change in the human voice.

Recent data on glucose and oxygen consumption measured by positron emission tomography (PET) show that both the motor and sensorimotor cortices are active in the neonate and the very young infant (Chugani *et al.* 1987). PET studies of glucose and oxygen consumption also indicate that the visual occipital cortical areas become active at around 10 weeks of life in infants born at term. It is not only conduction time in tracts but also maturation in interneuronal connectivity that should be considered. From the biochemical point of view, functional biochemical aspects of neural membranes, such as synaptic strengthening by learning, as well as neuromodulating factors are all important for the postural adaptations during the transition period as well as during the new postnatal start (Davies *et al.* 1989).

Postural development in the fetus and infant is most easily considered in a series of stages as described below. Observational studies on aborted fetuses reported by Hooker (1952) and Humphrey (1964) form the basis of the following discussion.
• *First flexor stage.*

Nine to 17 weeks gestation. During this period the fetus shows a predominant state of flexor tone, indicated by the retention of the flexed and adducted posture when suspended against gravity. There is loss of this muscle tone as asphyxia proceeds, showing that it is not simple elastic tissue recoil. If the limb is extended, resistance is felt and there is active flexor recoil back to the original position.

The flexor reflexes are easy to elicit and there is flexor withdrawal in all four limbs on nociceptive stimulation. Dermatome stimulation, by stroking over the flexor surface, will produce flexion of the limbs, particularly when the abdominal wall is stroked gently; the limb on that side flexes. No actual extension can be produced by stimulation over extensor surfaces as, for example, with trunk incurvation or Perez reflex.

Stroking of the palm at this stage produces flexion of the fingers and adduction of the thumb into a palmar grasp reflex (Fig. 1.8). Stroking of the foot causes extension of the big toe, but no fanning. There is a lot of spontaneous mass movement usually involving all four limbs. Perineal or oral stimulation produces a mass flexor response of all four limbs, whereas nociceptive stimulation of an individual limb produces more discrete flexor withdrawal of the limb. Perioral stimulation causes the head to turn, usually towards the stimulus, and the mouth to open. Fetuses show a rhythmic synchronous 2 per second flexion of both legs, which persists for several minutes when they are held suspended vertically.

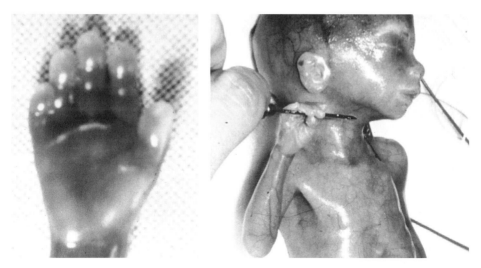

Fig. 1.8. *(Left)* Development of the hand at 10 weeks gestation with fingers and thumb well demarcated. *(Right)* Adduction of the thumb and flexion of fingers in response to traction across the palm, with primitive grasp reflex, at 12 weeks gestation.

At this stage the fetus also shows fine movements of the extremities, which are not seen again until much later in postnatal development. For example, pronation and supination movements are seen, as well as opening and splaying of the fingers, the latter being the most obvious extensor movement. Towards the end of this period, definite pursing of the lips can be produced by perioral stimulation. The ankle jerk appears and cross-reflexes can also be demonstrated, *e.g.* stimulation of the skin over one adductor surface caused a cross-adduction on the other side.

An anal reflex response can also be elicited at this stage. The bladder contains urine and micturition is seen by 12 weeks gestation.

• *First extensor stage.*

18–30 weeks gestation. Fetuses examined between the 18th and 24th weeks showed quite a marked change. Flexor tone is lost, the arms and legs stay extended, and spontaneous flexor and extensor movements, together with cycling movements and boxing movements, are observed. Dermatome to myotome responses were obtained over extensor surfaces, and the trunk incurvation reflex appeared. The asymmetrical tonic neck reflex (ATNR) also appears at about 18 weeks. Initially the ATNR shows an increasing flexion in the occipital limb, but by 20 weeks the full extensor pattern in the upper limbs ipsilateral to the jaw is present. Instead of mass flexion to stimulation there is now mass extensor spasm. Pressure over the nose or the perineum produces rigid extension of the legs with a spontaneous Babinski response. The grasp reflex is still present, but traction is now lost as the flexor tone has disappeared. When the arms are passively extended the mouth opens. Spontaneous movements (cycling movements, grasping, sucking movements) and rhythmic EEG waves appear at this time, suggesting that brainstem oscillatory circuits are beginning to operate.

Spontaneous movements are still both flexor and extensor; the latter may be rhythmic at 1 per second, and the fetus may appear to be shaking its fist. Incurvation of the trunk can readily be produced by stroking the paraspinal region, but the limb extension component of the reflex are seen only after the 22nd gestational week. The Moro, an extensor reflex (with abduction and extension of the arms and legs), is first seen fully at 22 weeks gestation. The phasic tendon reflexes, at the knee and ankle, are easy to elicit during this period. By 22 weeks, in addition to spontaneous sucking movements, the fetuses are noted to lick their lips, put out their tongue, and show definite rooting, cardinal points responses and crying. They may also stretch their arms above their heads and yawn. By 20 weeks, flexion, extension and fanning with a spontaneous Babinski response are seen. The plantar grasp can be weakly elicited. There is no observable mid-brain activity, such as eye movement artefact on the EEG, and pupils cannot be seen because the eyes are sealed. Flexor withdrawal and some of the dermatome to myotome flexor responses can still be elicited at this stage.

During the period from 23 to 30 weeks of gestation the brainstem matures to the point where it can support life outside the uterus, and the baby is considered viable. This therefore is the picture that we see in the very small preterm baby. All the reflexes already described together with homeostatic mechanisms regulating respiration, vasomotor tone and cardiac rate are present. Homeostasis is not complete and temperature control is unstable. Sucking and swallowing reflexes are present, although the infant cannot co-ordinate sucking and swallowing together with cessation of respiration and closure of the larynx as a sequential movement until about 32 weeks of gestation. Cardiac irregularities due to autonomic imbalance are also common. There may be intense vagal inhibition with stimulation of the nasopharynx. Periods of central apnoea are common, associated at times with sudden bradycardia. Respiration at this stage is of the Cheyne–Stokes type. The period 28–30 weeks is essentially the time when midbrain function develops. Although the muscle tone is basically very hypotonic there is a lot of spontaneous movement; the infant moves around the incubator and shows vigorous cycling and crawling movements.

• *Second flexor stage.*

30–44 weeks gestation. In this period flexor muscle tone returns (Fig. 1.9). Brown (1966) showed that lesions in the region of the red nucleus capsule, in the midbrain, result in a flexor rigidity. This appears to be the region of the brain that is developing, a view supported by the fact that anencephalic infants with an intact upper midbrain, but with no basal ganglia or cerebral cortex, will show the full picture of neonatal flexor tone by 40 weeks gestation.

At 30 weeks the legs begin to take up a flexed abducted posture, although they can be extended passively without too much resistance or recoil. At 35 weeks flexor tone gradually increases so that the legs return to the flexed posture when extended. Joint angles change so that there is a reduction in the range of abduction at the hip. Extension of the knee becomes restricted so that the popliteal angle decreases along with the ease with which the heels can be opposed to the ears or the nose. There is also an increase in the range of dorsiflexion of the foot. By term, the hips will not abduct more than 45° from the vertical. Extension of the knees, using the weight of the body as a guide to how much force to use,

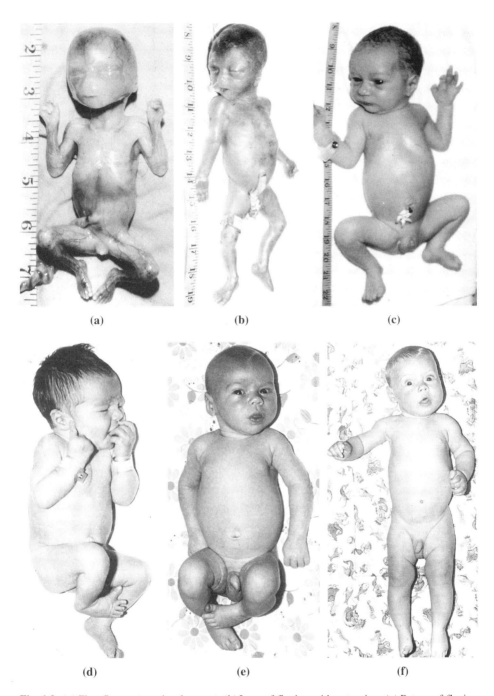

Fig. 1.9. *(a)* First flexor stage development. *(b)* Loss of flexion with extension. *(c)* Return of flexion without adduction. *(d)* Flexion with adduction. *(e)* Loss of flexion in the arms. *(f)* Loss of flexion in the legs in the second extensor phase.

23

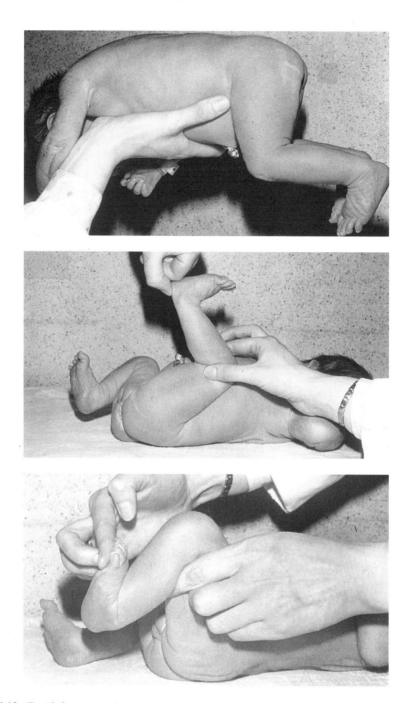

Fig. 1.10. *(Top)* Infant at term in ventral suspension. *(Middle)* The infant is at right angles at hip, knee and ankle. *(Bottom)* The popliteal angle is a right angle and the foot is dorsiflexed so that the dorsum of the foot approaches the tibia.

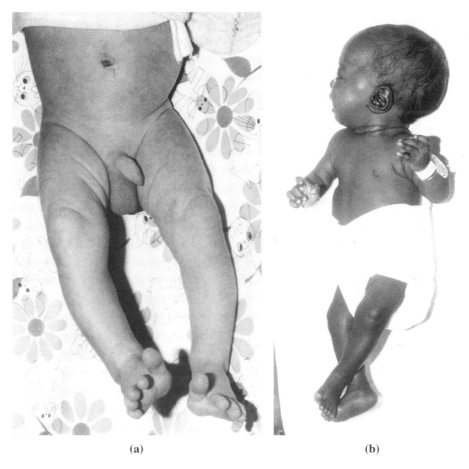

(a)   (b)

Fig. 1.11. *(a)* Extension in the second extensor phase is active, not just a loss of flexor tone, with bilateral spontaneous Babinski response. *(b)* Transient dystonia of preterm birth with the asymmetrical tonic neck reflex in an extensor posture which is reversible. This infant subsequently showed normal mobility with no evidence of cerebral palsy.

will not extend beyond the right-angle. The foot can be dorsiflexed completely so that the dorsum touches the tibia (Fig. 1.10).

Around 35 weeks gestation the arms begin to flex; this continues to increase and by 38 weeks there is quite good recoil in the arms. By term, when a grasp reflex is produced traction appears in the arms; that is, when one applies a force to the grasping fingers the arms flex and pull the baby upwards off the mattress, and the head also flexes forwards. The flexor component of the Moro reflex also appears, coinciding with increasing flexor tone of the upper limbs.

Adduction of the limbs occurs from 35 weeks onwards. It gradually appears in the legs, and by 38 weeks the knees should be adducted off the mattress. Also at 38 weeks the arms

(a)

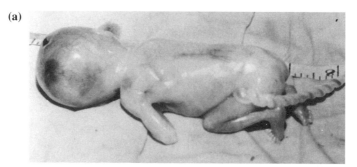

(b)

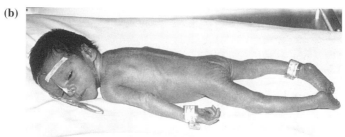

(c)

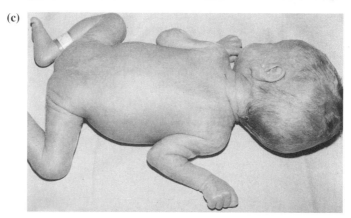

(d)

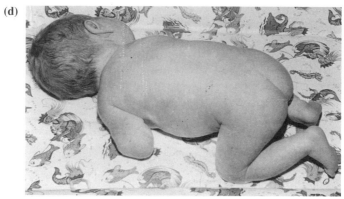

(e)

(f)

(g)

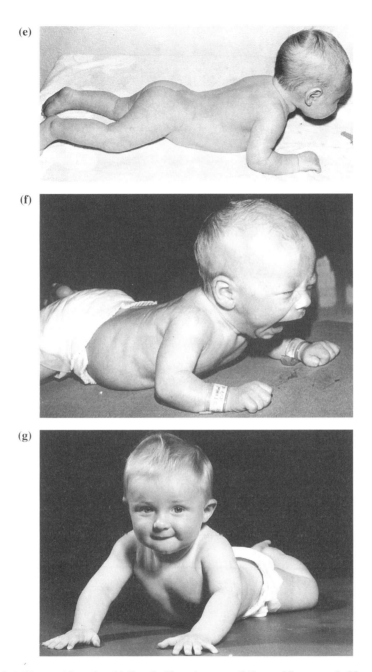

Fig. 1.12. *(a)* Fetus at 12 weeks with flexed adducted posture. *(b)* Loss of flexor tone in 26 week gestation infant. *(c)* Return of flexor tone with no adduction in 34 week gestation infant. *(d)* Term infant demonstrating flexion and adduction with the bottom high and the knees under the abdomen. *(e)* 10-week-old infant again showing extension of the head and hips. *(f)* 4-month-old infant with weight supported at forearms and face vertical. *(g)* 6-month-old infant taking weight on the forearms, chest wall clear of surface.

27

begin to adduct inwards and by term the infant should be not only flexed, but also adducted. When placed in the prone position, the knees are flexed under the abdomen showing that full adduction has occurred.

Any alerting influences such as mild hypoglycaemia, hunger or thirst will increase the basic tone. The infant therefore appears to show more traction response and to have stronger flexion/adduction when hungry.

• *Second extensor stage.*

Birth to 6 months. We do not intend to reiterate the pattern of normal infant development beyond pointing out that by about four weeks post-term the flexor tone in the infant's arms has again been inhibited so she lies with arms extended and legs flexed. The flexor traction response at the elbow is also less, although the grasp reflex in the hand, with flexion of the long finger flexors on traction, will stay until 3 months. By 6–8 weeks the legs also begin to extend when the infant is lying supine: this is an active extension and not simply inhibition of neonatal flexion. This is seen as a spontaneous Babinski response with extension of the big toes and fanning (Fig. 1.11a).

With prone suspension the head extends first and then the hips and knees. In prone lying the flexed hips and knees are gradually extended so that by 12 weeks the legs are fully extended from under the abdomen. The weight is at first on the flexed arms, and by 16 weeks the chest is clear from the surface with the face vertical and the legs extended at the hip. By 6 months the weight is on the fully extended forearms (Fig. 1.12). From 4 to 6 months the position dependent extension is gradually replaced by a more fluid pattern of muscle tone, *i.e.* flexion of one joint in a limb occurs independent of extension at another, so sitting becomes possible. If the extensor pattern persists as in cerebral palsy, independent sitting is impossible. Some preterm infants may show a very exaggerated physiological position dependent dystonic extension, similar to that seen in basal ganglia disorders or the dystonic phase of cerebral palsy, *i.e.* the transient dystonia of preterm birth (Fig. 1.11b).

With facilitation of extensor tone the ATNR, trunk incurvation and Moro reflexes, *i.e.* the extensor reflexes that had been inhibited by intense flexion at term, now return (Fig. 1.13). The ATNR shows a biphasic pattern of distribution, changing with the dominant pattern of muscle tone. It appears around gestational weeks 18–20, gets less towards term and then reappears after term. It normally disappears round about 5 months after birth. We emphasize this in an attempt to encourage neonatal neurologists to think in terms of patterns of maturation and to accept that individual reflexes by themselves are usually of significance only in that they relate to an underlying basic muscle tone pattern. These postural reflexes are usually subcortical in origin and are dependent on the infant's position in space (vestibular), the position of the infant's head (neck reflexes), contact with a surface (contact reactions) or pressure through the long axis. It is a neurological principle that most sensors make reflex connections at a lower level which have to be inhibited before the input from these sensors can be incorporated into higher cortical learned activity.

When a baby is pulled to the sitting position there is anticipation by the head and then by 4 months a voluntary pull up. Tilting the body sideways causes initially the head to right to the vertical and then by 5 months the trunk also, so that if the thighs are held the head and trunk can be kept vertical against gravity and thus prevent the infant falling over. By

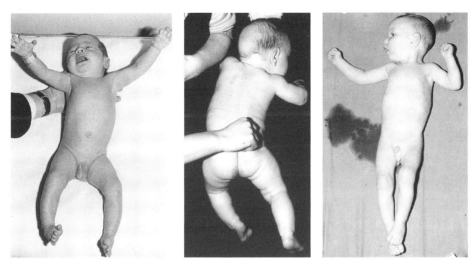

Fig. 1.13. *(Left)* Moro reflex in the extensor phase. *(Centre)* Trunk incurvation reflex, with the head turning to one side and the leg on the chin side showing abduction and extension, with the position of ATNR in the prone position. *(Right)* ATNR in the supine position is dependent purely on head position.

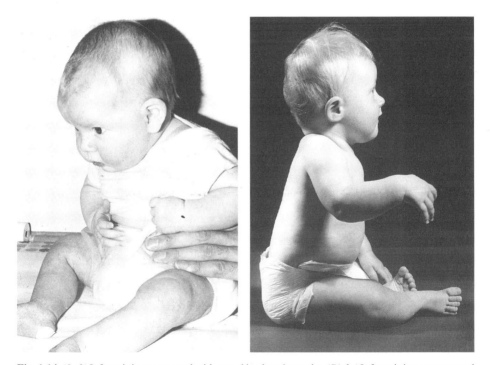

Fig. 1.14. *(Left)* Infant sitting supported with round back at 4 months. *(Right)* Infant sitting unsupported with straight back at 7 months.

6–7 months this is now automatic as sitting balance gradually improves (Fig. 1.14); lower limb righting develops and the improvement of balance enables the centre of gravity to be maintained at the level of the symphysis pubis. This permits independent standing. The protective or parachute responses appear from 5 months as a new reflex response to prevent falling over.

• *Cortical stage.*

At the cortical stage there is a fixed pattern of muscle control, either flexor or extensor. Posture does not depend on the position of the head or trunk or on contact. The infant can flex at one joint and extend at another in the same limb. At this stage the infant develops the capacity for standing balance and for progression. These involve righting reflexes, tilt reaction and the maintenance of the centre of gravity. At the same time, the infant begins to learn manual and postural skills. The development of standing, balance and propulsion, although interdependent, can be lost in isolation because they use different muscles and different CNS circuits.

SITTING

The head becomes stable with supported sitting. When displaced it is righted. This is followed, in the classical cephalocaudal progression described by Gesell and Amatruda (1941), by trunk righting and stability. As the extensor tone is inhibited the infant can flex at the hip, extend at the knee and turn the head without limb extension or trunk incurvation. This all allows the infant to be balanced with a rounded back and forward sitting by 4 months. The back gradually straightens, righting and balance improves, and by 7 months the child can sit with a straight back. Development of the lateral parachute responses in the arms prevents toppling over and allows tripod sitting (bottom and both arms). The age at which independent sitting occurs varies with the method of locomotion: in crawlers, 5–9 months (mean 7 months); in creepers, 6–12 months (mean 9 months); and in shufflers, 7–15 months (mean 12 months) (Holt 1977).

STANDING

The reflex standing seen at birth and during the first three months is due to a positive supporting reflex which is then lost and a period of so-called physiological ataxia is seen with legs that tend to bend and give way at about 4 months. Normal infants show awareness of the feet at about 6 months when they develop foot regard and suck their toes. They like to be stood up and take their weight on their legs, with good antigravity power, before the great bouncing age of 7 months. Pulling to stand is an important milestone occurring at a mean age of 10 months (7–13 months) in normal crawling infants; it is converted to independent standing as balance and righting responses develop. All infants who pull to stand, even those with cerebral palsy, should walk soon after. By 14 months they can bend down and pick up an object from the floor without falling over. They can also get into an unsupported standing position from lying supine or sitting, without any assistance from parent or furniture.

Balance continues to improve as the base required becomes narrower, *i.e.* tandem walking or walking on a beam. The child becomes able to stand on tiptoes with eyes open and then with eyes closed; this is followed by the ability to stand on one leg, and the final sophistication of standing on tiptoe on one leg with the eyes closed.

POSTURAL SKILLS
The combination of better balance and mobility allows the development of postural skills so that the child can transiently stand on one leg at 3 years, hop on the spot at 4 years and hop 5 metres at 5 years. Crouching is a good test of balance in the school age child, *i.e.* on tiptoe, straight back, hands on knees, eyes closed, and not falling over or touching the floor. Skills such as swimming, riding a bicycle and gymnastics depend very heavily on opportunity and teaching. The further acquisition of motor skills has been discussed by Connolly (1981).

Development of mobility

Frequent and active changes in fetal position may prevent adhesions between embryonic and extraembryonic membranes or between the different parts of the embryo (*e.g.* between the appendages and the trunk) and prevent local stasis of circulation, *i.e.* pressure sores in the fetal skin. Even when the mother is quietly resting, thereby preventing passive changes of fetal position, the fetus actively changes its position.

Spontaneous neuromuscular activity may be important for the normal differentiation of muscle and for the prevention of muscular atrophy arising from disuse (Pittman and Oppenheim 1979). Early fetal motility may play a role in shaping the skeletal system through mechanical effects on the growth of bones and joints. Immobilization leads to serious joint and bone defects such as ankylosis and club foot (Prechtl 1984). However, such embryonic activity is not essential for joint and muscle morphogenesis and is not a necessary antecedent of later motor behaviour.

The development of mobility begins with the spontaneous jerking and jumping of the first trimester, around 8–16 weeks. Then more rhythmic movements of individual limbs from about 12 weeks. These are gradually coordinated into a rhythmic swimming pattern with a cadence of about one per second. These movements are perceived by the mother as rhythmic kicking. They continue postnatally but are inhibited by 3 months. Mature walking then begins to emerge in the period 6–36 months. The development of mobility can thus be summarized into two phases: the antenatal, comprising (1) the myoclonic jerk, startle jump stage, (2) rhythmic movements of individual limbs, and (3) synchronized movements of all four limbs into swimming and hatching behaviour; and the postnatal, comprising (1) continuation of swimming movements in gradually more fragmented form, and (2) appearance of voluntary, supported walking after complete disappearance of the swimming pattern.

Development of fetal motor behaviour

The limb buds appear at about 30 days and by 42 days they are recognizable as arms and legs (Fig. 1.15). Sudden jerky movements appear soon after this, and startles with sudden flexor myoclonic jerks of the limbs and later the neck and trunk may be seen by 7 weeks. Using ultrasound, de Vries *et al.* (1984) documented slow extension and flexion movements

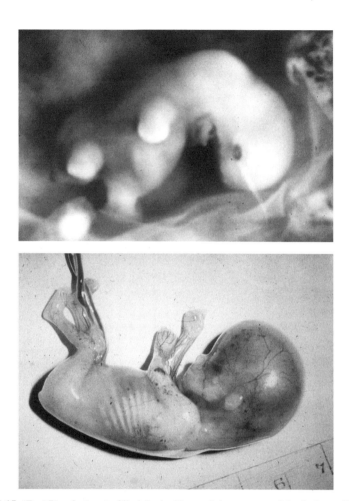

Fig. 1.15. *(Top)* Development of limb buds. *(Bottom)* Appearance of the limbs at 42 days.

of the spine by 7.5 weeks. From 8 weeks onwards, slow general movements and jerky startles can be observed. By 10 weeks, these generalized movements are followed by localized flexion and extension movements of an arm or leg. Movements of arms appear earlier than movements of legs. If the 12 week fetus is suspended it shows rhythmic symmetrical flexion movements of both legs. These will change the position of the fetus so that it appears to jump and then float upwards in the amniotic sac.

The localized limb movements may be either slow or fast. Overall activity increases rapidly during weeks 10–15 and many new movement patterns appear. The increase continues gradually and plateaus over the next 15–20 weeks; there is then a decline during the two to three weeks before birth (Edwards and Edwards 1971).

Paroxysmal jerky movements may also occur in the diaphragm as hiccups and are seen as an acute displacement of thoracic or abdominal contents on ultrasound (de Vries *et al.*

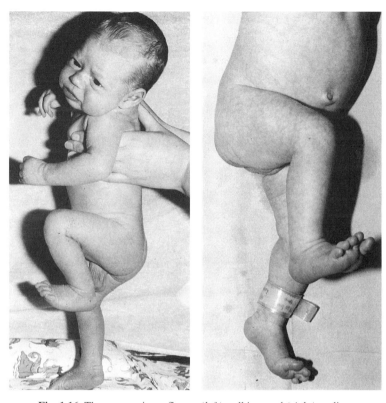

Fig. 1.16. The progression reflexes: *(left)* walking, and *(right)* cycling.

1984). They last several minutes and then stop. Breathing movements appear also at about 10 weeks gestation. Since the lungs are solid and noncompliant, respiration is paradoxical, that is, the chest goes in and the abdomen comes out.

Human hatching behaviour
The jerks, startles and stretches soon become organized into individual flexion–extension movements of a limb or rhythmic flexion of the legs. By the start of week 30 they have developed into a synchronous rhythmic reciprocal pattern of movement which will actually propel the fetus when it is submerged prone in water. Coughing and choking is inhibited. The arms and legs flex/extend rhythmically with side to side trunk flexion synchronized to leg flexion. The arm and leg extend on the same side, and then both flex as the contralateral arm and leg extend (McGraw 1945).

Many fetuses in the breech position two to three months prior to birth are found to have shifted spontaneously to the normal vertex position before birth (Braun *et al.* 1975). It has been suggested that the reflex facilitation of this pattern, which we see as reflex stepping and crawling movements that continue for a short while after birth, may also serve to position the fetus in the vertex position (Fig. 1.16).

33

The fetus swims into the vertex position and turns its head to the right at about 32 weeks gestation. Anything which interferes with swimming, such as oligohydramnios, an abnormal uterus, fibroids, neurological abnormality of the legs, neuromuscular disease or the presence of a twin, is likely to result in an abnormal breech presentation. After birth the infant still swims and shows a strong head-turning preference. It is thought that this prenatal swimming behaviour is organized at the level of the red nucleus in the midbrain. It may return later in childhood with brainstem release, *e.g.* with tentorial herniation. Vestibular connections develop as well as brain asymmetry at about the same time.

Orientation of fetal positions *in utero* show age-related preferences (de Vries *et al.* 1984) as follows.

(1) From 12 to 20 weeks the transverse orientation decreases considerably, while diagonal and longitudinal directions increase.

(2) The head up and rump down position shows a peak between 12 and 16 weeks at the expense of horizontal orientation. This preference disappears after 16 weeks and is thought to be due to the effects of gravity.

(3) From 10 weeks onward the most frequently observed postures are lateral and supine. Between 11 and 20 weeks, there is a steady increase in lateral posture at the expense of supine posture. The prone, upright and upside-down postures are less frequent.

Several classifications of fetal movements based on ultrasonographic studies have been proposed. The earliest classifications (Reinold 1971, Jouppila 1976) distinguished two classes: (1) strong and brisk movements involving the entire body that change its position in the amniotic cavity, and (2) slow and sluggish movements confined to the limbs after which the fetus retains its position in the amniotic cavity.

Babies born with motor defects such as limb paralysis are more likely to be in an abnormal position at birth and to suffer from positional abnormalities such as talipes or dislocated hips. Similarly, the decrease in spontaneous activity just before birth once the vertex position is adopted and the head engaged may serve to preserve the birth position from disruption. Preterm babies also show this increase in motor activity at about 32 weeks and a decrease after 37 weeks suggesting that this is an innate hatching behaviour pattern. Preterm infants born before 32 weeks are also much more likely to show abnormal birth presentation.

It is impossible to elicit fetal responses to vestibular stimulation. This suppression may denote a biologically protective mechanism preventing the fetus from responding to every maternal movement (Prechtl 1984). The vestibular apparatus will in fact impart a posture on the infant after 32 weeks; up to this time the fetal position in space does not seem to matter. After birth the vestibular system is activated not just because the infant is fully exposed to gravity for the first time, but because at birth there may be a change in the sensitivity of the vestibular receptor due to changes in partial oxygen tension or to neuroendocrine or other neuromodulating factors.

Postnatal mobility
NEONATAL MOVEMENTS
Walking, crawling, shuffling, commando crawling, etc. can all be regarded as fragments of cortical walking. The child will gradually acquire standing and balance but will walk

with support several months before she has the balance to walk alone. Only one cerebral hemisphere and the basal ganglia are required for walking.

Observations of the normal term infant demonstrate a myriad of movements at individual joints. These are often fragments of a movement pattern as already described and can be classified into groups (Weggemann *et al.* 1987). There are about 80 different individual movements which can be grouped together into the following patterns.

• *Progression movements.* These consist of alternating movements of flexion and extension of the limbs (*i.e.* they are remnants of the intrauterine swimming or hatching behaviour). Progression movements can be generalized, involving all limbs, or may involve both arms, both legs, or one arm and one leg on the same or contralateral side in a rhythmic fashion with or without movement of the head. These movements are really part of the walking, stepping, crawling or swimming movements seen on speeded ciné film.

• *Symmetrical movements.* These are slower than progression movements and are either flexor or extensor. If extensor they are synonymous with stretches when there is retroflexion of the neck, extension of the arms, rotation of the shoulders, extension of the legs with a spontaneous Babinski reflex of the big toe and fanning of the lesser toes.

In flexion the neck, trunk, arms and legs all flex, and the adducted hips and rounded back allow the infant to roll over like a rocking chair from supine to the side. This is the only way the neonate can change position when supine.

• *Startles.* A startle is a sudden brief flexor movement of head, trunk, arms and legs, the hands remaining closed. It is often confused with a Moro response which is predominantly extensor.

• *Reflex postures and movements.* If the baby spontaneously turns the head to one side, this may be followed by an ATNR. Likewise, if the baby suddenly falls over to one side or is exposed to a loud noise, then a spontaneous Moro reflex may occur. If during arm flexion the hand touches the mouth, rooting and sucking of fingers occurs. One reflex can inhibit part of another movement. For example, if while showing progression or symmetrical movements, one foot touches the side of the crib, this can result in either a flexor withdrawal reflex or a positive supporting reflex. All progression movements involving a leg will be inhibited as long as the foot is in contact with a hard surface, for example in the cliff edge reflex. Likewise if the hand is grasping at clothing the Moro reflex is inhibited by the grasp reflex.

• *Facial movements.* These consist of smiles, grimaces, frowns, opening and closing the eyelids, rapid and slow eye movements and bursts of sucking or tongue protrusion.

• *Athetoid movements.* These are represented by supination and pronation of the hand in combination with slow movements of the fingers from full extension to full flexion, flaring at the alae nasi, protrusion of the tongue, wide abduction of the toes and a spontaneous Babinski response (Fig. 1.17).

Description of typical clinical findings
Neonatal postural behaviour is closely related to the behavioural state of the newborn infant. The existence of an active posture can be best observed by its disappearance at the transition from the awake state to rapid eye movement (REM) sleep. The level of consciousness or

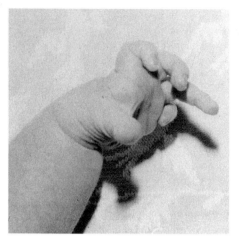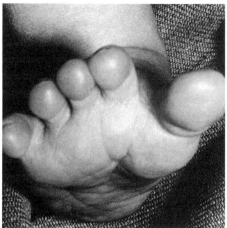

Fig. 1.17. Athetoid movements of *(left)* the fingers, and *(right)* the toes.

arousal is most easily divided into five states as follows: (a) hyperalert, the state of a hungry crying baby; (b) normoalert, the normal state of awareness; (c) hypoalert, the normal state after a feed; (d) active or REM sleep; and (e) quiet or non-REM sleep.

Immediately after a feed, the infant is awake in the hypoalert state. The eyes are open, bright and intermittently fixate and follow in a slow moving pattern with transient conjugation. The face is relaxed and does not smile or frown. A few slow progression movements occur, most commonly either in both arms or both legs. Generalized movements are less frequent. Sometimes there is hand to face contact in supination and flexion of the lower forearm, the movement originating from the elbow in the direction of the infant's face.

Bursts of non-nutritive sucking occur frequently. The nursing position is important as babies lying in the prone position soon go to sleep whereas those lying supine remain awake much longer. The baby then enters the first sleep state, when the eyes are closed or only intermittently open. There are frowns and bursts of non-nutritive sucking combined with irregular respiration. Rapid and slow eye movements can be seen under closed eyelids. Generally there is a loss of muscle tone so that the baby lies relaxed with the mouth open. A lot of athetoid finger and toe movements occur as well as myoclonic jerks. There are also quite a lot of single limb, isolated progression movements. Generalized movements are reduced, as are movements of both arms and both legs. Movements occur in bursts, sometimes slow and sometimes fast. Intermittent short bursts of vocalizing also occur. After a time, usually about 30 minutes, quiet or non-REM sleep occurs. Quiet sleep is characterized by regular respiration, no eye movement, much reduced activity with only a few movements, and sometimes athetoid hand movements or the opening and closing of the hand. All these movements occur more slowly than when awake. Bizarre postures of the arms or legs occur which are said to be due to increased muscle tone. During this period the infant is very sensitive to noise which can cause a sudden progression or startle movement. This sleep state is not altered by changing the position of the baby, in contrast to REM sleep when the child

36

quickly awakens. After 30 minutes, bursts of facial movements, followed by bursts of progression movements, show the change in sleep cycle, back to REM sleep. As time passes, the baby gets hungry and wakes. In the normoalert state there are a lot of isolated progression movements in the upper and lower limbs, which vary with the position of the child (prone, supine or lying on the side). During this state the upper limb progression movements involve the whole limb, starting with abduction of the shoulder and then flexion of the elbow, so that the hand describes a circle and finishes by touching the face with the palm or making a pincer grip at the ear. In the hyperalert state, when the child is extremely hungry, movements occur almost continuously. These can be generalized progression movements, especially when the baby is prone. Progression movements of both upper or lower limbs may occur at different speeds. When supine in the hyperalert state, progression movements, *i.e.* doggy paddling, may occur in the upper limbs while the lower limbs show rhythmic bilaterally synchronous flexion and extension movements reminiscent of the early fetus. The head turns from side to side, the body rocks and the infant often cries.

The development of cortical voluntary mobility
Rolling
Rolling is the first real means by which the child can voluntarily change position and move. The human baby differs greatly from the newborn of other mammals in that she is unable to turn from a supine to a prone position other than by accident as the rocking chair movement described above. The early rolling movements still display an automatic quality, the later purposive movements become incorporated into righting responses required for standing (McGraw 1945).

The head can be voluntarily turned to either side by 6 weeks (shoulder, trunk, hips and legs follow). Nearly all infants can roll from side to back by 4 months and from prone to back by 5 months, while the majority of 6-month-old infants are able to roll from back to stomach (Gesell 1930).

Prone progression
Before an infant can walk, she will usually develop some more primitive means of getting about by some form of prone progression. The commoner types of prone progression are hitching, crawling and creeping. Hitching means locomotion in a sitting position, crawling is any type of locomotion in which the body is prone, and creeping indicates locomotion in which the body is raised from the floor but remains roughly parallel with it, usually on hands and knees (Burnside 1927). A minority may shuffle and never crawl, a few simply 'stand up and walk', and some lie on their back and dig in their heels after flexing their legs and move by sudden extension. Following up infants to independent walking revealed that some never reach the stage of creeping, some never progress in the prone position, and some progress only in a sitting position (Touwen 1976).

The development of walking
Unpublished observations on a sample of normal Edinburgh children revealed that 50% could take five steps by their first birthday (range 10–14 months) and 97% were walking

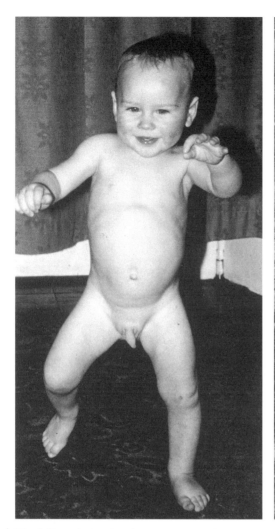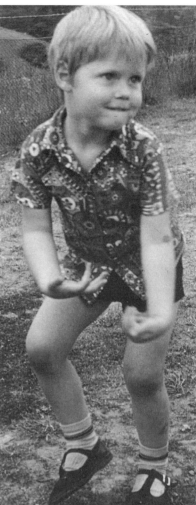

Fig. 1.18. *(Left)* Ataxic gait when the child first starts to walk. *(Right)* Continued postural immaturity with associated movements in the upper limbs dependent on the movements of the lower limbs (Fog test).

by the age of 18 months. There are three somewhat independent components to walking: antigravity support (standing), propulsion, and balance. Although interdependent they may be lost independently in disease, for example balance in ataxias. There is a close relationship between the mature phase of locomotion in the prone position and walking unsupported. Also, there is a close relationship between standing without support and the development of independent walking; the maturation of postural control mechanisms must precede independent walking. Supported walking or cruising normally precedes unsupported walking for a short period. At first support to the pelvis is required, then both hands, then one hand.

Walking around furniture or pushing a cart are part of the cruising phase, and in ataxic children this may last many months.

The attainment of unsupported walking is not the same as the achievement of a mature walking pattern. The initial form of independent walking shown by the infant is characterized by steps of variable length with a wide base, foot strike is flat footed, flexion of the hips and knees is maintained in stance, and the arms are held outstretched in abduction with the elbows in extension, *i.e.* the stage of physiological ataxia (Fig. 1.18). Typically, the movement pattern is staccato. From this initial phase the width of the base gradually diminishes, a reciprocal arm-swing appears, foot contact is by heel strike and then triple foot rocker, and both step length and walking speed increase. The staccato pattern gradually becomes smoother. A mature gait pattern is usually evident by the end of the third year (Sutherland *et al.* 1981).

THE NORMAL GAIT CYCLE

The gait cycle is customarily divided into stance and swing phases. In children there are three types of walking. The first type is the *shuffle gait*. Although there is heel strike with a triple rocker action of the foot there is little or no spring at the end of the rocker. This gait requires minimal energy, the feet are never both off the ground at the same time, and there is little bounce and hence little energy expenditure. There is no use of gravity to assist forward propulsion.

The second type of gait is known as *active propelled gait*. The body is actively thrown forwards into space by a strong contraction of the calf at toe off with a resultant fall into space and the prevention of actual fall by the swing through of the opposite leg as a forward parachute (or lateral parachute if the trajectory is to one side) which dampens the forward falling motion. This elongates the stride length by a greater amount than the distance between the feet. There is a lot of upward bounce and the energy requirements are higher.

The third type of gait is *running*. Here both feet are off the ground at the same time, the foot contact is in equinus, and the arms flex and stop swinging. There is more bounce and rotation of the trunk. Running is usually developed by 2 years of age.

The cadence, stride length and sequence of muscle activation is decided by the cerebral cortex and the basal ganglia in order to achieve the desired goal with minimal energy expenditure.

Conclusion

The brain develops in an orderly preprogrammed fashion under the influence of both genetic and nongenetic factors. The acquisition of skilled motor actions depends on the development of the brain, and findings from the neurological examination of children cannot be interpreted without some understanding of how the brain develops. What is normal, abnormal or delayed depends on the sequencing and timing of the various phases of brain development. The development of mobility begins early in the antenatal period, the first movements being evident by 8 weeks gestation. As the fetus develops, the complexity of movements, in both their kinematic and neurological aspects, increases. The combination of balance and mobility is the foundation on which further postural skills are based. Knowledge and understanding of brain development is the scientific basis of paediatric neurology: it encourages the concept of *developmental pathology* and of a developmental way of thinking generally.

REFERENCES

Ahlfeld, F. (1888) 'Über bisher noch nicht beschriebene intrauterine Bewegungen des Kindes.' *Verhandelungen der Deutchen Gesellschaft für Gynäkologie*, **2**, 203–210.
Annett, M. (1970) 'A classification of hand preference by association analysis.' *British Journal of Psychology*, **61**, 303–321.
Braun, F.H.T., Jones, K.L., Smith, D.W. (1975) 'Breech presentation as an indicator of fetal abnormality.' *Journal of Pediatrics*, **86**, 419–421.
Broca, P.P. (1861) 'Perte de la purole ramollissement chronique et destruction partielle du lobe antérieur gauche du cerveau.' *Bulletin of the Society of Anthropology*, **2**, 235–238.
Brodal, P. (1992) *The Central Nervous System: Structure and Function.* New York: Oxford University Press.
Brown, D. (1966) *The Cerebral Control of Movement.* Liverpool: Liverpool University Press.
Brown, M.C., Hopkins, W.G., Keynes, R.J. (1991) *Essentials of Neural Development.* Cambridge: Cambridge University Press.
Burnside, H.L. (1927) 'Co-ordination in the locomotion of infants.' *Genetic Psychology Monographs*, **2**, 279–372.
Casaer, P. (1993) 'Development of motor functions: a developmental neurological approach.' *In:* Kalverboer, A.F., Hopkins, B., Grenze, R. (Eds.) *Motor Development in Early and Later Childhood: Longitudinal Approaches.* Cambridge: Cambridge University Press, pp. 125–135.
Caviness, V.S. (1989) 'Normal development of cerebral neocortex.' *In:* Evrard, P., Minkowski, A. (Eds.) *Developmental Neurobiology. Nestlé Nutrition Workshop Series. Vol.12.* New York: Raven Press, pp. 1–10.
Chugani, H.T., Phelps, M.E., Mazziotta, J.C. (1987) 'Positron emission tomography study of human brain functional development.' *Annals of Neurology*, **22**, 487–497.
Clarke, E.L., Clarke, E.R. (1914) 'On the early postulation of the posterior lymph hearts in chick embryo: their relation to the body movements.' *Journal of Experimental Zoology*, **17**, 373–394.
Cockburn, F. (1995) 'The brain—which fat?' *Paper presented at the Symposium on Topical Paediatrics, Royal College of Physicians and Surgeons of Glasgow.*
Colamarino, S.A., Tessier-Lavigne, M. (1995) 'The axonal chemoattractant netrin-1 is also a chemorepellent for trochlear motor axons.' *Cell*, **81**, 621–629.
Conel, J.L. (1939–1967) *The Postnatal Development of the Human Cerebral Cortex.* Cambridge, MA: Harvard University Press. (8 volumes.)
Connolly, K.J. (1981) 'Maturation and the ontogeny of motor skills.' *In:* Connolly, K.J., Prechtl, H.F.R. (Eds.) *Maturation and Development: Biological and Psychological Perspectives. Clinics in Developmental MKedicine No. 77/78.* London: Spastics International Medical Publications, pp. 216–230.
Cowan, W.M., Fawcett, J.W., O'Leary, D.D.M., Stanfield, B.B. (1984) 'Regressive events in neurogenesis.' *Science*, **225**, 1258–1265.
Davies, S.N., Lester, R.A.J., Reymann, K.G., Collingridge, G.L. (1989) 'Temporally distinct pre- and post-synaptic mechanisms maintain long-term potentiation.' *Nature*, **338**, 500–503. *(Letter.)*
Davison, A.N. (1974) 'Myelination.' *In:* Berenberg, S.R., Carniaris, M., Masse, N.P. (Eds.) *Pre- and Postnatal Development of the Human Brain. Modern Problems in Paediatrics Vol.13.* Basel: Karger, pp. 116–122.
De Vries, J.I.P., Visser, G.H.A., Prechtl, H.F.R. (1982) 'The emergence of fetal behaviour. I. Qualitative aspects.' *Early Human Development*, **7**, 301–322.
—— —— —— (1984) 'Fetal motility in the first half of pregnancy.' *In:* Prechtl, H.F.R. (Ed.) *Continuity of Neural Functions from Prenatal to Postnatal Life. Clinics in Developmental Medicine No. 94.* London: Spastics International Medical Publications, pp. 46–64.
Dixon, J.E., Kintner, C.R. (1989) 'Cellular contacts required for neural induction in Xenopus embryos: evidence for two signals.' *Development*, **106**, 749–757.
Edwards, D.D., Edwards, J.S. (1970) 'Fetal movement: development and time course.' *Science*, **169**, 95–97.
Geschwind, N., Levitsky, W. (1968) 'Human brain: left–right asymmetries in temporal speech region.' *Science*, **161**, 186–187.
Gesell, A.L. (1930) *The Mental Growth of the Pre-school Child.* New York: Macmillan.

—— Amatruda, C. S. (1941) *Developmental Diagnosis: Normal and Abnormal Child Development.* London: Paul B. Hoeber.

Holt, K.S. (1977) *Developmental Paediatrics: Perspectives and Practice.* London: Butterworths.

Hooker, D. (1952). *The Prenatal Origin Of Behavior.* Lawrence, KA: University of Kansas Press.

Humphrey, T. (1964) 'Some correlations between the appearance of human fetal reflexes and the development of the nervous system.' *Progress in Brain Research*, **4**, 93–135.

Jacobson, M. (1978) *Developmental Neurobiology. 2nd Edn.* New York: Plenum Press.

Jessen, K.R., Mirsky, R., Morgan, L. (1987) 'Myelinated but not unmyelinated axons reversibly down-regulate N-CAM in Schwann cells.' *Journal of Neurocytology*, **16**, 681–688.

Jouppila, P. (1976) 'Fetal movements diagnosed by ultrasound in early pregnancy.' *Acta Obstetrica et Gynecologica Scandinavica*, **55**, 131–135.

Luria, A.R. (1966) *Higher Cortical Functions in Man.* London: Tavistock.

Marin-Padilla, M. (1988) 'Development of projection and local circuit neurons in neocortex.' *In:* Peters, A., Jones, E.G. (Eds.) *Cerebral Cortex, Vol.7: Development and Maturation of Cerebral Cortex.* New York: Plenum Press, pp. 133–166.

Marret, S., Gressens, P., Gadisseux, J-F., Evrard, P. (1995) 'Prevention by magnesium of excitotoxic neuronal death in the developing brain: an animal model for clinical intervention studies.' *Developmental Medicine and Child Neurology*, **37**, 473–484.

Martinez, M. (1989) 'Biochemical changes during early myelination of the human brain.' *In:* Evrard, P., Minkowski, A. (Eds.). *Developmental Neurobiology.* New York: Raven Press, pp 182–200.

McGraw, M.B. (1945) *The Neuromuscular Maturation of the Human Infant.* New York: Columbia University Press.

Molliver, M.E., Kostović, I., Van der Loos, H. (1973) 'The development of synapses in the cerebral cortex of the human fetus.' *Brain Research*, **50**, 403–407.

Oppenheim R. W., Chu-Wang, I.W. (1983) 'Aspects of naturally occurring motorneuron death in the chick spinal cord during embryonic development.' *In:* Burnstock, G., Vrobova, G. (Eds.) *Somatic and Autonomic Nerve–Muscle Interactions.* New York: Elsevier, pp. 57–107.

Penfield, W., Roberts, L. (1959) *Speech and Brain – Mechanisms.* Princeton, NJ: Princeton University Press.

Pittman, R., Oppenheim, R.W. (1979) Cell death of motoneurons in the chick embryo spinal cord. IV. Evidence that a functional neuromuscular interaction is involved in the regulation of naturally occurring cell death and the stabilization of synapses. *Journal of Comparative Neurology*, **187**, 425–446.

Prechtl, H.F.R. (1984) 'Continuity and change in early neural development.' *In:* Prechtl, H.F.R. (Ed.) *Continuity of Neural Functions from Prenatal to Postnatal Life. Clinics in Developmental Medicine No. 94.* London: Spastics International Medical Publications, pp. 1–15.

Preyer, W. (1885) *Specielle Physiologie des Embryo.* Leipzig: Grieben's Verlag.

Purpura, D.P., Bodick, N., Suzuki, K., Rapin, I., Wurzelmann, S. (1982) Microtubule disarray in cortical dendrites and neurobehavioral failure. I. Golgi and electron microscopic studies. *Brain Research*, **281**, 287–297.

Reinold, E. (1971) 'Beobachtung fetaler Aktivität in der ersten Hälfte der Gravidität mit dem Ultraschall.' *Pädiatrie und Pädologie*, **6**, 274–279.

Sanes, J.R. (1989) 'Extracellular matrix molecules that influence neural development.' *Annual Review of Neuroscience*, **12**, 491–516.

Sharpe, C.R., Fritz, A., De Robertis, E.M., Gurdon, J.B. (1987) 'A homeobox – containing marker of posterior neural differentiation shows the importance of predetermination in neural induction.' *Cell*, **50**, 749–758.

Sherrington, C.S. (1947) *The Integrative Action of the Nervous System.* Cambridge: Cambridge University Press.

Sidman, R.L., Rakic, P. (1974) 'Neuronal migrations in human brain development.' *In:* Berenberg, S.R., Caniaris, M., Masse, N.P. (Eds.) *Pre- and Postnatal Development of the Human Brain. Modern Problems in Paediatrics Vol.13.* Basel: Karger, pp. 13–43.

Sutherland, D.H., Olshen, R., Cooper, L., Woo, S.L-Y. (1981) 'The development of mature gait.' *Journal of Bone and Joint Surgery*, **62A**, 336–353.

Touwen, B.C.L. (1976) *Neurological Development in Infancy. Clinics in Developmental Medicine No. 58.* London: Spastics International Medical Publications.

Weggemann, T., Brown, J.K., Fulford, G.E., Minns, R.A. (1987) 'A study of normal baby movements.' *Child: Care, Health and Development*, **13**, 41–58.

Yakovlev, P.I., Lecours, A.R. (1967) 'The myelogenetic cycles of regional maturation of the brain.' *In:* Minkowski, A. (Ed.). *Regional Development of the Brain in Early Life.* Philadelphia: F.A. Davis, pp. 3–64.

41

2
THE IMPORTANCE OF FETAL MOVEMENTS

Heinz F.R. Prechtl

The history of fetal movement studies

It has long been known that spontaneous embryonic movements are present across the animal kingdom. The first reported observations go back to the 17th century, though the first systematic scientific investigations did not take place until the 19th century. Preyer, in his famous book *Spezielle Physiologie des Embryo* (1885), stated that human fetuses move from the age of 16 weeks onwards and suggested that movement might begin as early as 12 weeks. Preyer's comparative approach led him to fully accept the occurrence of spontaneous motor activity in the human fetus, an idea which was then lost for nearly a century. A similar fate befell Ahlfeld's (1888) observation of fetal breathing movements which met fierce opposition until they were confirmed in 1973 using ultrasound.

Around that time the growing influence of reflexology and behaviourism obscured knowledge concerning endogenously generated activity. This influence is evident in the first systematic neurological studies of exteriorized fetuses by Minkowski (1928). The same holds true for similar studies by the comparative anatomists Hooker and Humphrey [for an extensive summary see Hooker (1952) and Humphrey (1978)]. They also studied exteriorized fetuses who survived therapeutic abortions for a few minutes in a bath of isotonic fluid maintained at body temperature. 'Spontaneous' fetal movements were observed but apologetically explained as responses of which the 'eliciting stimulus is not yet known'. However, much was learned from their investigations of responses to stimulation with an aesthesiometer and this remained the basis for our knowledge of the prenatal development of neural functions until ultrasound studies were introduced. However, when Hooker's ciné recordings are compared with modern ultrasound recordings of intact and unstimulated fetuses, it becomes evident that the exteriorized fetuses were in a terminal condition and often did not show the normal pattern. Moreover, it must not be forgotten that the kind of stimulation provided in these experiments was artificial and does not occur in normal fetal life.

Another approach was followed in the 1940s and '50s by American psychologists who recorded fetal movements by mechanical means through the maternal abdominal wall. These techniques enabled the occurrence of movements to be detected although the pattern of these movements could not be discerned in any detail.

The real breakthrough in the analysis of fetal movement patterns was due to the introduction of high quality ultrasound equipment which enabled the observer to carry out realtime observations with sufficient dynamics and good image resolution. The capacity to store observations on video tape for subsequent off-line analysis was a further important factor which greatly facilitated the accuracy of the data.

Early ultrasound studies (Reinold 1971, 1976) were characterized by the description of movements according to their anatomical location. Birnholz *et al.* (1978) categorized motion 'according to a scheme suggested by Hooker and Humphrey with particular attention to extension of the head or limbs relative to the trunk, rotation or displacement of the torso, or individual phenomena related to specific limb, regional, or organ activity.' Although it remains difficult to relate their eight movement categories to Hooker's findings, it was the first attempt to classify observed fetal movements according to previous neurological investigations. The next step was carried out by the Italian obstetricians Ianniruberto and Tajani (1981). They related the observed fetal behaviour to motoscopic findings and were interested mainly in pattern analysis. Unfortunately, the descriptions were often too brief and interpretative and the authors did not specify what the fetus was actually doing (*e.g.* vermicular movements, creeping, climbing, hands exploring the uterine wall, etc.).

A different approach was followed when the movement repertoire of fetuses was systematically studied in the context of developmental neurology. The question was, what proportion of the fetal movements are similar to those seen in preterm and term infants and what proportion are different? To this end a study entailing the systematic observation and recording of spontaneous movements and postures was carried out on a carefully selected group of low risk preterm infants. These infants were selected as being comparable to fetuses from uncomplicated pregnancies. The study was based on two-hour direct observations with recordings made in each consecutive minute (Prechtl *et al.* 1979). The study was later replicated with off-line analysis of continuous video recordings (Cioni and Prechtl 1990) which confirmed the previous findings. We also examined the repertoire of spontaneous movements produced by term infants and how this changed during the first 18 weeks of postnatal life (Cioni *et al.* 1989, Cioni and Prechtl 1990). This was based on previous attempts to categorize patterns of spontaneous movements that occurred during the first five postnatal months (Hopkins and Prechtl 1984, Prechtl and Hopkins 1986).

These investigations did not reveal any fetal movement pattern which had not been seen postnatally. Although it came as a surprise to me, more than 12 years of detailed investigation of fetal movement failed to find any evidence of movement patterns which are restricted to the prenatal period.

How does the fetus move?

One of the first tasks in a longitudinal study of fetuses of carefully selected low risk pregnancies was to categorize the fetal movements. This work was undertaken with my co-worker Hanneke de Vries at the Department of Obstetrics in Groningen, the Netherlands. From the seventh week (postconceptional age) onwards these fetuses were recorded for one hour until 20 weeks and at 3–4 week intervals thereafter (de Vries *et al.* 1982; Prechtl 1988, 1989). The main findings can be summarized as follows. The very first movements seen in any fetus are slow extensions of the neck at 7–7.5 weeks. They are present for a few days and are then followed by the occurrence of startles and general movements (Fig. 2.1). While the first type consists of a rapid phasic contraction of all limb muscles, often with secondary involvement of neck and trunk muscles, the latter are complex movements involving neck, trunk and limbs. They vary in speed and are forceful but fluctuating in intensity. The

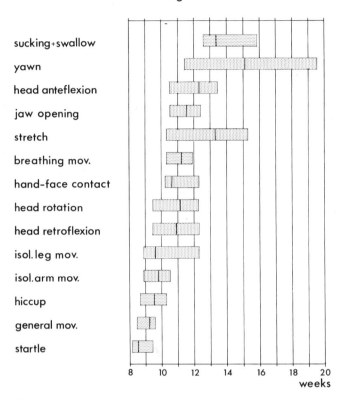

emergence of fetal movements

sucking+swallow
yawn
head anteflexion
jaw opening
stretch
breathing mov.
hand-face contact
head rotation
head retroflexion
isol. leg mov.
isol. arm mov.
hiccup
general mov.
startle

8   10   12   14   16   18   20
weeks

Fig. 2.1. Timetable of the emergence of the more important fetal movement patterns from 12 low risk fetuses studied longitudinally. The horizontal bars indicate the time period in which all fetuses started showing the particular movement patterns. The vertical line indicates the median. (Data from de Vries *et al.* 1982.)

temporal sequence of the moving parts is variable but they are by no means uncoordinated and unpatterned. Their fluent and complex character creates an impression of elegance and gracefulness. After the ninth gestational week the repertoire expands rapidly. Hiccups appear, often in series, for up to several minutes, and isolated arm and leg movements can be observed. This is remarkable in two respects. First, that the young fetus is able to perform isolated movements of one limb at an age when one would expect a longer period of diffuse and generalized motor activity. The second is the unexpected finding of the simultaneous onset of arm and leg movements, unexpected because of the long held principle of a cephalo-caudal development in spinal motor functions. After ten weeks, head movements of various types can be seen. They consist of lateral rotation of the head and overextension of the neck. These movements are carried out with moderate speed and occur in isolation. At about the same age, hand–face contact is seen for the first time. Usually, this is an accidental contact of a hand with the face or the mouth.

Between 10.5 and 12 weeks the fetus starts to make breathing movements. These are rhythmical contractions of the diaphragm, usually in a series of several movements although they may also occur in isolation. Such episodes of rhythmical breathing movements are paradoxical. Every contraction of the diaphragm leads to an expansion of the abdomen and a retraction of the thorax. Similar breathing patterns are seen regularly in the preterm infant but may occur during state 2 (REM sleep) even in the term infant.

At 11 weeks three new patterns, namely the opening of the jaw, bending forward of the head and complex stretch movements, are added to the repertoire. Somewhat later than the irregular jaw movements, yawns occur. These have the same pattern as in children and adults and hence are easily recognizable. The same holds true for the most complex stretches, which also retain an identical movement form into adult life.

At 13 weeks, rhythmical sucking movements, often followed by swallowing, occur in bursts. The rate of these sucking movements at 14 weeks is already about the same as in term infants during breastfeeding. Fetal drinking regulates the amount of amniotic fluid.

After fetal eye movements were discovered by Bots *et al.* (1981), Birnholz (1981) reported the onset of slow, rolling eye movements at 16–18 weeks, followed by rapid eye movements at 20–22 weeks which include also nystagmoid movements. To what extent prenatal and postnatal eye movements are comparable has been discussed by Prechtl and Nijhuis (1983). The quantitative developmental course of fetal eye movements throughout pregnancy has been studied by Inoue *et al.* (1986).

During the second half of pregnancy hardly any new movement patterns emerge. In a personal study (unpublished) in which mothers were monitored while lying recumbent on a bed which could be pushed around on wheels, no vestibular responses could be elicited in the fetus by accelerating and turning the mothers. This is biologically a meaningful adaptation because it prevents fetal responses to every maternal movement which would be most inappropriate.

With the rise of P_aO_2 during lung ventilation after birth, the vestibular system begins to function, as has been found in animal experiments (Schwartze and Schwartze 1977). The limp condition of newborn infants before respiration begins corroborates these observations in the human.

How often does the fetus move?

From our one-hour video recordings it is possible to produce actograms, an example of which is given in Figure 2.2. Such a display contains all the information concerning the variety of different movement patterns and their time course of occurrence during the observation period. Every attempt to find a mutual relationship between the occurrence of the different movements was unsuccessful, and I am forced to conclude therefore that the different movement types are generated independently of each other by separate modules. These modules represent several central pattern generators which endogenously generate the various movement types at different rates.

What is especially noteworthy about fetal movements is the fact that right from the beginning they are patterned into recognizable forms. There is no stage of amorphic and random movements. This may seem surprising; however, in the light of recent studies of embry-

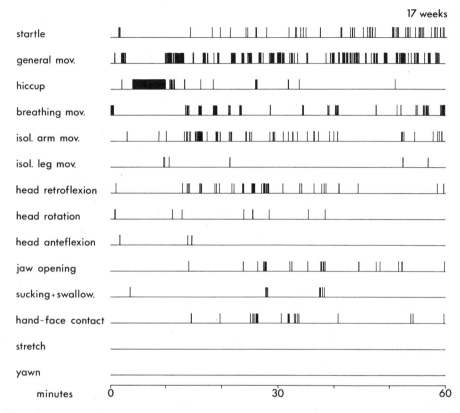

Fig. 2.2. Actogram of the various movement patterns shown by a 17-week-old fetus during a one hour recording.

onic neuronal tissue culture, the order as well as the endogenous generation of the fetal movements become understandable. Stafström *et al.* (1980) have worked with reaggregated cultures of fetal rat brain which had been mechanically dissociated into single cells. Extracellular recordings indicated spontaneous bioelectrical activity which was occasionally rhythmic and was autogenic in origin. In another most elegant experiment, Droge *et al.* (1986) cultured spinal cord tissue of 13- to 14-day-old mouse embryos in a monolayer cell culture on a printed chip. This enabled them to record simultaneously from many separate cells. The authors found not only tonic and phasic firing patterns, but also a considerable temporal ordering into rhythmical bursts with a rate of 2.5–7 cycles per minute. It is clear that such simple neural networks without any sensory input are able to generate ordered activity. There is a big leap from these preparations to the intact neural structures *in vivo*, but they nevertheless indicate important elementary properties of the developing nervous system which are consistent with the observations of the intact embryo and fetus.

In order to provide sound data on normal development, the temporal course of the various movement patterns has been studied extensively (de Vries *et al.* 1985, 1987, 1988;

46

Roodenburg *et al.* 1991). The frequently occurring patterns have a clear developmental course in that the general movements show an increase in incidence from 8 to 10 weeks, reaching a plateau at about 15% of the recording time. At the end of pregnancy there is a decline from about 32 weeks onwards. Previous studies concerning gross fetal body movements during the last 10 weeks of pregnancy (Patrick *et al.* 1982) have not differentiated between the various movement patterns and hence are not comparable with our data.

Startles were found to be the most frequent pattern at 9 weeks and to show a gradual decline until 36 weeks. In contrast to these tendencies of gross body movement the incidence of eye movements increases gradually from 20 to 36 weeks. A particularly interesting feature has been observed in the breathing movements of the fetus. Their incidence increases from 11 weeks onwards to a maximum at 32 weeks and decreases thereafter. Of special interest is the interval distribution of breathing movements. At 10 and 11 weeks the mode of the interval between consecutive breathing movements is between 2 and 3 seconds. Afterwards a gradual shift is seen toward shorter intervals but with a much wider distribution. This is an indication that in the beginning the central respiratory pattern generator works autonomously, and only later is it influenced and modulated, leading to more irregular breathing patterns and consequently to a wider scatter of the interval distribution.

Isolated arm movements increase considerably during the first half of pregnancy, while isolated leg movements increase up to 15 weeks gestation and decline thereafter until 20 weeks. Unfortunately, there are not yet any quantitative data available for the second half of pregnancy.

In those movement patterns which have a relatively infrequent incidence such as jaw movements, hand–face contact, head rotations and head retroflexion there is hardly any trend detectable during the second half of pregnancy (Roodenburg *et al.* 1991).

The trends mentioned above were identified in groups of fetuses studied longitudinally; plainly of great interest is the question of how consistent they are in individuals. It appears that intra-individual as well as interindividual differences are considerable from recording to recording. These large variations make quantitative measurements a poor marker for individual characteristics of fetuses, even if 60-minute ultrasound observations are made. This is in contrast to the data obtained on fetal movements from studies of pregnant women. Sadovsky *et al.* (1974) believed that 'Each fetus has its own rhythm and rate of movements and their perception by the mother depends on her subjective reactions to them.' Our own ultrasound studies could not confirm this claim. When the most frequently occurring movement pattern is compared between the first and second halves of pregnancy, the rank order of individuals is inconsistent. Those fetuses with a low or high incidence of movement during the first half of pregnancy may not show a corresponding incidence in the second half (Figs. 2.3, 2.4). As all these recordings have been carried out at the same time of the day, circadian rhythms could not account for the differences. Circadian rhythms do have an influence on the incidence of fetal movements, and there is a well known increase in movements during the night (de Vries *et al.* 1987).

What is the functional significance of fetal movements?
The rich repertoire of different distinct fetal movement patterns raises of course the question

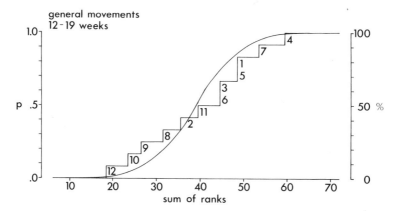

Fig. 2.3. Cumulative sum of ranks for general movements of 12 fetuses from 12 to 19 weeks. Numbers indicate case number per individual (from de Vries *et al.* 1988).

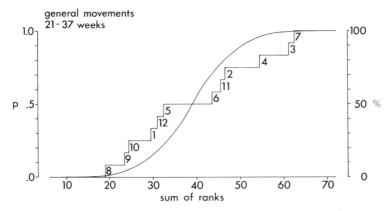

Fig. 2.4. Cumulative sum of ranks for general movements from 21 to 37 weeks, from the cases shown in Figure 2.3 (from de Vries *et al.* 1988).

of their meaning and function. It is hard to imagine that all these movements are simply an epiphenomenon of the developing neural structures. This is the more so as movements of the embryo have been found throughout the animal kingdom, including invertebrates. If such activity has been preserved throughout evolution it is likely that it reflects a fundamentally important function, and there is accumulating evidence of the significant role this activity plays in the development of the nervous system and the muscles. Not only is it important for the regulation of the natural cell death in the brain and spinal cord, but it also modulates the fine tuning of the connectivity in the nervous system. Hence, this activity appears crucial for the development of most parts of the nervous system. This explains the long period of anticipation of final postnatal function, as seen in the examples of fetal breathing movements or fetal eye movements.

Not all movements observed in the fetus belong to the category of anticipation of post-natal functions. The human fetus frequently changes its position in the uterus. There are specific movement patterns to bring this about: rotation of the body along the longitudinal axes, as well as alternating leg movements which, if proper contact is made with the uterine wall, lead to somersaults. The latter pattern lingers on for the first two months after birth and is known as neonatal stepping; it plainly represents a fetal adaptation and not a post-natal locomotor pattern.

The prenatal emergence of behavioural states

Many fetal movement patterns continue virtually unchanged in form and shape after birth. Another aspect of the continuity from pre- to postnatal life is seen in the behavioural states of sleep and wakefulness. States are mutually exclusive, distinct modes of neural activity which are relatively stable over time and which are separated from each other by synchronized transitions of the state variables. They do not represent a continuum of arousal as they are characterized by state-specific changes of the input–output relations of responses to stimulation by the different sensory modalities (for a detailed discussion of behavioural states in the neonate, see Prechtl 1974). These behavioural states of the newborn infant have a prenatal history. They emerge between 35 and 37 weeks of gestation when the state transitions become synchronized and all variables start to change in concert (Nijhuis *et al.* 1984). Similar findings have previously been obtained from preterm infants (Parmelee *et al.* 1967). In the younger fetuses and preterm infants these states are poorly organized. A clarification of this condition came from our introduction of the concept of coincidence (Nijhuis *et al.* 1982, 1984). If the state variables are in line with the criteria for state 1 (*i.e.* stable heart rate, no eye movements, only rarely body movements), this condition is called C1F (coincidence 1 fetal). If the heart rate is fluctuating between movements, eye movements are present and gross body movements occur repeatedly, this is called C2F and is equivalent to the neonatal state 2. There are awake states in the fetus as well: the rarely occurring C3F with eye movements, stable heart rate but no body movements; and the more often present C4F with continual body movements and high heart rate. The fetus does not have a crying state, and even the crying face has so far never been observed with ultrasound. The important point which makes episodes of coincidence different from true behavioural states is the lack of synchronized transitions. The variables do not yet change in concert. These synchronizing mechanisms are gradually coming into action after 30 weeks gestation (Visser *et al.* 1987) but reach stability only by the beginning of the last four weeks of pregnancy.

All parts of the recording which do not meet the criteria of coincidence F1 to F4 are called noncoincident. This provides a simple measure of the degree of maturation of behavioural states in the individual fetus. This approach gained special importance in studies of the compromised fetus, *e.g.* cases of intrauterine growth retardation, the fetuses of diabetic mothers and cases where maternal alcohol intake is high. In these cases the emergence of states is often delayed (see Nijhuis 1992).

The qualitative assessment of general movements: a window into the brain

Assessment of the integrity of the fetal nervous system is a major task in obstetrics. There have been many attempts to achieve this goal although most have concentrated on risk factors which could impair the nervous system. Signs of hypoxia as reflected in the fetal heart rate and heart rate variability, pulse oximetry and Doppler measurements of cerebral blood flow have raised great interest, but no direct assessment of the functional condition of the fetal nervous system was considered. Divon *et al.* (1985) have suggested a fetal neurological examination by eliciting a startle response with a vibroacoustic stimulus. It is clear that this approach ignores the complexity of the problem.

The extensive studies of the quantity of fetal movements and the installation of movement-counts as a widely used clinical test failed to detect neurological defects. It has been convincingly shown that in preterm infants with brain damage the incidence of motility is not different from that of low risk controls (Prechtl and Nolte 1984, Ferrari *et al.* 1990). There is no reason to believe that this would be different in the fetus and in fact it is not. What turned out to be different in fetuses, preterm infants and term infants with neural dysfunction is the quality of their general movements (Prechtl 1990, 1994). General movements were chosen because of their complex character and their frequent occurrence. It is easy to collect in relatively short ultrasound recordings of fetal movements sufficient samples of general movements the quality of which can be judged on video replay. Normal general movements are complex, fluent and graceful, and variable in speed and amplitude. There is a waxing and waning in the strength of movements and they last from several seconds up to a minute or so. If the fetal nervous system is impaired, characteristic changes in the quality of general movements can be detected. They lose their fluent appearance and become monotonous and repetitive, and may also become very short, jerky and abrupt or last only a few seconds and be fragmented.

In a series of systematic studies on the fetus, the experience gained from observations of brain damaged preterm infants (haemorrhages, leukomalacia) (Ferrari *et al.* 1990) was applied to the fetus. This had the great advantage that the same criteria could be employed in the functional assessment of the integrity of the nervous system during pre- and postnatal life. One of the first questions was whether a purely mechanical restriction of movements has an impact on the quality of fetal movements. This is the case in pregnancies with premature rupture of the membranes and consequently oligohydramnios (Sival *et al.* 1990). However, although their amplitude and later also their speed decreased, their complexity did not change. This indicates a preservation of their integrity despite unfavourable external mechanical factors. The situation changes if the fetus suffers from intrauterine growth retardation, with or without oligohydramnios. In many cases the complexity is reduced and general movements become fragmented, especially after the fetal heart rate shows signs associated with hypoxia (Bekedam *et al.* 1985; Sival *et al.* 1992*a,b*). Fetuses with prenatally acquired leukomalacia, as documented after birth by cystic abnormalities of their brain which must have occurred at least ten days earlier, have shown the abnormal pattern of general movements before birth (personal observations).

The most striking abnormalities of general movements have been observed in cases with brain malformations (Visser *et al.* 1985). In the more severe cases, no patterned movements were recognizable, a fact which had already been reported by Preyer (1885) who mentioned the abnormal character of fetal movements in anencephaly.

Interscoring reliability

The question of interobserver agreement on these judgements needs careful attention (Prechtl 1990). Using a test tape with 20 cases (ten normal and ten abnormal preterm infants in random order), ten scorers (neonatologists, neuropaediatricians, developmental neurologists) with varying experience in the assessment of motor activity were compared. None had prior training on the specific task with preterm infants. The average agreement for the 20 cases was 90%, with a range of 75–100% (Prechtl 1990). This result was very similar to that of a previous test employing obstetricians judging normality or abnormality of the movements of ten fetuses which produced an 89% agreement average (Bekedam *et al.* 1985). Hence, this method can be considered highly reliable and robust.

Fetal movements have a rich repertoire which develops mainly during the first half of pregnancy. It must be seen as an adaptive mechanism, insuring the proper development of the organism and especially of the nervous system and its function after birth. Seen in the context of a continuum of neural functions from pre- to postnatal life, we have gained a new understanding of early human development. In conclusion it can be claimed that a neurological assessment of the integrity of the fetal nervous system is now at hand and doubts about the feasibility of this can be refuted.

REFERENCES

Ahlfeld, F. (1888) 'Über bisher noch nicht beschriebene intrauterine Bewegungen des Kindes.' *Verhandlungen der Deutschen Gesellschaft für Gynäkologie*, **2**, 203–210.
Bekedam, D.J., Visser, G.H.A., de Vries, J.J., Prechtl, H.F.R. (1985) 'Motor behaviour in the growth retarded fetus.' *Early Human Development*, **12**, 155–165.
Birnholz, J.C. (1981) 'The development of human fetal eye movement patterns.' *Science*, **213**, 679–681.
—— Stephens, J.C., Faria, M. (1978) 'Fetal movement patterns: a possible means of defining neurologic developmental milestones in utero.' *American Journal of Roentgenology*, **130**, 537–540.
Bots, R.S.G.M., Nijhuis, J.G., Martin, C.B., Prechtl, H.F.R. (1981) 'Human fetal eye movements: detection in utero by ultrasonography.' *Early Human Development*, **5**, 87–94.
Cioni, G., Prechtl, H.F.R. (1990) 'Preterm and early postterm behaviour in low-risk premature infants.' *Early Human Development*, **23**, 159–191.
—— Ferrari, F., Prechtl, H.F.R. (1989) 'Posture and spontaneous motility in fullterm infants.' *Early Human Development*, **18**, 247–262.
de Vries, J.I.P., Visser, G.H.A., Prechtl, H.F.R. (1982) 'The emergence of fetal behaviour. I. Qualitative aspects.' *Early Human Development*, **7**, 301–322.
—— —— —— (1984) 'Fetal motility in the first half of pregnancy.' *In:* Prechtl, H.G.R. (Ed.) *Continuity of Neural Functions from Prenatal to Postnatal Life. Clinics in Developmental Medicine No. 94*. London: Spastics International Medical Publications, pp. 46–64.
—— —— —— (1985) 'The emergence of fetal behaviour. II. Quantitative aspects.' *Early Human Development*, **12**, 99–120.
—— —— Mulder, E.J.H., Prechtl, H.F.R. (1987) 'Diurnal and other variations in fetal movement and heart rate patterns at 20–22 weeks.' *Early Human Development*, **15**, 333–348.
—— —— Prechtl, H.F.R. (1988) 'The emergence of fetal behaviour. III. Individual differences and consistencies.' *Early Human Development*, **16**, 85–103.
Divon, M.Y., Platt, L.D., Cantrell, C.J., Smith, C.V., Yeh, S-Y., Paul, R.H. (1985) 'Evoked fetal startle response: a possible intrauterine neurological examination.' *American Journal of Obstetrics and Gynecology*, **153**, 454–456.
Droge, M.H., Gross, G.W., Hightower, M.H., Czisny, L.E. (1986) 'Multielectrode analysis of coordinated, multi-site, rhythmic bursting in cultured CNS monolayer networks.' *Journal of Neuroscience*, **6**, 1583–1592.
Ferrari, F., Cioni, G., Prechtl, H.F.R. (1990) 'Qualitative changes of general movements in preterm infants with brain lesions.' *Early Human Development*, **23**, 193–231.

Hooker, D. (1952) *The Prenatal Origin of Behavior.* Lawrence, KA: University of Kansas Press.

Hopkins, B., Prechtl, H.F.R. (1984) 'A qualitative approach to the development of movements during early infancy.' *In:* Prechtl, H.F.R. (Ed.) *Continuity of Neural Functions from Prenatal to Postnatal Life. Clinics in Developmental Medicine No. 94.* London: Spastics International Medical Publications, pp. 179–197.

Humphrey, T. (1978) 'Function of the nervous system during prenatal life.' *In:* Stave, U. (Ed.) *Perinatal Physiology.* New York: Plenum, pp. 651–683.

Ianniruberto, A., Tajani, E. (1981) 'Ultrasonographic study of fetal movements.' *Seminars in Perinatology,* **5,** 175–181.

Inoue, M., Koyanagi, T., Nakahara, H., Hara, K., Hori, E., Nakano, H. (1986) 'Functional development of human eye movement in utero assessed quantitatively with real-time ultrasound.' *American Journal of Obstetrics and Gynecology,* **155,** 170–174.

Minkowski, M. (1928) 'Neurobiologische Studien am menschlichen Fötus.' *Handbuch der biologischen Arbeitsmethoden,* **5** (5B), 511–618.

Nijhuis, J.G. (1992) (Ed.) *Fetal Behaviour. Developmental and Perinatal Aspects.* Oxford: Oxford Medical.

—— Prechtl, H.F.R., Martin, C.B., Bots, R.S.G.M. (1982) 'Are there behavioural states in the human fetus?' *Early Human Development,* **6,** 177–195.

—— Martin, C.B., Prechtl, H.F.R. (1984) 'Behavioural states of the human fetus.' *In:* Prechtl, H.F.R. (Ed.) *Continuity of Neural Functions from Prenatal to Postnatal Life. Clinics in Developmental Medicine No. 94.* London: Spastics International Medical Publications, pp. 65–78.

Parmelee, A.H., Wenner, W.H., Akiyama, Y., Schultz, M., Stern, E. (1967) 'Sleep states in premature infants.' *Developmental Medicine and Child Neurology,* **9,** 70–77.

Patrick, J., Campell, K., Carmichael, L., Natale, R., Richardson, B. (1982) 'Patterns of gross fetal body movements over 24-hour observation intervals during the last 10 weeks of pregnancy.' *American Journal of Obstetrics and Gynecology,* **142,** 363–371.

Prechtl, H.F.R. (1974) 'The behavioural states of the newborn infant (a review).' *Brain Research,* **76,** 185–212.

—— (1988) 'Assessment of fetal neurological function and development'. *In:* Levine, M.I., Bennett, M.J., Punt, J. (Eds.) *Fetal and Neonatal Neurology and Neurosurgery.* Edinburgh: Churchill Livingstone, pp. 33–41.

—— (1989) 'Fetal behaviour.' *In:* Hill, A., Volpe, J.J. (Eds.) *Fetal Neurology.* New York: Raven Press, pp. 1–16.

—— (1990) 'Qualitative changes of spontaneous movements in fetus and preterm infant are a marker of neurological dysfunction.' *Early Human Development,* **23,** 151–158.

—— (1994) 'Abnormal movements are a marker of brain impairment in fetuses and preterm and fullterm infants.' *In:* Lou,, H.C., Greisen, G., Falck Larsen, J. (Eds.) *Brain Lesions in the Newborn. Hypoxic and Haemodynamic Pathogenesis.* Copenhagen: Munksgaard, 37, 314–326.

—— Hopkins, B. (1986) 'Developmental transformations of spontaneous movements in early infancy.' *Early Human Development,* **14,** 233–238.

—— Nijhuis, J.G. (1983) 'Eye movements in the human fetus and newborn.' *Behavioural Brain Research,* **10,** 119–124.

—— Nolte, R. (1984) 'Motor behaviour of preterm infants.' *In:* Prechtl, H.F.R. (Ed.) *Continuity of Neural Functions from Prenatal to Postnatal Life. Clinics in Developmental Medicine No. 94.* London: Spastics International Medical Publications, pp. 79–92.

—— Fargel, J.W., Weinmann, H.M., Bakker, H.H. (1979) 'Postures, motility and respiration of low-risk preterm infants.' *Developmental Medicine and Child Neurology,* **21,** 3–27.

Preyer, W. (1885) *Spezielle Physiologie des Embryo.* Leipzig: Grieben.

Reinold, E. (1971) 'Fetale Bewegungen in der Frühgravidität.' *Zeitschrift für Geburtshilfe und Perinatologie,* **174,** 220–225.

—— (1976) *Ultrasonics in Early Pregnancy. Diagnostic Scanning and Fetal Motor Activity. Contributions to Gynaecology and Obstetrics, Vol. 1.* Basel: Karger.

Roodenburg, P.J., Wladimiroff, J.W., van Es, A., Prechtl, H.F.R. (1991) 'Classification and quantitative aspects of fetal movements during the second half of normal pregnancy.' *Early Human Development,* **25,** 19–35.

Sadovsky, E., Yaffe, H., Polishuk, W.Z. (1974) 'Fetal movement monitoring in normal and pathologic pregnancy.' *International Journal of Gynaecology and Obstetrics,* **12,** 75–79.

Schwartze, H.P., Schwartze, P. (1977) *Physiologie des Fötal-, Neugeborenen- und Kindesalters.* Berlin: Academie Verlag.

Sival, D.A., Visser, G.H.A., Prechtl, H.F.R. (1990) 'Does reduction of amniotic fluid affect fetal movements?' *Early Human Development,* **23,** 233–246.

—— —— —— (1992a) 'The effect of intrauterine growth retardation on the quality of general movements in the human fetus.' *Early Human Development*, **28**, 119–132.

—— —— —— (1992b) 'The relationship between the quantity and quality of prenatal movements in pregnancies complicated by intra-uterine growth retardation and premature rupture of the membranes.' *Early Human Development*, **30**, 193–209.

Stafström, C.E., Johnston, D., Wehner, J.M., Sheppard, J.R. (1980) 'Spontaneous neural activity in fetal brain reaggregate cultures.' *Neuroscience*, **5**, 1681–1689.

Visser, G.H.A., Laurini, R.N., de Vries, J.I.P., Bekedam, D.J., Prechtl, H.F.R. (1985) 'Abnormal motor behaviour in anencephalic fetuses.' *Early Human Development*, **12**, 173–182.

—— Poelmann-Weesjes, G., Cohen, T.M.N., Bekedam, D.J. (1987) 'Fetal behavior at 30 to 32 weeks of gestation.' *Pediatric Research*, **22**, 655–658.

3

POSTURE CONTROL IN CHILDREN: DEVELOPMENT IN TYPICAL POPULATIONS AND IN CHILDREN WITH CEREBRAL PALSY AND DOWN SYNDROME

Dafne Mattiello and Marjorie Woollacott

Throughout life our ability to move through our environment and to manipulate objects is dependent upon the successful control of posture. Early signs of postural development are apparent even in the fetus. The first decade of life represents a dynamic period during which maturation of body systems and environmental interaction play a role in the achievement of mature postural control. Congenital problems such as those seen in children with cerebral palsy and Down syndrome can significantly affect this process.

The development of posture control can be thought of as the evolution of a set of 'rules' which couple sensory inputs with motor actions. These actions control the variables which form the infrastructure of posture control. They include generation of antigravity forces, control of intersegmental relationships, and the maintenance of equilibrium. A child moves from the newborn state of minimal head and trunk control to independent standing and locomotion via increasingly sophisticated interactions between these variables.

Although it is generally agreed that the central nervous system plays a role in the control of posture, the specific control mechanisms are still the subject of debate. While traditional approaches focus on CNS maturation as the basis for postural development, more contemporary theories suggest that the interaction of many body systems along with environmental and task-related factors is instead responsible.

The aim of this chapter is to acquaint the reader with concepts and research related to the development of posture control in the developing infant and young child. We will also consider the implications of impaired postural development in children with cerebral palsy and Down syndrome.

Nearly all motor skills have an underlying stability component. Think of a baby reaching for a toy. The baby would need to control its stability by maintaining its trunk and head within the base of support of the legs in order to successfully reach in sitting. Only then could the upper extremities be oriented appropriately to obtain the object. It is through the control of these two components that body position in space is modulated. As illustrated in the reaching baby example, we obtain stability by controlling our body's center of mass within a base of support.

Once stability is achieved, the relative orientation of body segments can be organized to carry out the movement task. Therefore, posture control can be thought of as the coordination of stability and body orientation in space for the purpose of executing movement tasks (Shumway-Cook and Woollacott 1993).

Let us now consider the importance of posture control in the newborn infant. At birth, it may appear that babies have little ability to coordinate the use of their eyes and upper extremities. They may seem to be at the mercy of early reflexes such as the Moro or startle reflex. However, it has been shown that when these infants are well supported, more mature responses begin to emerge. When they are not required to control the head and trunk, infants are able to use vision to attend to faces and can coordinate beginning reaching behaviors. Primitive reflexes also appear less dominant (Amiel-Tison and Grenier 1980). Based on these findings, posture control can be considered a rate-limiting factor upon which the development of upper extremity skill and reflex integration is dependent.

The stages of motor development occurring in infants and young children have been well documented (McGraw 1932, Gesell 1946). The observation that these changes occur in a predictable sequence led Gesell to formulate the 'principles of developmental morphology'. One of his principles, that of developmental direction, suggests that development occurs in predominantly cephalocaudal and proximal–distal directions. This notion is supported by his observations that infants first acquire control of cephalic structures such as the lips, mouth and eyes. This control then progresses in a caudal direction with the trunk, legs and feet being the last structures brought under control. Within the extremities, mastery of proximal joint control occurs first, followed by increasing control in the distal joints. For example, in the first four to six weeks after birth, infants gain the ability to coordinate oculomotor pursuits for tracking. In the next 16–18 weeks reaching behaviors emerge as head and arm control develops. During the 28–40 weeks period hand and trunk control leads to object manipulation and independent sitting. Between 40 and 52 weeks the infant gains control of the legs and feet, as well as fine control of the hands, for ambulation and refined grasp.

In order for these developmental sequences to occur successfully, concurrent development of posture control must also take place.

Reflex/hierarchical model

Traditionally, developmental theorists have focused on maturation of the CNS to provide an explanation for motor skill development. In this reflex/hierarchical model of control, the emergence of increasingly mature postural reflexes and responses is dependent upon the maturation of higher CNS structures. The emergence of motor skills occurs as the result of sensory input into the CNS where 'hard-wired' central programs are located. It is these central programs that mediate the execution of posture and equilibrium responses. Viewed in this way, the postures and movement patterns seen in young infants are controlled by primitive reflexes which are organized at the spinal cord and brainstem levels. The tendon jerk and asymmetrical tonic neck reflex are examples of reflexes controlled at these levels. As maturation of the CNS ascends to the midbrain level, righting reactions become apparent. Mature equilibrium responses are seen with maturation of cortical brain areas. Motor skills also progress from low levels of reflexive movement to stereotypic reactions at the brainstem level, automatic movements at the midbrain level and finally voluntary skills controlled at the cortical level. Based on the reflex/hierarchical model, reflexes and responses seen at lower levels disappear as control is taken over by higher centers. The integration of lower level responses into more mature ones, and the inhibition exerted on lower levels by higher centers explains the disappearance of primitive responses with maturation.

According to the reflex/hierarchical model lower-level responses persist only in conditions of CNS pathology, such as cerebral palsy. Abnormal maturation of higher centers is thought to be responsible for the retention of primitive patterns in these cases. When higher CNS levels do not mature, there is resultant lack of inhibition of the lower centers, allowing primitive patterns to dominate (Horak 1992).

Another assumption of the reflex/hierarchical theory is that the development of equilibrium must always progress in the following order: supine, prone, sitting, all-fours and standing. If a child does not obtain stability in one posture, control of equilibrium in subsequent positions cannot emerge.

Systems model of posture control

Although the reflex/hierarchical model of control has been generally accepted and has formed the basis for many types of therapeutic intervention, research in the past decade has yielded results which directly challenge the assumptions of this model. For example, Jouen (1988) found that infants as young as 3 or 4 days old demonstrated compensatory head movements in response to visual flow that mimicked head sway. It is also difficult to explain, on the basis of reflex/hierarchical theory, the apparent re-emergence of primitive reflexes in adults without CNS pathology. In particular circumstances, such as stepping on a sharp object, the flexor withdrawal reflex may emerge, functioning to protect the foot from injury. This demonstrates that although primitive reflexes are no longer obligatory movement patterns in the normal adult, they do not 'disappear' as reflex theory would suggest.

According to the systems model of motor control, movement and posture control do not occur solely as the result of sensory input eliciting predetermined movement patterns. Instead, they emerge from the interaction of multiple body systems with the task and with the environment. This interaction is flexible in nature and allows for adaptation to changing physical, environmental and task constraints. Posture control develops in a continuous fashion as the various systems mature coincidentally. Individual systems mature at different rates, with particular ones having been identified as 'rate limiters' to the development of posture control. Based on the cumulative research in this area, Shumway-Cook and Woollacott (1993, 1995) identify the rate-limiting processes of posture control as including the following: (1) the individual development of the visual, vestibular and somatosensory systems, along with maturation of central sensory processing which organizes inputs from these senses for body and limb orientation; (2) changes in musculoskeletal attributes such as structural and soft tissue morphology and muscle strength development; (3) the emergence of muscular synergies which maintain stability involving the head, trunk and legs; (4) the ability to adapt sensory and motor processes in response to changes in the task and environment; (5) the ability to anticipate destabilization and modify sensory and motor processes.

In summary, the systems model suggests that the predictable sequence seen in motor development (the so-called motor milestones) is not dependent only on the progression of CNS development from lower to higher levels. Instead, new behaviors emerge from the interrelation of maturing systems. These new behaviors may seem to appear suddenly as one or more of the rate-limiting systems reaches a threshold level for function (Horak 1991).

Development of head control

Several researchers have compiled descriptive accounts of observed behaviors in infants from the newborn stage to independent sitting (McGraw 1932, Gesell 1946, Campbell 1994). This progression of behaviors reflects the attainment of new skills which occurs as the ability to control posture develops. When well supported in the upright position, newborn infants have the ability to bring the head to vertical from full flexion or extension and maintain this position briefly. The head typically wavers and oscillates, suggesting that smooth synergic coordination of the flexors and extensors is not yet present. By 2 months, the infant is able to maintain the head in midline in supported sitting although a face-vertical orientation is not consistent. At 4 months, the infant has gained smooth synergic control of the neck musculature, and with it, the ability to sustain a face-vertical orientation while turning the head side-to-side (Campbell 1994). An important question with respect to the development of head control systems is how does the maturation of individual sensory and motor systems correlate with the progression of head control? What are the rate-limiting factors for development of head control?

Motor coordination

Prechtl (1986) studied the emergence of head control in the first few weeks after birth. His findings led him to the view that infants under 2 months of age lack both the coordination and the muscular strength needed for head control. The notion of immature neural connections acting as a rate limiter of head control is supported by the work of Myklebust *et al.* (1986). They recorded muscle activity in the dorsiflexors and plantarflexors in infants in response to an Achilles tendon tap and found that in infants younger than 2 months of age activation of both muscle groups was elicited. Infants older than 2 months demonstrated only agonist activation in response to Achilles stretch. These findings support the notion that incorrect neuromuscular connections characterize the early stages of motor development and these are replaced by appropriate connections as the infant matures.

Role of muscle tone and antigravity force generation

The predominance of flexor muscle tone can be observed in newborn infants. As the infant gains strength and begins to move against gravity, head control develops as the result of increased force generation in the flexor and extensor muscles. What role does this increased ability to generate force play in the development of posture control? Schloon *et al.* (1976) examined the ability of neonates to generate muscular force against gravity. When they tilted infants on a platform in the prone and supine positions, they found that infants younger that 2 months of age did not show muscular responses to the perturbation. They suggested

57

that infants cannot respond to this type of perturbation until they gain the capacity to generate sufficient muscular force to move against gravity, which usually occurs between 2 and 3 months.

Mapping of sensation to action
Jouen (1988) examined the role of vision in posture control in infants. Using a moving light display to provide visual flow and create the illusion of head movement, he documented head and neck muscle responses via transducers in the supporting surface. He found that infants as young as 3–4 days old responded to the pseudo-perturbation, although not with consistent directional correctness. By the age of 2 months the infants' responses were directionally appropriate in all perturbations. It appears, therefore, that infants under 2 months do not have the correct neuromuscular maturity needed to respond in a directionally specific manner. These behavioral findings correlate well with those of Myklebust *et al.* (1986).

The fact that infants in Jouen's study showed muscular activation in response to visual input suggests that the mapping of vision on to motor systems occurs early in development. Another experiment revealed that infants were better able to maintain a midline head orientation in conditions where visual input was also available (Jouen 1984; Jouen *et al.*, in press). In one experiment preterm infants (32–34 weeks gestation) were supported in an infant seat while the examiners positioned the head in midline. The infants were tested both with and without goggles (vision present and absent), and movements which occurred as the examiners released the head were recorded. They found that infants were better able to reorient to the midline with visual input than without.

Other studies indicate that infants are able to respond to vestibular and somatosensory inputs shortly after birth (Tibbling 1969, Eviatar *et al.* 1974, Jouen 1984, Hirschfeld 1994). Jouen (1984) explored the relationship of the visual and vestibular systems in infants aged 1–7 months. He found that all were able to respond to vestibular stimulation (tilting) with some degree of neck righting responses. However, responses were stronger when visual information was also present. The older infants showed stronger responses compared with the younger in all conditions. From these results the author suggested that the visual system shows an effect on the vestibular system beginning early in development. He also proposed that the stronger responses seen in infants in the older group were a consequence of their having more experience with head control.

These studies lend support to the notion that single-sense control of posture develops early with respect to all three sensory systems (visual, vestibular and somatosensory), and that the visual system may be dominant in pre-sitting and newly-sitting infants.

Development of trunk control
As with the development of head control, the progression which occurs as infants achieve transition to independent sitting is characterized by predictable behavioral stages. Gaining control in the sitting position is a predominant focus of infants aged 5–6 months. Behavioral studies have shown that intersegmental control of the head and trunk are emerging and the infant is able to sit when placed in the propped position, or with the arms held high for balance.

In prone the face-vertical position is easily sustained with the arms flexed forward from the trunk and propped in full extension. Rolling to and from the supine position then emerges. By 8–9 months the infant sits easily with the arms free for exploration; control of the lower trunk and pelvis is developing and mobility in the prone and sitting positions is achieved. Control of the legs is emerging, which coupled with increases in pelvic control leads to transitions in and out of various positions using long-axis rotation (McGraw 1932, Gesell 1946, Campbell 1994).

The transition to and attainment of independent sitting has been the focus of a number of studies designed to answer questions such as: when do children gain the ability to respond to postural perturbations and how are these responses organized in terms of sensorimotor coordination? As infants develop the ability to sit independently, they must learn to control the postural sway which occurs as the result of movements of the head, trunk and upper extremities. Control of this type of spontaneous sway must be in place before the infant can reach for and manipulate objects in the environment while maintaining sitting. It has been documented that the control of spontaneous sway as well as compensatory responses to induced perturbation develop simultaneously around 6–7 months (Shumway-Cook and Woollacott 1995).

Motor coordination

Moving platform experiments are commonly used to investigate postural responses to perturbation. The moving platform can be used to induce a translatory displacement in the anterior or posterior direction, causing forward or backward sway in the child (Fig. 3.1). Some platform apparatuses also have the capability to induce rotational displacements, causing a toes-up or toes-down displacement in standing and legs-up or legs-down displacement in sitting. These rotations can be used as external perturbations, or can be set to move with the child thus eliminating proprioceptive cues from the feet and ankles. Other equipment which confounds vestibular and visual input has also been used along with the perturbation platform to explore the role of the various sensory systems in posture control. Researchers have focused on the acquisition of sitting posture control and response to platform perturbation in different studies, with similar results (Woollacott *et al.* 1987, Hirschfeld and Forssberg 1994).

Hirschfeld and Forssberg (1994) sought to determine when muscular response patterns begin to emerge in the pre-sitting infant, when they become coordinated, and whether responses differ with perturbation direction. They examined the organization of these patterns in the early and later stages of emergent sitting, comparing them with those seen in the adult.

Both pre-sitting (5–7 months) and independently sitting children (7–8 months) were given seated anterior and posterior translational platform perturbations, while EMG responses of the head, trunk and leg muscles were recorded. The pre-sitting infants were supported at the waist, and released just prior to perturbation. Children in the pre-sitting group were found to activate ventral muscles in response to forward translation in 60% of the trials. Only one or two muscles responded to the perturbation in most of the trials, with all three muscles (neck flexors, abdominals and hip flexors) active in 25% of the trials. All combinations of ventral muscle firing sequences were seen in these children. The responses of the independently sitting children were similar in temporal structure to those of adults, although with generally slower onset latencies. These children demonstrated consistent activation of ventral muscles with inhibition of dorsal muscles in response to forward translation. The sequence of ventral muscle activation typically progressed in a caudal to rostral fashion, beginning in muscles closest to the support surface and moving up (hip flexors firing first, followed by the abdominals and neck flexors). Although bursts of muscle activity were recorded with backward translation (anterior sway), responses were not consistent in any of the children. Interestingly, adults tested in the same paradigm also showed less response in the anterior sway condition. The authors surmised that this asymmetry may be due to the large differences in the sitting support surface. Since individuals are less likely to lose their balance with anterior sway because of the large base of support provided by the legs, they feel less threatened by backward perturbation; consequently, less muscular activation occurs. It is evident from the results of this experiment that infants as young as 5 months respond with some muscular activation in response to sitting perturbation, although well coordinated responses are not present until 7–8 months.

Mapping of sensation to action
Woollacott *et al.* (1987) also studied the role of visual, vestibular and proprioceptive input in sitting posture responses. Infants 4–5 months old were given seated perturbations, inducing anterior or posterior body sway both with and without vision (goggles on or off). The authors found that this group of infants had more consistent directionally specific responses to perturbation in the vision-absent condition. They concluded that sitting posture responses can be elicited via input from the vestibular and somatosensory systems in the absence of vision in infants learning to sit, but that vision may be dominant in normal vision-present conditions. However, the absence of vision may actually enhance the infant's ability to use vestibular and somatosensory information for postural responses. We have seen that the visual, vestibular and somatosensory systems all play a role early in the development of posture control. It also appears that as children move to independent sitting they acquire the ability to map information from all three sensory systems to motor actions.

The dominance of the visual system in the development of posture control has been of particular interest. Woollacott *et al.* (1987) have shown that by the time infants are sitting well independently, the ability to mediate consistent, directionally specific responses to sitting perturbations is present both with and without vision. Hirschfeld and Forssberg (1994) used rotational platform perturbations to differentiate the relative contributions of the visual, vestibular and somatosensory systems in trunk posture control. In comparing translational and forward rotational perturbations they found that children showed similar muscle activation responses to both. However, kinematic analysis of the resultant body movements with these perturbations reveals that although the pelvis rotates in the same direction with both perturbations, the head moves anteriorly with rotation and posteriorly with translation. They concluded that it is proprioceptive information from the pelvis that triggers the postural response in these children rather than visual or vestibular input. Nevertheless, when visual information is available it seems to exert a modulatory effect on postural responses to perturbation.

Development of posture control in stance

As with early development, milestones and movement characteristics related to the transition to standing, the development of stance control and progression to ambulation have been well documented (Campbell 1994). At 8–9 months, environmental exploration is the activity of choice for the infant. Creeping on all fours is well established and pull-to-stand behaviors are appearing. Transitions between positions are developing with the infant moving in and out of sitting and 'all fours' swiftly and with ease. Qualitative changes in movement patterns are evident, with increases in speed and smoothness of reciprocal patterns seen almost daily. The infant begins to stand at stable objects, and lateral cruising emerges as selective control of the lower extremities improves on an ever more stable trunk and pelvis. As infants gain confidence in their new abilities, they practice controlled lowering to the floor and bouncing. Finally, they attempt independent standing and progress to walking. The months that follow the advent of independent walking are dedicated to refinement of the ambulation pattern and development of posture adaptation skills. With increasing control of upright posture, the ability to adapt to perturbations, both intrinsically and extrinsically induced, emerges.

How children develop control in standing is a topic of great interest. Investigations carried out on adults indicate that upright posture control is characterized by the distinct organization of muscle activation patterns or synergies which are used in response to spontaneous sway as well as induced perturbations (Nashner and Woollacott 1979). These muscular response synergies are directionally specific, with anterior muscles (anterior tibialis, quadriceps and abdominals) responding to forward perturbations or posterior sway, and posterior muscles (gastrocnemius, hamstrings and trunk extensors) responding to backward perturbations or anterior sway. These activation patterns are temporally organized, with activation progressing from distal to proximal muscles. Ankle muscles are activated first, with muscles in the thigh and trunk responding in turn.

These findings in adults have led researchers to explore the development of such synergies in children. The next studies we will discuss focus on several questions: When do children begin to show muscular responses to perturbations in standing? How are these responses organized? Does the organization of responses change with development?

Motor coordination

Several studies which focus on the emergence of standing posture muscle synergies in children have yielded interesting results (Sveistrup *et al.* 1990; Woollacott and Sveistrup 1992; Sveistrup and Woollacott, in press). In these investigations the development of muscle response synergies was studied longitudinally in children from 2 to 18 months. The children were classified according to behavioral levels of development: pre-sitting (2–6 months), early pull-to-stand (7–8 months), pull-to-stand (9–10 months), independent stance (10–12 months), independent walkers (12–14 months) and late independent walkers (14–16 months). Their responses to anterior and posterior platform perturbations were examined through EMG recordings of the lower extremity and trunk musculature (Fig. 3.1).

The authors reported that the children did not demonstrate coordinated muscle responses to standing platform perturbations in the pre-sitting stage. In the early pull-to-stand stage, directionally appropriate muscular responses emerged in the ankle musculature (gastrocnem-

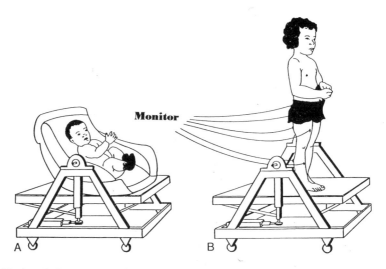

Fig. 3.1. Moving platform apparatus used to study postural responses in children: (A) sitting; (B) standing. (Adapted from Shumway-Cook and Woollacott 1995.)

ius and anterior tibialis), but coordinated responses in more proximal muscles were not seen. As the children gained more experience with pulling-to-stand, responses in the thigh and trunk muscles were noted along with those at the ankle. However, these multiple-muscle responses were not consistently organized with respect to temporal sequencing. By the time the children were standing independently temporal organization between the responding muscles was more consistent, with the activation sequence progressing in a distal to proximal fashion as is seen in adults. As the children began to walk independently, their muscular responses became even more consistent, and appeared very similar to those seen in adults (Fig. 3.2).

Studies focusing on the evolution of these muscle synergies have demonstrated that changes with respect to the magnitude and latency of responses to perturbations can be seen as children mature. Shumway-Cook and Woollacott (1985b) observed that children in the 15–36 month age range showed larger response amplitudes, increased response latencies and longer duration of responses compared with adults. It is interesting to note that the anterior sway condition produced the longer response latencies and durations in the children, but responses for the posterior sway condition were similar to those of adults. These results are similar to those found by Hirschfeld and Forssberg (1994) in connection with perturbation responses in sitting. Forssberg and Nashner (1982) reported longer latencies for responses in children of this age group and they also noted that these children demonstrated larger excursion in sway and more oscillations compared with adults.

Shumway-Cook and Woollacott (1985b) tracked the changes in muscle synergy characteristics in older children from 4 to 10 years of age. They found that 4- to 6-year-old children showed increased latency of responses compared with both the 15- to 36-month-olds and the 7- to 10-year-olds. The 4- to 6-year-olds were also more variable in their responses.

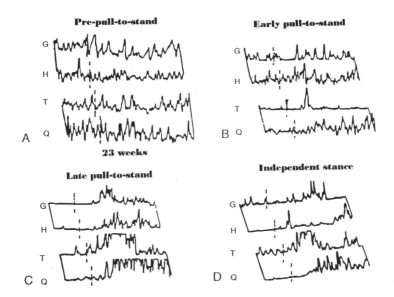

Fig. 3.2. EMG responses from one child in: (A) pre-pull-to-stand stage; (B) early pull-to-stand stage; (C) late pull-to-stand stage; and (D) independent stance. G = gastrocnemius, H = hamstring, T = tibialis anterior, Q = quadriceps muscles. (Adapted from Sveistrup and Woollacott 1993.)

Why would this apparent regression in upright posture control occur in 4- to 6-year-old children? Shumway-Cook and Woollacott have speculated that the regression may be linked to the significant morphological changes which occur in children at this age.

In summary, we can see that standing muscular responses are present in children who are just entering the pull-to-stand stage. These responses become organized into synergies, with maturing temporal organization as the child moves to independent standing. Response characteristics related to response onset latency, magnitude and duration also undergo dynamic changes as the child develops.

Speculation on the factors which contribute to the development of these organized synergies has implicated muscle strength, neurological changes and experience.

Role of muscle strength
It has been suggested that muscle strength may be a rate-limiting factor in the development of stance posture control (Thelen and Fisher 1982). Studies in which the weight-bearing abilities of infants were examined have shown that infants are able to generate ground reaction forces in standing that are more than adequate for sustaining their body weight against gravity by the age of 6 months (Roncesvalles and Jensen 1993; Jensen and Bothner, in press).

Thus it appears that muscle strength may not be critical in the development of upright posture control since children can generate levels which are adequate to support stance in the transition to pull-to-stand.

Morphological changes

Studies have described the relationship between body morphology and control of upright posture in children from infancy through the teenage years (Taguchi and Tada 1988, McCollum and Leen 1989). It appears that young children sway at a faster rate in response to upright postural displacements due to their configuration of body mass. Compared with older children and adults, young children have more mass in the head, arms and trunk segment versus the legs. This accentuates the 'inverted pendulum' action which occurs when the body begins to sway. As body morphology changes this effect is decreased, and children show sway velocities which are similar to those of adults by the age of 12–15 years. This relationship between body mass configuration and rate of sway may partially explain why young children respond to perturbations with increased magnitude and duration of responses. If the body is swaying at an increased rate, greater correction would be necessary to counteract the displacement.

Some researchers have speculated that the apparent regression of standing posture responses seen in 4- to 6-year-old children may be related to the fact that they are in the process of modifying their postural strategies in order to adapt to changing anthropometric characteristics (Shumway-Cook and Woollacott 1985b). In contrast, there is evidence that suggests morphology may not significantly affect body movement in response to platform perturbations in 4- to 9-year-old children. Kinematic analysis of body movement in a study of 4- to 6-year-old and 7- to 9-year-old children revealed no significant differences between the two groups or in comparison with adults (Woollacott *et al.* 1988).

Role of experience

We have seen that children at the pull-to-stand stage of development exhibit muscular activation in response to perturbations in standing before having much experience in this position. Sveistrup and Woollacott (in press) have examined the effects of experience on standing posture responses in children at this developmental level. In their experiment children were divided into a control and a practice group and given pre- and post-tests on a perturbation platform with EMG muscle responses recorded for both forward and backward displacements. Children in the practice group received 300 perturbations over a three-day period between the pre- and post-test measures, while the control group children participated only in pre- and post-testing. Results comparing pre- and post-tests for the practice group showed that there were no differences in the onset latencies due to training. However, the children in the practice group showed an increased probability of muscular responses, with better temporal organization compared with those in the control group. From these results the authors concluded that experience can influence the relationship between sensation and action for these responses, but that experience is not a rate-limiting factor in their maturation.

Mapping of sensation to action

It appears that children are able to utilize information from the visual, proprioceptive and vestibular systems in postural responses at the stage of independent sitting. Lee and Aronson (1974) developed a method for testing children in situations of sensory conflict. Using a mobile 'room' (walls and ceiling but not floor) which when moved forward or backward

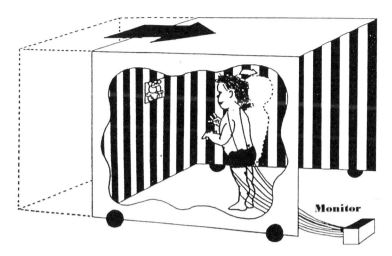

Fig. 3.3. Moving room paradigm used in visual flow experiments. (Adapted from Sveistrup and Woollacott 1993.)

provided the illusion of postural sway when none was occurring (Fig. 3.3), they found that newly standing children (13–16 months old) stepped, staggered or fell with movement of the room. They thus concluded that children in this age group depend heavily on vision for posture control in standing. From this experiment it appears that new walkers are not able to integrate information from different sensory systems. When does this ability emerge?

Research by Brandt *et al.* (1976) looked at the effects of a rotating visual display on postural sway and showed that children's postural sway was not affected by erroneous visual cues until they had learned to stand. However, more recent research has shown that vision has an effect on posture control in very young infants as well. Foster *et al.* (1996) examined the effects of visual flow on posture control in infants sitting independently (5–8 months) and those pulling to stand (8–10 months) as well as older children. They used a moving room paradigm similar to Lee and Aronson's. When the room was moved, the children (in standing or supported stance) received input from vision which signaled that a postural perturbation was occurring, while vestibular and somatosensory inputs gave no such signal. The frequency with which the children swayed in response to the visual perturbation, how they responded to the induced sway and muscle activation patterns were monitored. The results indicated that the probability of eliciting a sway response to the pseudo-perturbation was highest in the 5- to 8- and 8- to 10-month-olds compared with the older children. These children were also the most likely to show a step, stagger or falling as a result of the sway. However, even the youngest children were able to show directionally specific muscular responses to the induced sway.

Both distal-to-proximal and proximal-to-distal muscle activation patterns were seen in the 5- to 8- and 8- to 10-month-old children. However, children in the latter group showed a predominance of the distal-to-proximal pattern, while the 5- to 8-month-olds showed both patterns with equal frequency.

65

These outcomes lend support to the notion that children can detect and process visual flow information, contributing to stance posture control, as early as 5 months. They also appear able to interpret this information as sway, and mediate muscular responses. However, it is not until 8–10 months that they become more consistent in showing mature proximal-to-distal response patterns to visual flow. It is also evident that although children who are not yet walking are beginning to learn to deal with conflicting sensory conditions, these abilities are far from mature.

In the same experiment, Foster *et al.* also tracked the changes in intersensory integration which occur as children mature. They tested children at the new-walker stage (11–14 months) and three groups of experienced walkers. The experienced walkers were classified by the amount of experience in independent walking. The groups consisted of 2- to 3-year-old, 4- to 6-year-old, and 7- to 10-year-old children respectively. The results revealed that children in the new-walker group had the largest magnitudes of sway responses, as well as the highest number of resulting falls compared with the older children. However, there was a significant decrease in response magnitude and likelihood of falls in children in the older groups beginning with the 2- to 3-year-olds. This led to the conclusions that children are most visually dominant as new walkers, and that they are beginning to integrate intersensory inputs in conflict situations by age 2–3 years.

Sensory adaptation
In studies focusing on multisensory integration, Forssberg and Nashner (1982) and Shumway-Cook and Woollacott (1985b) examined the ability of children to produce appropriate motor responses in conditions of intersensory conflict. A platform apparatus capable of confounding somatosensory cues was used in these experiments. In the study by Shumway-Cook and Woollacott, children from 3 to 10 years of age were tested in four experimental conditions; eyes open with firm surface, eyes closed with firm surface, eyes open with sway-referenced surface and eyes closed with sway-referenced surface. In the sway-referenced conditions the platform surface moved to match the spontaneous sway of the child, thus giving the illusion that no movement was occurring at the ankle joints. This condition was paired with the vision present or absent condition to invoke sensory conflict conditions.

The results indicated that 4- to 6-year-old children were beginning to mediate compensatory responses in conditions of intersensory conflict, although their abilities were far from mature. When the authors compared the amount of sway elicited in 4- to 6-year-old and 7- to 9-year-old children with that found in adults, they found that the 4- to 6-year-olds demonstrated the greatest amount of sway and variability of responses in all four sensory conditions (Fig. 3.4). The 7- to 9-year-olds' responses were much more like those of the adults, with much less variability and less sway. The authors suggested that until age 7, children are not able to balance effectively in conditions using only vestibular input (somatosensory and vision removed), or in conditions where sensory inputs from one or more sensory systems are in conflict.

Forssberg and Nashner (1982) also found that although children under 7 years showed consistent responses with respect to automatic postural adjustments, they were unable to reconcile and adapt to conflicting sensory information. What is the mechanism by which

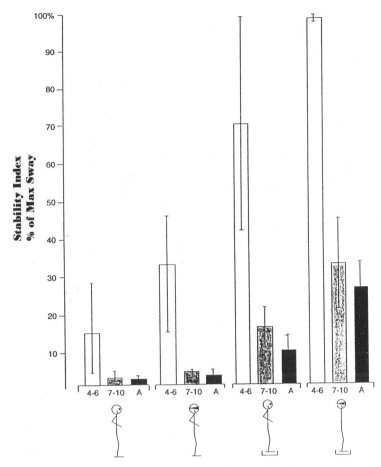

Fig. 3.4. Comparison of body sway in four sensory conditions for 4- to 6-year-olds, 7- to 10-year-olds and adults: (A) firm surface with eyes open; (B) firm surface with eyes closed; (C) confounded surface with eyes open; (D) confounded surface with eyes closed. Graph shows mean and standard deviation across children in each age group. (Adapted from Shumway-Cook and Woollacott 1985b.)

older children and adults resolve conflicting sensory inputs and mediate correct postural responses? The authors proposed that the resolution and integration of conflicting sensory information occurs through the relative weighting of information related to the movement context. This involves the ability to identify the information which is confounded and utilize it less, while focusing on the correct input provided from the remaining sensory systems.

Anticipatory posture control
Several researchers have explored the relationship between posture control and active voli-tional movement (Forssberg and Nashner 1982, Nashner *et al.* 1983). In these studies,

EMG activity of postural muscles was monitored to see if preparatory postural adjustments occur in advance of volitional upper extremity movements in the standing position. It was shown that children activate postural muscles in anticipation of potentially destabilizing upper extremity movements by 1 year of age (Forssberg and Nashner 1982).

In a study by Woollacott and Shumway-Cook (1986) children were asked to pull on a moveable lever while standing. The results showed that they made anticipatory postural adjustments similar to those seen in adults by age 4–6 years. Comparing these results with those found in studies testing postural responses to perturbation, we can see that the ability to adjust to an anticipated destabilization develops simultaneously with the ability to react to externally generated destabilizing forces in normally maturing children.

Impaired development of posture control

Cerebral palsy

Cerebral palsy (CP) is a term commonly used to label deficits ascribed to an injury to the cerebral cortex. It has traditionally been used in reference to an insult to the immature brain, occurring sometime during the perinatal period. However, the term cerebral palsy is nonspecific in that the manifestations of injury are extremely variable depending upon a variety of factors including etiology, location, timing and severity of injury. As a pathological entity, CP is unique in that it involves a static lesion upon which maturation and development are superimposed. The etiology of CP is also variable. Injury may occur through several mechanisms, the most common being anoxic or hypoxic encephalopathy, intracerebral hemorrhage, and CNS neuropathy resulting from malformation (Olney and Wright 1994).

Children with CP may have a conglomeration of clinical symptoms affecting sensori-motor systems. Classifications designating different types of CP are based largely on these clinical symptoms, along with morphological distribution patterns. Although description of all the different classifications is beyond the scope of our discussion, we will describe three types: spastic hemiplegia, spastic diplegia and ataxia. Children with hemiplegia demonstrate dysfunction on one side of the body, while children with diplegia show the most involvement bilaterally in the lower extremities. Spasticity describes the muscular abnormality of hyperactive reflexes and increased stiffness, which is a common feature of these disorders. Ataxia refers to the coordination dysfunction which may also be seen in children with CP. Although children may show more than one type of movement dysfunction, such as spasticity along with ataxia, we shall not consider these cases.

ROLE OF THE STRETCH REFLEX

The fact that children with CP manifest hyperactive stretch reflexes is undisputed. However, the functional significance of this finding is the subject of debate. Several studies focusing on this issue have failed to find a significant correlation between stretch reflex abnormalities and functional ability. This has led some researchers to question the role of the stretch reflex in posture control (Nashner *et al.* 1983).

Nashner and co-workers conducted a study in which postural perturbations were induced in children with spastic hemiplegia and diplegia who showed hyperactive stretch reflexes in the ankle plantarflexor muscles on clinical examination. Standing perturbations causing forward sway and toes-up rotation were given with the intention of delivering a quick stretch to the plantarflexor muscles. Because these muscles were hyperactive when the children were tested clinically, the expected response to these perturbations was that the stretch reflex would be activated. Instead, the plantarflexors of the children with CP showed a delayed response to the perturbations (150 ms compared with a normal response of 95–110 ms). This led the authors to surmise that the monosynaptic stretch reflex does not play a role in the ankle posture responses of children with CP.

The systems perspective is based on the idea that posture control evolves through the interaction of many subsystems within the context of the task and the environment. In this view, the dysfunctions seen in posture control development in children with CP do not result solely from the retention of primitive patterns or reflex and muscle tone abnormalities. Instead, the interactions of multiple systems which are maturing in parallel within the context of a neurological insult must be considered (Fig. 3.5).

Studies in which children with spastic diplegia have undergone selective dorsal rhizotomy (to normalize muscle tone) have brought to light several important factors which appear to have significant implications related to the movement and postural dysfunction seen in these children (Giuliani 1991). It has been shown that children with spastic diplegia do not show normal movement patterns and posture control after dorsal rhizotomy. The fact that these children are not able to control posture normally in the absence of spasticity supports the systems view of posture control. As a result researchers have begun to study the role of musculoskeletal constraints and sensorimotor abnormalities related to posture control in children with CP.

SITTING POSTURE CONTROL

Children with CP often have difficulty maintaining stable sitting postures, which makes functional use of the upper extremities and hands difficult. In an effort to better understand the basis of these difficulties, researchers have examined how children with CP respond to sitting perturbations compared with unaffected children. These investigations have yielded interesting results related to differences in motor coordination in these children.

In one study, Brogren (1995) used a perturbation platform to compare sitting motor coordination patterns of seven children with spastic diplegia with those of age matched controls. In response to posterior sway the children with CP showed two types of activation patterns in the ventral muscles: a cephalocaudal activation with the neck flexors responding first followed by the trunk and hip musculature, and a simultaneous activation pattern involving all of the ventral muscles responding at once. In contrast, children in the control group demonstrated a consistent caudocephalad pattern with the muscles nearest the support surface responding first. In response to anterior sway, children in the control group again showed muscles closest to the support surface (the hamstrings) responding first. These children seldom activated the trunk extensors in response to this perturbation, and the neck extensors were typically inhibited. Comparatively, the responses of the children with CP were highly variable. These children demonstrated a high degree of neck extensor activation combined with hamstring activation and inhibition of the trunk extensors. From these results we can

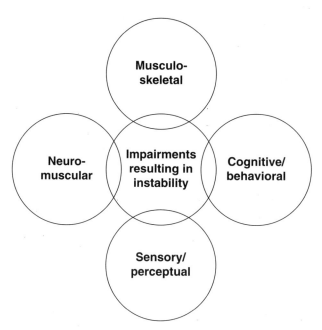

Fig. 3.5. Impairments in different systems can lead to constraints on posture control development. (Adapted from Shumway-Cook and Woollacott 1995.)

see that children with spastic diplegic CP demonstrate disordered motor coordination in response to sitting posture perturbations.

STANDING POSTURE CONTROL

The findings of Brogren *et al.* are supported by other work in which investigators have examined muscle activation patterns in children with CP in response to standing posture perturbations. Woollacott *et al.* (in press) studied the responses of seven children with spastic diplegia and seven normally developing children. Since they were interested in posture control from a developmental perspective, the children in this experiment were grouped and matched with control subjects by developmental level rather than age. Three groups of children participated in the study: a pull-to-stand group (2 CP, 2 normal), a young walker group (2–4 years walking experience: 2 CP, 2 normal) and an experienced walker group (8–14 years walking experience: 3 CP, 3 normal). The children were exposed to translational platform perturbations in standing (or supported standing for those in the pull-to-stand group). EMG activity of the trunk and lower extremity musculature was recorded. Analysis focused on EMG responses of the posterior muscles in response to anterior sway, with respect to onset of muscle activation and temporal organization patterns.
• *Temporal organization.* The typically developing control children generally demonstrated distal to proximal activation patterns in response to anterior sway, with the plantar-flexors responding first, followed by the hamstrings and trunk extensors. Control children

70

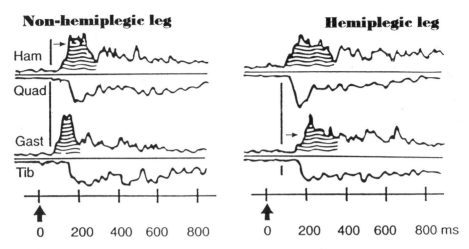

Fig. 3.6. Reversal of normal temporal muscle activation pattern in the involved and less-involved legs of a child with hemiplegic cerebral palsy. Ham = hamstring, Quad = quadriceps, Tib = tibialis anterior. (Adapted from Nashner *et al.* 1983.)

in the pull-to-stand group did show occasional disorganization of this pattern and agonist/ antagonist coactivation was seen in a small number of trials. However, the consistency of the activation patterns increased with experience, with children in the older groups showing no disorganization or coactivation.

In contrast, the children with CP showed agonist/antagonist coactivation and temporal disorganization at all developmental levels. The children with CP in the pull-to-stand group demonstrated a proximal to distal muscle activation pattern in more than half of the trials, with the hamstring muscles typically responding first (Fig. 3.6). The children with CP also did not show the same degree of pattern refinement seen in the control children. This is illustrated by the fact that children in the older groups continued to show the 'reversed' pattern, along with a persistence of agonist/antagonist coactivation. In fact, the children with CP in the experienced walker group showed the most coactivation in response to perturbations compared with children in the other groups.

• *Onset of muscle activation.* The children with CP demonstrated onset latencies that were generally similar to those of the typically developing children. However, the children with CP did not have clear onset and offset of muscle activation and the duration of muscle responses was prolonged compared with the control children. While there was a trend among the control children for decreased duration of muscle activation as the patterns became more refined, responses in the children with CP remained prolonged even in those with the most walking experience.

In summary, children with spastic diplegia demonstrate a consistent pattern of disorganization with respect to muscle activation patterns in response to both sitting and standing postural perturbations. These children also seem to retain immature postural response characteristics seen in typically developing children of younger ages.

Woollacott *et al.* (in press) were also interested in the effects of musculoskeletal abnormalities on motor coordination in standing. Many children with spastic diplegia develop muscle and joint contractures throughout the lower extremities, resulting in a crouched standing posture. This crouched posture is characterized by increased hip and knee flexion with either equinus or excessive dorsiflexion at the ankle.

To test the effects of the crouched position on muscular responses, children with no neurological dysfunction were positioned in a crouched posture and subjected to standing postural perturbations while EMG activity was recorded in the lower extremity musculature. Analysis of their muscular responses showed increased antagonistic activity and disorganization of temporal sequencing. When in the crouched position, these children activated their muscles in a proximal to distal fashion, showing the reversals typical in children with spastic diplegia. Sienko-Thomas *et al.* (1996) found similar results in a study where children with no neurological dysfunction were videotaped in a crouched position during gait (*i.e.* with knees bent and trunk inclined forward). Analysis of their walking patterns also revealed muscle activation abnormalities characteristic of those seen in children with CP having similar musculoskeletal limitations.

From these findings, it is clear that musculoskeletal constraints can play a significant role in the coordination of posture and moment. These results lend support to the argument that the study of postural and movement dysfunction in children with CP should be approached from the systems perspective.

SENSORY ADAPTATION AND ANTICIPATORY CONTROL

We have discussed the deficits in motor coordination related to posture control seen in children with CP. Are the functional deficits seen in these children the result of motor dysfunction alone, or are sensory systems also involved?

Nashner *et al.* (1983) explored this question by testing children with different types of CP and age-matched controls under various sensory conditions. Included in the CP group were three subjects with hemiplegia, three with diplegia and three with ataxia. The children stood on a moveable platform, while lower extremity and trunk muscle EMG recordings were taken during six spontaneous sway conditions. The first three conditions included a stable support surface with vision, with no vision or with vision confounded. The second three conditions included confounded proprioceptive input (the support surface swayed with the child) and vision, no vision or confounded vision. Analysis focused on the organization of muscle response patterns in the children with different types of CP, as well as their ability to balance under the various sensory conditions.

• *Sensory adaptation.* All of the children with CP had more difficulty maintaining balance in the first set of sensory conditions than the control children. However, the ataxic children had more difficulty compared with the others, particularly in the vision-confounded condition.

In the second set of sensory conditions, all of the children (cerebral palsied and control) had more difficulty maintaining balance than under the first three conditions. None of the control children lost balance in the three proprioception-confounded conditions, even when vision was also confounded. The children with hemiplegia had more difficulty under these conditions than the control children, and one lost balance in the vision- and proprioception-confounded condition. However, the children with ataxia had the greatest difficulty in the proprioception-confounded conditions, two of them losing their balance when both vision and proprioception were confounded.

• *Muscle activation patterns.* The muscle response patterns of all the children were examined in response to anticipated postural perturbation when pulling a moveable lever in standing. EMG activity was recorded in the lower extremity, trunk and arm musculature. The control children demonstrated a distal to proximal muscle activation pattern, with muscles in the lower extremities and trunk responding before those in the upper extremities. In contrast, the children with hemiplegia and diplegia exhibited a reversal of this pattern with activation progressing in a proximal to distal fashion. In addition, the children with CP often failed to use anticipatory activation of postural muscles; the upper extremity muscles were often activated first in these children.

From these results the authors hypothesized that children with CP (especially ataxia) have difficulties with sensory organization systems as well as motor systems. They speculated that these sensory deficits may be a result of delayed or disrupted development of sensory organization systems, along with abnormalities in peripheral sensory inputs.

In summary, it appears that children with CP have deficits which encompass both sensory and motor systems, resulting in functional difficulties in seated and standing postural control, and control of locomotion as well as sensory adaptation and anticipatory postural control.

Down syndrome

It has been well established in the literature that children with Down syndrome are delayed in their motor development, demonstrating particular difficulties with static and dynamic balance (Shumway-Cook and Woollacott 1985a, Woollacott and Shumway-Cook 1986). Children with Down syndrome typically display hypotonia throughout all the body musculature, and they have difficulties with coordination.

Using platform posturography, researchers have examined the responses of children with Down syndrome to postural perturbations and sensory conflict conditions. Shumway-Cook and Woollacott (1985a) studied children with Down syndrome from 1 to 6 years of age in order to track their posture control development. These children were exposed to forward and backward translational perturbations in standing while EMGs from the trunk and legs were monitored. The older children (4–6 years of age) were also tested under four altered sensory conditions; normal surface with eyes closed and eyes open, and stabilized surface with eyes closed and eyes open. In the stabilized surface conditions, the platform surface rotated proportionally to the sway of the child thus confounding the proprioceptive input.

The authors found that the responses of the children with Down syndrome in the 1–3 year age range were inconsistent, poorly organized and slow compared with those of control children of similar age. In contrast, children with Down syndrome in the 4–6 year range demonstrated muscular responses to perturbation which were directionally appropriate and

73

normally organized. However, their responses were delayed in terms of onset times. When these children were tested under the different sensory conditions they were able to mediate appropriate postural responses. However, they had greater amounts of sway in three of the conditions, and increased variability of responses in all four conditions compared with children of the same age. The children with Down syndrome were also unable to adapt their responses over successive trials in the various sensory conditions, while control children adapted by attenuating their responses within 15 trials.

What factors are responsible for the posture control dysfunction seen in children with Down syndrome? Since hypotonia is a prominent characteristic in these children, does muscle strength play a role?

ROLE OF MUSCLE STRENGTH

Davis and Kelso (1982) tested the ability of individuals with Down syndrome to generate and voluntarily modulate muscle stiffness. They found no difference in these parameters compared with normal control subjects. These findings would suggest that the ability to generate muscular force is not associated with decreased postural control in individuals with muscle hypotonia due to Down syndrome. However, it is difficult to relate the ability to voluntarily control muscle stiffness to the generation of muscular force in automatic postural responses (Woollacott and Shumway-Cook 1986).

Summary

We have summarized the development of posture control in the infant and young child from the stage of emerging head control to refinement of stance and systems perspectives related to this developmental process.

The systems model of posture control suggests that new behaviors emerge as the result of increasingly sophisticated interactions between multiple body systems in the context of the movement task and environment.

Research suggests that the ability to relate sensory input to motor output forms the basis of posture control development. As the infant learns to sit and stand the rules linking sensory and motor systems are extended to the trunk and legs.

Single sense control of posture emerges first in young infants, with vision being dominant in the pre-sitting and newly sitting infant. As the infant gains experience in sitting, reliance on vision decreases, and postural responses appear to be initiated through somatosensory input, with vision playing a modulatory role. A reliance on vision is again seen during transitions, such as to independent standing and walking. Children begin to integrate multisensory inputs before the emergence of independent walking; however, the ability to mediate correct motor responses in sensory conflict situations does not emerge until later.

Rules which characterize the development of postural responses in sitting include the following: (a) children respond earlier and more consistently in response to posterior sway; (b) onset latencies and variability in sequencing of muscular responses decrease with maturation, with caudal to rostral patterns becoming dominant.

Rules which characterize the development of postural responses in pre-standing and standing include: (a) an increase in response probability and consistency with response organization in a distal to proximal fashion; (b) onset latencies, response magnitudes and response duration decrease, and muscle activity is more appropriately scaled to the amount of induced sway. Sensory adaptation, a process of 'relative weighting' of information from different sources, matures by age 7. The ability to adjust to anticipated destabilization appears to develop simultaneously with the ability to react to externally generated forces in typically developing children.

Children with CP demonstrate postural responses in sitting and standing which are both immature and disorganized. Musculoskeletal constraints contribute to this dysfunction. Children with spastic CP show a reversal of the normal muscular sequencing patterns along with unclear onset and offset of muscle activation. They also demonstrate deficits in anticipatory posture control. Children with ataxia show the most difficulty in adaptation to sensory conflict situations.

Children with Down syndrome are delayed in their development of automatic postural responses. However, these responses are directionally specific and normally organized once they emerge. These children also demonstrate difficulty with adaptation in varying sensory conditions, although they generally do not demonstrate the degree of instability seen in children with CP under similar conditions.

ACKNOWLEDGEMENT

This work was supported by a grant from the National Science Foundation, #BNS 9110897, to Dr Marjorie Woollacott.

REFERENCES

Amiel-Tison, C., Grenier, Q. (1980). *Évaluation Neurologique du Nouveau-né et du Nourrisson (Neurological Evaluation of the Human Infant).* Paris: Masson.
Brandt, T., Wenzel, D., Dichgans, J. (1976). 'Die Entwicklung der visuellen Stabilisation des aufrechten Standes bein Kind. Ein Refezeichen in der Kinder-neurologie.' *Archiv für Psychiatrie und Nervenkrankheiten,* **223**, 1–13.
Brogren, E. (1995) 'Postural adjustments in sitting children with spastic diplegia.' *In: Proceedings of the International Sven Jerring Symposium: Children with Functional Disabilities. Stockholm, June 11–15,* pp. 73–75.
Campbell, S.K. (1994) 'The child's development of functional movement.' *In:* Campbell, S.K. (Ed.) *Physical Therapy for Children.* Philadelphia: W.B. Saunders, pp. 3–37.
Davis, W., Kelso, J.A.S. (1982) 'Analysis of "invariant characteristics" in the motor control of Down's syndrome and normal subjects.' *Journal of Motor Behavior,* **14**, 194–212.
Eviatar, L., Eviatar, A, Naray, I. (1974) 'Maturation of neurovestibular responses in infants.' *Developmental Medicine and Child Neurology,* **16**, 435–446.
Forssberg, H., Nashner, L.M. (1982) 'Ontogenetic development of postural control in man: adaptation to altered support and visual conditions during stance.' *Journal of Neuroscience,* **2**, 545–552.
Foster, E.C., Sveistrup, H., Woollacott, M.H. (1996) 'Transitions in visual proprioception: a cross-sectional developmental study of the effect of visual flow on postural control.' *Journal of Motor Behavior,* **28**, 101–112.
Gesell, A. (1946) 'The ontogenesis of infant behavior.' *In:* Carmichael, L. (Ed.) *Manual of Child Psychology.* New York: Wiley, pp. 335–373.
Giuliani, C. (1991) 'Dorsal rhizotomy for children with cerebral palsy: support for concepts of motor control.' *Physical Therapy,* **71**, 248–259.
Hirschfeld, H. (1992) 'On the integration of posture, locomotion and voluntary movements in humans: normal and impaired development.' Stockholm: Nobel Institute of Neurophysics, Karolinska Institute. *(Dissertation.)*
Hirschfeld, H., Forssberg, H. (1994) 'Epigenetic development of postural responses for sitting during infancy.' *Experimental Brain Research,* **97**, 528–540.

Horak, F. (1992) 'Motor control models underlying neurologic rehabilitation of posture in children.' *In:* Forssberg, H., Hirschfeld, H. (Eds.) *Movement Disorders in Children.* Basel: Karger, pp. 21–32.

Jensen, J.L., Bothner, K.E. (in press) 'Revisiting infant motor development schedules: the biomechanics of change.' *In:* van Praagh, E. (Ed.) *Anaerobic Performance During Childhood and Adolescence.* Champaign, IL: Human Kinetics.

Jouen, F. (1984) 'Visual–vestibular interactions in infancy.' *Infant Behavior and Development*, **7**, 135–145.

—— (1988) 'Visual–proprioceptive control of posture in newborn infants.' *In:* Amblard, B., Berthoz, A., Clarac, F. (Eds.) *Posture and Gait: Development, Adaptation and Modulation.* Amsterdam: Elsevier Science, pp. 13–22.

—— Lepecq, J.C., Gapenne, O. (in press) 'Early visual vestibular relations in newborns.' *Child Development.*

Lee, D., Aronson, E. (1974) 'Visual–proprioceptive control of standing in human infants.' *Perception and Psychophysics*, **15**, 529–532.

McCollum, G., Leen, T.K. (1989) 'Form exploration of mechanical stability limits in erect stance.' *Journal of Motor Behavior*, **21**, 225–244.

McGraw, M.B. (1932) 'From reflex to muscular control in the assumption of an erect posture and ambulation in the human infant.' *Child Development*, **3**, 291–297.

Myklebust, B.M., Gottlieb, G.L., Agarwal, G.C. (1986) 'Stretch reflexes of the normal infant.' *Developmental Medicine and Child Neurology*, **28**, 440–449.

Nashner, L., Woollacott, M. (1979) 'The organization of rapid postural adjustment of standing humans: an experimental–conceptual model.' *In:* Talbott, R.E., Humphrey, D.R. (Eds.) *Posture and Movement.* New York: Raven Press, pp.243–257.

—— Shumway-Cook, A., Marin, O. (1983) 'Stance posture control in selected groups of children with cerebral palsy: deficits in sensory organization and muscular coordination.' *Experimental Brain Research*, **49**, 393–409.

Olney, S.J., Wright, M.J. (1994) 'Cerebral palsy.' *In:* Campbell, S. (Ed.) *Physical Therapy for Children.* Philadelphia: W.B. Saunders: pp.489–523.

Prechtl, H.F.R. (1986) 'Prenatal motor development.' *In:* Wade, M.C., Whiting, H.T. (Eds.) *Motor Development in Children: Aspects of Coordination and Control.* Dordrecht: Martinus Nijhoff, pp. 53–64.

Roncesvalles, N.C., Jensen, J. (1993) 'The expression of weight-bearing ability in infants between four and seven months of age.' *Sport and Exercise Psychology*, **15**, 568. *(Abstract.)*

Schloon, H., O'Brien, M.J., Scholten, C.A., Prechtl, H.F.R. (1976) 'Muscle activity and postural behaviour in newborn infants. A polymyographic study.' *Neuropädiatrie*, **7**, 384–415.

Shumway-Cook, A., Woollacott, M.H. (1985a) 'Dynamics of postural control in the child with Down syndrome.' *Physical Therapy*, **65**, 1315–1322.

—— —— (1985b) 'The growth of stability: postural control from a developmental perspective.' *Journal of Motor Behavior*, **17**, 131–147.

—— —— (1993) 'Theoretical issues in assessing postural control.' *In:* Wilhelm, I.J. (Ed.) *Clinics in Physical Therapy: Physical Therapy Assessment in Early Infancy.* New York: Churchill Livingstone, pp. 161–171.

—— —— (1995) *Motor Control: Theory and Practical Applications.* Baltimore: Williams & Wilkins.

Sienko-Thomas, S., Moore, C.A., Kelp-Lenane, C., Norris, C. (1996) 'Simulated gait patterns: the resulting effects on gait parameters, dynamic electromyography, joint moments, and physiological cost index.' *Gait and Posture*, **4**, 100–107.

Sveistrup, H., Woollacott, M.H. (1993) 'Systems contributing to the emergence and maturation of stability in postnatal development.' *In:* Savelsbergh, G.J.P. (Ed.) *The Development of Coordination in Infancy.* Amsterdam: Elsevier, pp. 319–336.

—— —— (in press) 'Practice modifies the developing automatic postural response.' *Experimental Brain Research.*

—— —— Shumway-Cook, A., McCollum, G. (1990) 'A longitudinal study on the transition to independent stance in children.' *Neuroscience Abstracts*, **16**, 893.

Tibbling, L. (1969) 'The rotatory nystagmus response in children.' *Acta Oto-Laryngologica*, **68**, 459–467.

Taguchi, K., Tada, C. (1988) 'Change of body sway with growth of children.' *In:* Amblard, B., Berthoz, A., Clarac, F. (Eds.) *Posture and Gait: Development, Adaptation and Modulation.* Amsterdam: Elsevier, pp. 59–65.

Thelen, E., Fisher, D.M. (1982) 'Newborn stepping: an explanation for a "disappearing reflex".' *Developmental Psychology*, **18**, 760–775.

Woollacott, M., Shumway-Cook, A. (1986) 'The development of the postural and voluntary motor control systems in Down's syndrome children' *In:* Wade, M.G. (Ed.) *Motor Skill Acquisition of the Mentally Handicapped: Issues in Research and Training.* Amsterdam: Elsevier Science, pp. 45–71.

—— Sveistrup, H. (1992) 'Changes in the sequencing and timing of muscle response coordination associated with developmental transitions in balance abilities.' *Human Movement Science,* **11,** 23–36.

—— Debû, B., Mowatt, M. (1987) 'Neuromuscular control of posture in the infant and child: is vision dominant?' *Journal of Motor Behavior,* **19,** 167–186.

—— Rösblad, B., von Hosten, C. (1988) 'Relation between muscle response onset and body segmental movements during postural perturbations in humans.' Experimental Brain Research, **72,** 593–604.

—— Burtner, P., Jensen, J., Jasiewicz, J., Roncesvalles, N., Sveistrup, H. (in press) 'Development of postural response during standing in healthy children and children with spastic diplegia.' *Acta Paediatrica.*

4
NEUROBIOLOGY OF NORMAL AND IMPAIRED LOCOMOTOR DEVELOPMENT

Hans Forssberg and Volker Dietz

Many movement behaviours are automatized, allowing our brain to deal with complex mental processes while we are moving. The development of some of these automatic behaviours is constrained to species-specific movement patterns that are expressed even under abnormal conditions. Other less constrained behaviours show quite extensive variation within the same species. To the former category belong vital functions that are crucial for fitness. Locomotion, which is strongly canalized during development, is one such function. Respiration, mastication and swallowing are other examples of species-specific patterns. This category of movements is controlled by neural networks in the spinal cord and brainstem. The networks appear to be well preserved during phylogeny, retaining the properties of the nerve cells, synaptic transmission and connection to other networks.

The human body constitutes a multisegmented musculoskeletal system of great complexity. Each joint is spanned by several groups of mono- and biarticular muscles. This implies that a particular motor task, *e.g.* locomotion, can be performed in a variety of trajectories and by various muscle activation patterns. Yet, the locomotor movements and the underlying muscle activation are similar for all nonimpaired persons. Bernstein (1967) was one of the first to discuss this problem of *motor equivalence* from a neural control/dynamics perspective. He argued that the motor system has too many degrees of freedom to be controlled by a single controller and proposed that the CNS solves this complex problem by organizing the motor command signals for muscle synergies rather than for individual muscles. The grouping into synergies would greatly reduce the complexity of the control systems. Bernstein also suggested that the motor control systems are organized in a hierarchical structure with the muscle synergies at a lower level, while centres at higher levels, informed by an evaluator system (decision maker), plan the motor action.

The first section of this chapter describes the neurobiological basis for locomotion, including the central pattern generating networks which are the basis for the locomotor synergy; the interaction between central and sensory mechanisms, the descending control systems which initiate and adapt the locomotor activity, and the development of human locomotion in healthy children and in children with early brain damage leading to cerebral palsy are also described.

Central pattern generators

Central pattern generators (CPGs) underlie a wide variety of rhythmic motor behaviours, such as feeding (rooting, sucking, mastication, swallowing), locomotion and respiration. The CPG consists of neuronal networks that for the most part are capable of generating rhythmical signals to the muscles without phasic sensory input from the moving body part. Bickel (1897) and Hering (1897) were the first to demonstrate in frogs, dogs and monkeys that movements could be produced after dorsal root transection, *i.e.* without any afferent information from the legs. Brown (1911) showed in cats that the deafferented spinal cord could generate alternation between a pair of antagonistic muscles similar to the locomotor rhythm. He postulated that reciprocal inhibition between antagonistic neurons (or groups of neurons) was responsible for the rhythmic activity. This CPG network could only generate a simple pattern with alternation between flexor and extensor muscles while the fine tuning and details of the locomotor pattern were shaped by interaction of peripheral reflexes. In later experiments in which all dorsal roots were cut some complexity of the motor pattern remained, indicating that the central networks could generate a more specific pattern (Grillner and Zangger 1979). Indeed, studies in invertebrates and lower vertebrates have shown that complex motor patterns can be produced by the isolated CPG networks, *e.g.* the crustacean stomatogastric network (Selverston and Moulins 1987) or locomotion in the lamprey (Grillner *et al.* 1995).

The isolated spinal cord of the lamprey can be maintained in a Petri dish over a period of several days, with spontaneous or induced activity of the locomotor CPG network. The application of modern techniques in studies of these *in vitro* preparations has allowed a detailed analysis of the network, with identification of transmitters and intrinsic cellular properties. Modulatory substances can modify the type, number and properties of various ion channels located in the membrane and thereby change the excitability of the cell. Consequently, a single neuron can display a variety of intrinsic activity patterns, switching between them depending on the modulatory influence. Basically, the lamprey spinal CPG network contains: (i) excitatory (glutamate) interneurons that project to ipsilateral interneurons and motoneurons, and (ii) inhibitory (glycinergic) interneurons projecting to the contralateral side (Fig. 4.1). The locomotor network is turned on by excitatory amino acids (EAAs), while the fine tuning of the movements is accomplished by a dopamine–serotonin system which changes the network properties.

The CPG networks are also located in the spinal cord in higher vertebrates. In several species, like the eel or dogfish, the networks are released after a spinal cord transection and the creatures continue to swim. In several mammals, locomotion can be induced immediately after a spinal transection by injecting monoaminergic substances intravenously, *e.g.* clonidine, a noradrenergic agonist (Forssberg and Grillner 1973). Locomotion can also be induced in chronic spinal* animals (Forssberg *et al.* 1980a). The locomotor movements in chronic spinal cats improve by training, *i.e.* by letting the hindlimbs walk on a treadmill belt. The loco-motion is also improved by administration of clonidine or serotonergic antagonists (Barbeau *et al.* 1987, Barbeau and Rossignol 1991). An *in vitro* brainstem/spinal cord preparation, similar to the lamprey preparation, has been developed in the neonatal rat (Cazalets *et al.* 1992). Robust locomotor activity can be induced by infusing serotonin or EAA into the

---

*'Spinal' in this context implies spinal transection performed experimentally (*i.e.* vivisection).

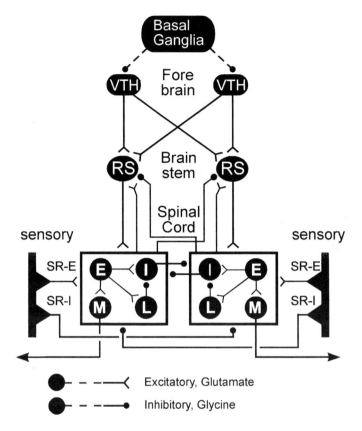

Fig. 4.1. Schematic representation of the neuronal network that coordinates locomotion in the lamprey. The reticulospinal glutaminergic brainstem neurons (phasic, R_{ph}; tonic, R_t) project to the spinal cord and excite all the spinal neurons that are depicted within the black box. The excitatory interneurons (E) excite all types of spinal neurons within the box, that is, inhibitory glycinergic interneurons (I) that cross the midline and inhibit all neurons within the contralateral box, the lateral interneuron (L), which inhibits the I interneuron, and motoneurons (M), which are cholinergic. The stretch-receptor neurons are of an excitatory (SRE) type that excites neurons within the ipsilateral box and an inhibitory (SRI) type that inhibits all neurons within the contralateral box. Synapses that are shown to terminate on the frame of the box indicate effects that are common to all neurons within the box. Note that only one cell of each type is indicated in the scheme although each cell represents a group of cells. (Reproduced by permission from Grillner *et al.* 1995.)

solution surrounding the isolated preparation, while GABA suppresses the locomotor activity. Plateau-like membrane properties, critical to induce the rhythmicity, have also been found in the cat. Thus, there seems to be a strong conservation during evolution, and transmitter systems and cell properties, as well as spinal CPG networks, are retained in mammals.

Recent evidence suggests that L-dopa can trigger 'fictive locomotion' in the spinal marmoset, a low level primate (Hultborn *et al.* 1993). Several groups have recently been able to induce locomotion in humans after incomplete spinal lesions (Fig. 4.2). The locomotor

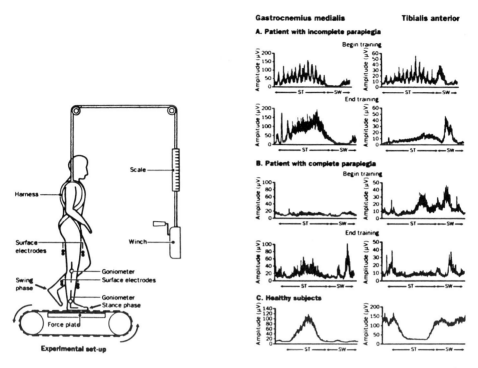

Fig. 4.2. *(Left)* Experimental set-up. *(Right)* Rectified and averaged EMG of lower-leg muscles during locomotion (around 1–3 km/h) of patients with incomplete (A) and complete (B) paraplegia, respectively, and group averages of five healthy subjects (C). (Reproduced by permission from Dietz *et al.* 1994a.)

capacity improves by training on a treadmill with the body suspended in a harness supporting part of the body weight (Fung *et al.* 1990; Barbeau *et al.* 1992; Dietz *et al.* 1994a, 1995). A locomotor pattern can also be induced and trained in completely paraplegic patients. However, the amplitude of the induced leg muscle activity is so small that the legs have to be moved by external forces (Dietz *et al.* 1994a, 1995). By analogy with the results from cats and marmosets, one would expect that noradrenergic activation would also improve the locomotor capacity in humans with spinal lesions. Clonidine administered intravenously has shown such effects in some studies (Fung *et al.* 1990, Rossignol and Barbeau 1993), while intrathecal administration of small doses leads to flaccid paresis (Dietz *et al.* 1995).

Motor–sensory interaction
Modulation of the CPG network
Animals and humans are remarkably adept at altering their movements in response to changing demands from the external environment. Still, the CPG network controlling locomotion must be sufficiently robust to avoid disruption of the locomotor activity. At the same time, the CPG network must be flexible so that the movements can be modified. On a cellular basis this can be achieved by various modulatory transmitter systems changing the

membrane properties of the neurons included in the CPG network. It can also be achieved by modulating the transmission (e.g. the transmitter release) in the synapses.

In the lamprey, there are excitatory and inhibitory sensory stretch-receptor neurons that sense the lateral bending movements occurring during locomotion and which act on the CPG interneurons and contribute to burst termination (see Fig. 4.1) (Grillner *et al.* 1995). Indeed, they may be regarded as a part of the CPG network. That such sensory feedback systems are organized at a spinal level also in mammals, is supported by the walking hindlimbs of spinal cats which closely follow the speed of the treadmill belt (Forssberg *et al.* 1980a). At lower velocities the limbs alternate, as during walking or trotting, while they may change the coordination between the limbs to gallop at higher speed. The temporal structure of the locomotor cycle is adjusted in a similar way in humans, *i.e.* the stance phase is decreased while the swing phase remains unchanged as speed increases. Concurrently, extensor bursts are enhanced in amplitude and reduced in duration. The switch from trot (out of phase) to gallop (in phase coordination) in spinal cats also shows that the interlimb coordination can be controlled by spinal sensory mechanisms. This has been further explored by letting the spinal cats walk on split belts moving at different speeds (Forssberg *et al.* 1980b). Each limb followed its own belt with respect to stance duration, while the same rhythm was maintained by prolonging the swing phase of the fast walking limb. Similar adaptations of the locomotor cycle take place in healthy human adults (Dietz *et al.* 1994b) and infants (Thelen *et al.* 1987b) walking (or stepping) on split belts. This behaviour can be explained by two CPG networks, one for each side, mutually interacting with each other (same rhythm) and driven by the sensory information from the ipsilateral side.

Some sources of the sensory feedback influencing the CPG network have been described for the cat, *i.e.* the hip and the ankle muscles. If a hindlimb of a walking spinal cat is not allowed to extend during stance, the activity in the extensor muscles continues and does not cease until the hip joint is extended (Grillner and Rossignol 1978). In other experiments, when a spinal cat is immobilized and the CPG network pharmacologically activated, the movements of the hip can entrain the rhythm of the CPG network (Andersson *et al.* 1978). The onset of flexor muscle activity at the end of the stance phase can also be prevented by loading the ankle extensors (Duysens and Pearson 1980). During normal cat locomotion the maximal load of these muscles occurs in the beginning of stance, while the load is decreased during later parts. Thus, in cats there are feedback systems associated with the position and movement of the hip joint and the ankle muscle force that influence the duration of the stance phase. So far there is no evidence of similar feedback systems in humans, but probably there are similar mechanisms of sensory–motor interaction.

Reflex modulation
The spinal cord also has the capacity to compensate for unexpected perturbations of the limbs during walking. If the forward swinging limb of a walking spinal cat meets an unpredicted obstacle, a brisk flexion lifting the foot above the obstacle is elicited (Fig. 4.3). This corrective movement is achieved by a brisk flexor activation superimposed on the ongoing locomotor activity. Depending on whether the perturbation is induced in the beginning or at the end of the swing phase, the size of the reflex activation is modulated, *i.e.* phasic gain

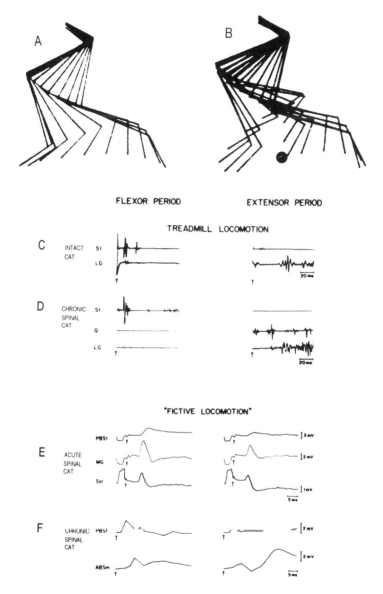

Fig. 4.3. Movement analysis in an intact cat walking on the treadmill during: (A) a normal swing phase; (B) a stumble corrective reaction elicited by a stick inserted in front of the limb during the swing phase. At the top, the movement of the left limb is displayed with stick diagrams at 30 ms intervals (limb moves from right to left). In C–F reflex responses are evoked by an electrical pulse (1 mA, 0.5 ms–5 mA, 5 ms) applied to the dorsum of the paw during different periods of locomotor activity in different preparations. (C, D) Single reflex responses from EMG recordings. In E and F, the responses are intracellularly recorded, and averaged from motoneurons. The stimulus is indicated by an arrow. St = semitendinosus; LG = lateral gastrocnemius; Q = quadriceps; PBSt = posterior biceps semitendinosus; MG = medial gastrocnemius; Sol = soleus; ABSm = anterior biceps semitendinosus. (Reproduced by permission from Forssberg 1979b.)

control. If the same tactile stimulus occurs during stance, it evokes an extensor reaction, *i.e.* reflex reversal (Forssberg *et al.* 1977). By this dynamic control of the muscle response, corrective movements can be adapted to be functionally meaningful in each phase of the step cycle. This illustrates that sensorimotor pathways are not hard-wired reflex circuits dedicated to a stereotyped motor response but can be modulated by central mechanisms. Central reflex modulation is a feature common to most rhythmic behaviours. The same cellular mechanisms seem to underlie the modulation or gating during locomotion in several species, including cat, rat, bullfrog tadpoles and lamprey. In principle, the synaptic transmission can be modulated by the activity of the CPG network at four major synaptic sites along the reflex pathway (Sillar 1991). Probably the most important feature is the presynaptic inhibition by which the release of neurotransmitter from the terminals of primary afferents can be modulated. A similar modulation of the corrective reflexes occurs in the intact walking cat (Prochazka *et al.* 1978, Forssberg 1979, Duysens and Loeb 1980), indicating that the spinal gating mechanisms are well integrated in the normal locomotor behaviour.

During human locomotion the threshold and amplitude of the gastrocnemius–soleus H-reflex is strongly modulated over the entire step cycle, with maximal facilitation during the end of the stance phase and maximal inhibition during the swing phase and beginning of the stance phase (Capaday and Stein 1986). Similarly, the quadriceps H-reflex and the short latency stretch reflex are greatest at the impact of the foot and then continuously decrease in amplitude during the stance phase (Dietz *et al.* 1990a,b). This modulation of the stretch reflex is not caused by the cyclic variation of the excitability level of the motoneurons, but presumably by modulation of the presynaptic inhibition of the primary afferent terminals (Capaday and Stein 1986). Reflexes mediated by group I afferents represent only a part of the reflex system, and primary afferents from leg and foot muscles are not likely to play a dominant role in mediating compensatory leg muscle responses (Berger *et al.* 1984b, Dietz *et al.* 1987). Still, the modulation of the group I afferent input during locomotion may have some functional implications. The facilitation of the stretch reflex at foot impact assists in controlling yielding at the knee and helps support the body weight at the beginning of the stance phase (Dietz *et al.* 1990a,b). The gastrocnemius–soleus stretch reflex facilitation at the end of the stance phase contributes to the compensation for ground irregularities and assists during the push-off phase, while the depression during the swing phase prevents the occurrence of extensor stretch during ankle dorsiflexion (Capaday and Stein 1986).

A modulation of cutaneous reflex responses is also present in walking humans, although the effects are smaller than in other animals and the EMG responses do not produce prominent corrective movements. Cutaneous stimulation of the leg by electrical stimuli evoke distinct EMG responses, which are modulated depending on the phase in which the stimulus is delivered (Crenna and Frigo 1984, Duysens *et al.* 1990, Yang and Stein 1990). Compensatory polysynaptic responses evoked by perturbation during stance and gait are probably mediated by muscle proprioceptive input from group II afferents (Lundberg et al. 1987). These proprioceptive spinal reflex mechanisms have several similarities to the phasic modulation of the cutaneous reflexes during locomotion in humans. The polysynaptic reflex system does not behave as a simple stretch reflex mechanism, rather its function depends on multisensory afferent information and on supraspinal influences. The behaviour of these stretch reflexes during locomotion has to subserve the complex situation for a multivariable control that designates a certain goal to numerous individual parameters (Ito 1982). During perturbations of stance and gait the body's centre of mass is the main parameter to be constrained within the base of support and therefore represents the variable to be controlled by the compensatory responses, with the purpose of preventing falling.

Supraspinal control

Although the spinal cord controls many aspects of locomotion, crucial functions are either completely lacking or greatly reduced after spinal transection. Functionally, the supraspinal control can be divided into three systems. First, locomotion (the CPG network) has to be initiated and the speed has to be controlled. Second, the locomotion has to be directed wherever the individual wishes to go, the feet have to be placed properly, and obstacles must be avoided. And third, equilibrium has to be maintained during the movement of the body.

Locomotor driving systems

In the lamprey, glutaminergic reticulospinal neurons in the brainstem provide an excitatory drive to the spinal CPG networks and can thereby induce swimming (Grillner *et al.* 1995). The reticulospinal neurons can be activated from rostral brainstem structures and by a variety of sensory stimuli, including the lateral line system which carries information from the body surface. Some reticulospinal cells are tonically active, and others receive feedback from the spinal cord that results in a phasic modulation of the driving activity.

A similar organization of locomotor driving systems has been demonstrated in the cat by delivery of brief electrical pulses through small electrodes to various areas of the brainstem (Shik *et al.* 1966, Orlovsky 1969). One such area is located within the subthalamic nucleus and another just ventral to the inferior colliculus in the mesencephalon (mesencephalic locomotor region, MLR). Weak stimulation produces a slow walk while stronger intensity increases the speed; eventually the interlimb coordination may be changed into a gallop. Microinjections of orthograde and retrograde tracers into the MLR have shown that it receives afferent projections from a number of sources including the basal ganglia, the sensorimotor cortex and the limbic system (Garcia-Rill 1986). During rest, MLR is under inhibitory control from the basal ganglia (Jones and Mogenson 1980). When the individual wants to initiate locomotion, this inhibition is released and at the same time excitatory influence from the motor cortex is induced. The akinesia and the difficulty in initiating walking in subjects with Parkinson's disease support the view that a similar organization is also maintained in humans. Parkinson's disease is secondary to degeneration of dopaminergic neurons projecting from the pars compacta of the substantia nigra to the striatum. The net effect of the dopaminergic degeneration is an increased inhibition of the MLR from the basal ganglia and difficulty in releasing this inhibition when locomotion should be initiated.

There seem to be at least two different routes from the MLR to the CPG network in the mammalian spinal cord. One is through the medial reticular formation and the reticulospinal tract in the ventrolateral funicle of the spinal cord (Steeves and Jordan 1980,

Garcia-Rill *et al.* 1983). An alternative route is constituted by the pontine locomotor strip, a system of fibres oriented longitudinally from the MLR via the pons and medulla down to the upper cervical cord, and through which the signals are propagated polysynaptically (Shik and Yagodnitsyn 1977). This system continues down into the spinal cord in a similar chain of propriospinal neurons (Kazennikov *et al.* 1985).

There is another system which controls the postural tone and the force during locomotion (Mori *et al.* 1988). It originates from medial medullary structures and decreases the threshold to initiate locomotion by MLR stimulation. It also enhances the power of the locomotor bursts in the extensor muscles in the walking cat and increases the propulsive force.

There is some evidence that humans and primates have a similar descending control of spinal locomotor circuits and that the same brainstem structures and descending pathways are involved. Lesions of medial reticular systems produce serious locomotor deficits in monkeys (Lawrence and Kuypers 1968). Electrical stimulation of the subthalamic nucleus and a brainstem region similar to the MLR induces locomotion in monkeys lesioned just above the thalamus (Eidelberg *et al.* 1981). The locomotor drive seems to be conveyed through the ventrolateral quadrant of the spinal cord, since locomotion is abolished after selective lesions of the cord.

Adaptive systems
In addition to the segmental mechanisms explained earlier, supraspinal systems adapt the locomotion to the environment. In contrast to the spinal mechanisms, this control can anticipate the changes and modify the motor pattern in advance. Locomotion is practically always performed in relation to an external frame of reference, and thus visual coordination of the locomotor movements is crucial. Many cortical and subcortical areas are engaged in the processing and transformation of the visual information into functional motor adjustments. Data from experiments on primates suggest that the visual signal passes from primary visual cortical areas to parietal and temporal cortex, from where it passes progressively to premotor cortex and finally to the primary motor cortex (Georgopoulos 1991). Human experiments have shown that intermittent visual information is sufficient to allow a subject to judge distance and to modify step length in order to attain a target. The only structure which has been subjected to detailed study during locomotion is the primary motor cortex in the cat (area 4), sending motor commands to the spinal cord via the corticospinal and other pathways (Drew 1991). Electrophysiological recording from single corticospinal neurons in freely walking cats has shown an increased discharge above that seen during normal locomotion, when the cat suddenly adjusts the placement of a foot or avoids an obstacle. The adjustment is normally integrated in the locomotor movements so that the animal may continue its forward progression with minimal disruption. This is achieved by the descending motor command from the motor cortex being distributed through interneuronal networks that are influenced by or may even form part of the CPG network.

The cerebellum seems to have a crucial role in the adaptation of the locomotor movements. Normally, descending motor pathways are rhythmically active in phase with the step cycle. Following cerebellectomy of the cat, this rhythmic activity vanishes and the movements become less coordinated. The cerebellum receives detailed information about the state of spinal motor centres and of the environment. It selects essential data concerning both the activity of the CPG network and afferent activity from the moving limbs (Arshavsky and Orlovsky 1985). This means that the cerebellum receives an efferent copy of the activity generated by the CPG, which fits with Bernstein's framework and von Holst's reafference principle (von Holst and Mittelstaedt 1950). The cerebellum can act as a comparator between the programmed movement and the actual movement and then transmit the corrective signals to the spinal cord via appropriate descending systems. The cerebellar contribution to motor control can be achieved by presetting and adjustment of the gain of proprioceptive reflexes and the sequencing of programmed responses (Hore and Vilis 1985). The influence of the cerebellum on the dynamic modification of stretch reflexes is certainly not limited to individual muscles but rather is concerned with an alliance of stretch reflexes in various muscles for the regulation of posture and locomotion.

Equilibrium control

While much information has been accumulated about postural control during static conditions (see Chapter 3), less is known about the dynamic demands controlling equilibrium in moving humans. The space orientation system, which controls the posture both at rest and during locomotion, plays a crucial role in spatial orientation. The vertical direction of the force, the horizontal surface of the earth, and sunlight are the essential features of the external world for each living being, and effective sensory systems have been developed to continuously monitor these modalities both in animals and humans. Gravity is normally the most reliable reference for orientation, and therefore the gravity system (vestibulospinal system) has evolved to perfection in vertebrates. This causes problems during space flights when no gravity is present. In the simple vertebrate model of the lamprey it has been possible to identify a posture control system in the brainstem consisting of otolith afferents of the vestibular organ, which are activated by a tilt (Grillner *et al.* 1995). They activate reticulospinal neurons which in turn activate spinal interneurons producing a corrective motor response restoring the normal body position. Stimulation of light from one side elicits a positional bias by affecting the reticulospinal pathway.

Head stabilization during human locomotion depends on an intact vestibular system (Assaiante and Amblard 1990, Pozzo *et al.* 1991). The contribution of the vestibular system to the control of stance and locomotion is, however, a matter of controversy. Some investigators have suggested that vestibulospinal reflexes contribute to the compensations induced by external displacements of the body, whereas others claim that vestibular receptors underlie the genesis of sway stabilization. This controversy arises, to a large extent, because the function of the vestibular system is difficult to investigate during natural movements without having a mixture of afferent signals. All experiments using displacements of the feet activate both muscle proprioceptive and vestibular receptors.

Irrespective of the receptors activated by an external displacement of the body, the induced motor pattern is always directed to hold the centre of mass over the base of support. One consequence is that the selection of afferent input by the central mechanisms must correspond to the actual requirements for body stabilization. Furthermore, neuronal signals of muscle stretch or length alone are insufficient for the control of upright posture. Only a combination of afferent inputs can provide the information needed to control body equilibrium. Some of these complex interactions between afferent inputs have been partially revealed in recent years: the functions of proprioceptive reflexes and of the otoliths depend on contact forces or load receptors within the leg extensor muscles, which include information about the position of the body's center of gravity relative to the feet. This leads to the question of how so much information can be processed within a short time. Some interesting hypotheses have been put forward, all with a similar basis: error detection by comparison of the ongoing movement with a central reference pattern. In 1950, von Holst and Mittelstaedt proposed the reafference principle. A similar organization for the adjustment of an ongoing movement to a central representation (the body schema) for postural stabilization was suggested by Gurfinkel *et al.* (1988).

Development of locomotion in humans

Phylogeny

Humans have a bipedal, plantigrade gait, which is unique. Analysis of hominid skeletons (Lovejoy 1988) and preserved footprints (White 1980) suggests that the evolution of plantigrade gait occurred about three million years ago. Although modern apes can walk on two legs, their musculoskeletal system, their muscle activation pattern and their movement trajectories during locomotion differ significantly from those of humans.

The adaptation of the musculoskeletal system to the upright position has resulted in a unique gait pattern, although many of the basic characteristics of locomotion are the same as in quadrupedal gait. There are several determinants of the bipedal plantigrade gait (Table 4.1) which distinguish it from other forms of quadrupedal or bipedal gait (Saunders *et al.* 1953, Forssberg 1985). These determinants contribute to saving energy expenditure during walking by reducing the vertical oscillation of the body and increasing the step length. The development of a prominent heel strike is of special significance. It is provided by an active dorsiflexion of the foot during the end of the swing phase, produced by contractions of the pretibial muscles and inhibition of the calf muscle. The pretibial muscle has a second major burst around heel strike, to resist the extending torque around the ankle. The propulsive force is mainly generated by a push-off movement about the ankle joint through a forceful contraction of the calf muscle in the second half of the stance phase. Activity in the quadriceps group at heel strike guarantees extension at the knee joint and controls flexion of the knee during the weight bearing stance phase.

Ontogeny

Children go through several phases during their locomotor development (Table 4.2). The first locomotor-like movements occur in the fetus at 10–12 weeks of gestation, and have been observed *in utero* by means of real-time ultrasonography (de Vries *et al.* 1984). The alternating leg movements are spontaneously induced in episodes until birth. The existence of this rhythmic behaviour, before most descending supraspinal systems have developed, strongly supports a spinal origin of the activity. Interestingly, it has been suggested that the fetal locomotor-like movements may play a role in positioning the fetus with the head in the birth canal prior to delivery (Oppenheim 1981).

TABLE 4.1
Plantigrade determinants

1. Foot movement: heel strike – push off
2. Knee movement: flexion of supporting leg
3. Intralimb coordination: joint movements out of phase
4. Pelvic movement: rotation, tilt, translation
5. Muscle activity: specific temporal pattern

TABLE 4.2
Stages of human locomotor development

1. Fetal locomotor-like movements
2. Infant stepping
3. Supported locomotion
4. Free walking
5. Transformation to plantigrade gait

Prechtl (1984; and Chapter 2) has shown that fetal motor behaviours are maintained after birth, and that there is a continuity of neural function from prenatal to postnatal life. The postnatal continuation of the fetal locomotor-like movements is the infant stepping which can be elicited a few minutes after birth when the child is held erect over a horizontal surface and slowly pulled forwards (Peiper 1963). The infant stepping pattern differs markedly from the plantigrade pattern of adult gait (Forssberg 1985). One important feature is the lack of segment-specific movements, *i.e.* the leg tends to flex–extend as one unit. The leg is relatively flexed during the whole step cycle, rotated forwards during the swing phase by hip flexion and backwards during the stance phase by hip extension (Fig. 4.4). Other features are the lack of heel strike and the uniform EMG pattern with pronounced antagonistic coactivation. Flexor and extensor muscles tend to fire simultaneously, with their larger bursts at foot contact and foot-off. The activity of the calf muscles prior to foot contact plantar-flexes the foot and contributes to a digitigrade gait, *i.e.* there is no heel strike and instead the toes or the forefoot contact the ground first. After foot contact, a large EMG peak often occurs, more pronounced in extensor than in flexor muscles (Berger *et al.* 1984a, Leonard 1991a). The latencies are quite variable, but usually it occurs about 20–30 ms after foot contact, indicating a short-latency segmental reflex triggered by the foot contact. The wide distribution of the reflex effects, to both flexor and extensor muscles, is in agreement with a similar reflex antagonistic coactivation when myotatic reflexes are elicited during this early period (Myklebust *et al.* 1986, Leonard *et al.* 1991b). It probably reflects an immature organization of the reflex pathways and lacks supraspinal control (*cf.* Berger *et al.* 1984a). In essence, kinematic analysis of the infant stepping movements shows that all the plantigrade determinants of adult gait are lacking, although the basic alternating movements are similar.

The stepping movements can be elicited during the neonatal period, and deteriorate in most infants after a couple of months. The deterioration may be delayed by daily training, *i.e.* by letting the child step for some minutes several times every day (Zelazo 1983), the same effect as when cats or humans with spinal lesions are trained by means of treadmill

89

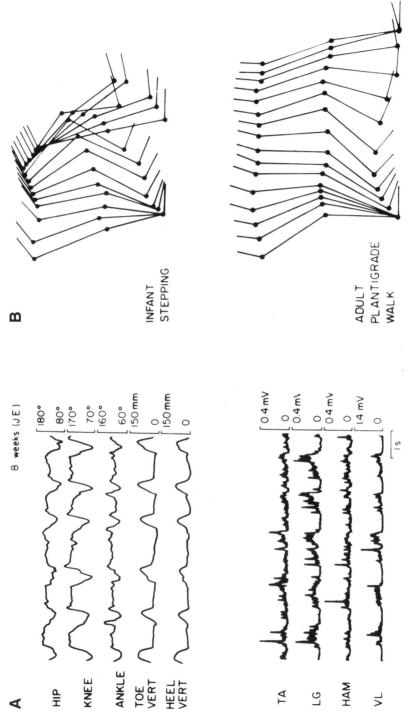

Fig. 4.4. (A) Kinematics and EMG patterns of an 8-week-old infant. The angular rotations in the sagittal plane around the hip, knee and ankle joints are plotted with extension upwards and flexion downwards for five consecutive stride cycles. Surface EMGs (recorded simultaneously with the movements) are shown after rectification and filtering. (B) Stick diagrams of gait patterns from a 6-week-old infant (*top*) and from an adult with plantigrade walk (*bottom*). (Reproduced by permission from Forssberg 1985.)

walking. It supports the view that these early locomotor-like movements are generated by a spinal CPG network, in which the excitability level can be enhanced by frequent training.

Supported locomotion emerges at 7–9 months of age. The movements during supported locomotion appear to be voluntarily elicited and goal directed, whereas infant stepping is externally induced by pulling the child slowly forward, *i.e.* by sensory stimulation of the CPG network from the moving limb. During supported locomotion, the child can support its body weight with one leg but still needs assistance to maintain equilibrium (during infant stepping weight support is also required). Between 9 and 18 months the child starts to walk independently, *i.e.* without any external support. This event is often mentioned as a 'milestone', and is used clinically to monitor the progress of locomotor development. Probably, it has nothing to do with the CPG networks or the descending control systems, but rather with the development of the postural control system and early and polysynaptic reflexes (Berger *et al.* 1984a).

Throughout all these phases, the infant has an immature locomotor pattern, *i.e.* lacking all the plantigrade determinants (Forssberg 1985). Flexor and extensor muscles are coactivated producing synchronized flexion–extension movements in all joints of the leg. The calf muscles are activated during the end of the swing phase, plantarflexing the foot before contact with the ground. This produces a gait in which the toes or the fore part of the foot are placed on the ground (digitigrade gait) first. Following foot contact there are short-latency EMG bursts in several muscles, reflecting hypersensitive early stretch reflexes and a wide distribution of the reflex effects, as during infant stepping. Development of the locomotor EMG pattern is characterized by the appearance and function of polysynaptic spinal reflexes and the disappearance of early stretch reflexes (Berger *et al.* 1984a, 1985). The character of the movements starts to change towards a more mature gait pattern during supported locomotion, and after the establishment of independent walking there is a lengthy period during which the gait is gradually transformed into the plantigrade pattern.

During the early stage of independent walking there is some regression towards the infantile pattern, *i.e.* antagonistic coactivation and simultaneous bursting of flexor–extensors with a lack of ankle–knee coordination (Okamato and Goto 1982). After some months the quality of walking develops and the step length and the duration of single support increases almost linearly up to the age of 3 years (Sutherland *et al.* 1980). Several of the plantigrade determinants emerge before the child is 2 years old. There is a successive delay of the calf muscle activity. As a consequence, the heel is placed first on the ground between 18 and 24 months in most children, while a prominent heel strike, including an active dorsiflexion until heel strike, does not occur until after the age of 2. The uniform muscle activation with antagonistic coactivation is shaped and tuned to a more specific muscle activation pattern, and the joint movements are desynchronized with the ankle getting out of phase with the proximal joints. The reflex EMG potentials following foot contact disappear when long-latency reflex activity becomes established, with great functional significance (Berger *et al.* 1984a, 1985). The maturation of the gait pattern is mainly completed by 4 years, but measurements have shown that children up to the age of 12 expend more energy than adults. This might indicate that the final development may take even more time.

In summary, children are born with an immature locomotor pattern, in which flexor and extensor muscles are contracted together with simultaneous flexion–extension of hip, knee and ankle joints. This early pattern is probably generated by an autonomous spinal CPG network. A seemingly voluntary and goal directed bipedal locomotor behaviour (supported locomotion) develops around 7–9 months. This probably reflects the maturation of locomotor centres in the brainstem and the fact that these have established control over the spinal locomotor CPG network via reticulospinal pathways. At about 9–18 months, children start to walk independently, due to maturation of the postural control system. The slow and gradual transformation of the locomotor pattern after the onset of independent walking suggests that the original neural networks can be used and that they are gradually more and more influenced by other neural and biomechanical mechanisms changing the locomotor pattern. The nature of these underlying mechanisms is not clear. Thelen and co-workers (Thelen and Cook 1987, Thelen *et al.* 1987a) have suggested that there is an ensemble of different subsystems, which during a dynamic period of practice are organized to achieve the most efficient pattern, and that the changes are functionally imposed from 'outside–in' on the developing nervous system and not the other way around. No doubt, the interaction with the environment and the sensory information from the moving limbs are important and necessary factors contributing to locomotor development. However, it is likely that the major parts of the locomotor control system described in lower vertebrates have been conserved during phylogeny, and that development also depends on the maturation of these specific neural mechanisms.

Locomotion in children with spasticity syndromes

Spasticity produces numerous physical signs such as exaggerated reflexes, clonus and muscle hypertonia. Lance (1980) defined spastic hypertonia as a resistance of passive muscle to stretch in a velocity-dependent manner following activation of tonic stretch reflexes. On the basis of the clinical signs a widely accepted conclusion was drawn up for the pathophysiology and treatment of spasticity. Exaggerated reflexes were thought to be responsible for muscle hypertonia, and consequently for the movement disorder. However, in reality the physical spastic signs, including exaggerated reflexes, have little relationship to the patient's disability.

The neural activation of the leg muscles is transformed into a functionally modulated muscle tension by the mechanical muscle fibre properties (Gollhofer *et al.* 1984). The functional deficit, *e.g.* the gait impairment in children with cerebral palsy (CP), is thus a result of disturbances of central mechanisms generating the motor activation patterns, and also of muscle properties.

Exaggerated reflexes and muscle tone

It has been suggested that neuronal reorganization occurs after a central lesion in the cat (Mendell 1984) and in humans (Carr *et al.* 1993). This includes: (1) novel connections, *e.g.* sprouting, functional strengthening of already available connections, derepression of previously inactive connections; (2) changes in the strength of inhibition; and (3) denervation hypersensitivity. However, recent observations indicate that following a spinal cord lesion sprouting of primary afferents does not cause spasticity in the cat (Nacimiento *et al.* 1993) or in humans (Ashby 1989). Changes in the reduction of presynaptic inhibition of group Ia fibres occur (Burke and Ashby 1972) which correlate with the enhanced excitability of tendon tap reflexes. There exists, however, no correlation between decreased presynaptic inhibition of Ia terminals and the degree of spasticity measured by Ashworth's scale (Faist *et al.* 1994).

The treatment of spasticity is usually directed to reducing stretch reflex activity because it was thought that exaggerated reflexes are responsible for increased muscle tone and, consequently, for spastic movement disorder. These studies on muscle tone and reflex activity were, however, usually done under *passive* motor conditions (*cf.* Thilmann *et al.* 1990, 1991). In the latter condition increased elbow torque following a displacement was associated with increased EMG activity in the flexor muscles of the spastic side compared to the unaffected one in patients with spastic hemiparesis (Ibrahim *et al.* 1993).

Spastic movement disorder
The pattern of muscle activation and the development of muscle tone in spasticity is basically different in an *active* motor condition, compared to the clinical testing of the *passive* muscle. Extensive investigations on functional movements of leg (Dietz and Berger 1983, Berger *et al.* 1984b) and arm (Dietz *et al.* 1991) muscles did not reveal any causal relationship between exaggerated reflexes and motor dysfunction. In adult patients, the reciprocal mode of leg muscle activation during gait is preserved in spasticity. Exaggerated stretch reflexes in spasticity are associated with an absence or reduction of the functionally essential polysynaptic (or long-latency) reflexes. Tension development during functional movements (Berger *et al.* 1982, 1984c) does not depend on exaggerated stretch reflexes. The overall leg muscle activity is reduced in patients with spasticity.

In patients with spastic hemiparesis due to a cerebral lesion, the strength of EMG activity on the affected leg is reduced compared to the unaffected leg, the difference corresponding with the degree of paresis (Berger *et al.* 1984c). Corresponding to a loss of EMG modulation during gait in these subjects, a fast regulation of motoneuron discharge, which characterizes the normal muscle, is absent in spasticity (Rosenfalck and Andreassen 1980, Dietz *et al.* 1986). A lack of both, inhibition of monosynaptic and facilitation of polysynaptic spinal reflexes, is present also in healthy young children (see below). Inhibition and facilitation of spinal reflexes obviously depend on supraspinal control, which is impaired in spasticity and has yet to mature in young children.

Locomotion in cerebral palsied children
The main feature of the early gait pattern consists of a coactivation of antagonistic leg muscle during the stance phase, associated with a reduced and tonic mode of leg extensor muscle activation (starting before ground contact), and the appearance of large, isolated potentials just after ground contact. The latter probably represent monosynaptic (or oligosynaptic) stretch reflex potentials, mediated by group I afferents, as they appear with a short latency (20–30 ms) following onset of gastrocnemius stretch. This pattern closely resembles the pattern described for newborn stepping by Forssberg (1985). From 4 years of age on, the monosynaptic reflex potentials disappear, the polysynaptic potentials become more

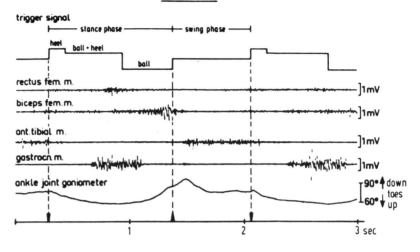

Normal child

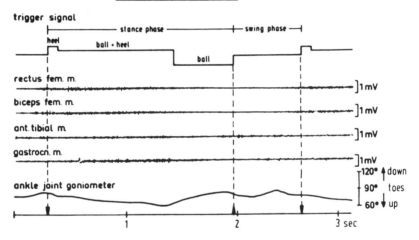

Child with spastic diplegia

Fig. 4.5. Typical record for a step cycle from a normal child *(above)* and from a child with spastic diplegia *(below)* during slow gait. From *top* to *bottom*: electrical switch signals (trigger) from the heel and the ball of the foot, rectus femoris, biceps femoris, tibialis anterior and gastrocnemius EMGs and potentiometer signal of ankle joint. Vertical lines indicate touch down and lift up of the foot. (Reproduced by permission from Berger *et al.* 1982.)

phasic and stronger, and a reciprocal mode of leg muscle activation becomes established. These changes represent a shift from the predominance of the rigid and functionally ineffective monosynaptic stretch reflexes to polysynaptic spinal reflexes.

The leg muscle activity during locomotion in children with a supraspinal lesion of the motor system acquired at an age before normal gait is established, shows characteristic signs of impaired maturation of the normal gait pattern (Berger *et al.* 1982, Leonard *et al.* 1991a).

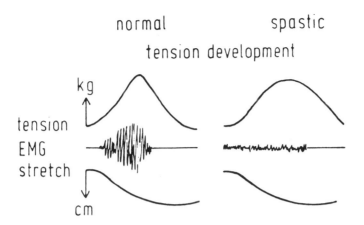

normal   spastic

tension development

kg

tension
EMG
stretch

cm

Fig. 4.6. Schematic illustration of tension development in a leg muscle during locomotion. *(Left)* Normal behaviour: increase in tension is closely correlated to muscle activation. *(Right)* Spastic muscle paresis: increase in tension is closely correlated to the stretching phase of the slightly tonically activated muscle. This change of tension development in spastic paresis is explained by the transormation of the motor units with their muscle fibres. (Reproduced by permission from Dietz *et al.* 1987.)

The pattern recorded in children with CP around 10 years of age mainly consists of a coactivation of antagonistic leg muscles during the stance phase of a gait cycle and a general reduction in amplitude of EMG activity. Kinematically, this is connected with the persistence of the early-stage leg movements, *i.e.* a non-plantigrade gait pattern (Fig. 4.5).

In contrast to this, when the cerebral lesion is acquired at a later stage and the reciprocal mode of leg muscle activity is already established (*i.e.* around the age of 4), a reciprocal activation of antagonistic leg muscles is preserved during spastic gait.

Muscle EMG activity and spastic muscle tone
In patients with spastic paresis acquired at an early or later stage, an essentially different tension development of triceps surae takes place during the stance phase of gait (Dietz and Berger 1983, Berger *et al.* 1984c) (Fig. 4.6). In the unaffected leg, the tension development correlates with the modulation of EMG activity (the same is true in healthy subjects), while in the spastic leg, tension development is connected to the stretching period of the tonically activated (with small EMG amplitude) muscle. There is no visible influence of monosynaptic reflex potential on muscle tension. A similar discrepancy between the resistance to stretch and the level of EMG activity is described for the flexor muscles of the upper limb in spastic patients (Lee *et al.* 1987, Powers *et al.* 1989).

Spastic muscle tone during functional movements can hardly be explained by an increased activity of motoneurons. Instead, a transformation of motor units occurs in muscle. Such a transformation is functionally meaningful, because it enables the patient to support the body weight during gait. However, fast active movements become impossible. It is misleading to uncritically apply findings from animal studies to pathophysiological and therapeutic considerations, because there are basic differences in the development of muscle tone:

an acute rigor appears in the decerebrate cat, while in patients with an acute supraspinal lesion connected with paresis, muscle tone develops slowly over a period of weeks.

There are additional findings which support the suggestion that changes in the mechanical muscle fibre properties occur in spasticity: (a) contraction times in hand muscles and in the triceps surae are prolonged (Young and Mayer 1982, Dietz and Berger 1984); (b) torque motor experiments applied to upper and lower limb muscles indicate a major non-reflex contribution to the spastic muscle tone in the antigravity muscles, *i.e.* in the leg extensors and elbow flexors (Hufschmidt and Mauritz 1985, Ibrahim *et al.* 1993, Sinkjaer *et al.* 1993); and (c) histochemistry and morphometry of spastic muscle reveal neurogenic-looking changes of muscle fibres (Edström 1970, Dietz *et al.* 1986). The latter comprise (a) increased levels of muscle fibre atrophy, especially type II; (2) a predominance of type I fibres during later stages, when spasticity is established; (3) structural changes, such as the appearance of target fibres, mainly type I fibres.

The alteration to a simpler regulation of muscle tension following paresis due to a spinal or a supraspinal lesion is basically advantageous: it enables the patient to support the body during gait and, consequently, to achieve mobility. However, rapid movements are no longer possible due to the missing modulation of muscle activity. Following a severe spinal or supraspinal lesion, these transformative processes can overshoot with unwelcome sequelae, *i.e.* painful spasms and unvoluntarily induced movements.

Little is known about the natural history of CP over the life span. There is even a dearth of controlled studies documenting the positive effect of treatment and training. It appears that children with CP have a quite normal developmental history during the early stages of infant stepping and supported locomotion, but fail to develop plantigrade gait (Leonard *et al.* 1991a). In adults with a brain lesion, changes in mechanical muscle fibre properties occur in the leg extensors after a few weeks (Dietz *et al.* 1986). The structural changes of the spastic muscle become most evident a year or more after acute brain damage (Hufschmidt and Mauritz 1985).

REFERENCES

Andersson, O., Grillner, S., Lindquist, M., Zomlefer, M. (1978) 'Peripheral control of the spinal pattern generators for locomotion in cat.' *Brain Research*, **150**, 625–630.

Arshavsky, Y.I., Orlovsky, G.N. (1985) 'Role of the cerebellum in the control of rhythmic movements.' *In:* Grillner, S., Stein, G.S., Douglas, G., Forssberg, H., Herman, R.M. (Eds.) *Neurobiology of Vertebrate Locomotion. Wenner–Gren International Symposium Series, Vol. 45.* Stockholm: Wenner–Gren Center, pp. 677–689.

Ashby, P. (1989) 'Discussion I.' *In:* Emre, M. Benecke, R. (Eds.) *Spasticity. The Current Status of Research and Treatment.* Carnforth: Parthenon, pp. 68–69.

Assaiante, C., Amblard, B. (1990) 'Head stabilization in space while walking: effect of visual deprivation in children and adults.' *In:* Brandt T., Paulus, W., Bles, W., Dieterich, M., Krafczyk, S., Straube, A. (Eds.) *Disorders of Posture and Gait, 1990. Xth International Symposium of the Society for Postural and Gait Research, München, September 2–6, 1990.* Stuttgart: Thieme, pp. 229–232.

Barbeau, H., Rossignol, S. (1991) 'Initiation and modulation of the locomotor pattern in the adult chronic spinal cat by noradrenergic, serotonergic and dopaminergic drugs.' *Brain Research*, **546**, 250–260.

—— —— (1994) 'Enhancement of locomotor recovery following spinal cord injury.' *Current Opinion in Neurology*, **7**, 517–524.

—— Julien, C., Rossignol, S. (1987) 'The effects of clonidine and yohimbine on locomotion and cutaneous reflexes in the adult chronic spinal cat.' *Brain Research*, **437**, 83–96.

—— Dannakas, M., Arsenault, B. (1992) 'The effects of locomotor training in spinal cord injured subjects: a preliminary study.' *Restorative Neurology and Neuroscience*, **12**, 93–96.

Berger, W., Quintern, J., Dietz, V. (1982) 'Pathophysiology of gait in children with cerebral palsy.' *Electroencephalography and Clinical Neurophysiology*, **53**, 538–548.

—— Altenmueller, E., Dietz, V. (1984a) 'Normal and impaired development of children's gait.' *Human Neurobiology*, **3**, 163–170.

—— Dietz, V., Quintern, J. (1984b) 'Corrective reactions to stumbling in man: neuronal co-ordination of bilateral leg muscle activity during gait.' *Journal of Physiology*, **357**, 109–125.

—— Horstmann, G., Dietz, V. (1984c) 'Tension development and muscle activation in the leg during gait in spastic hemiparesis: independence of muscle hypertonia and exaggerated stretch reflexes.' *Journal of Neurology, Neurosurgery and Psychiatry*, **47**, 1029–1033.

—— Quintern, J., Dietz, V. (1985) 'Stance and gait perturbations in children: developmental aspects of compensatory mechanisms.' *Electroencephalography and Clinical Neurophysiology*, **61**, 385–395.

Bernstein, N. (1967) *The Co-ordination and Regulation of Movements.* Oxford: Pergamon.

Bickel, A. (1897) 'Ueber den Einfluss der sensibelen Nerven und der Labyrinthe auf die Bewegungen der Thiere.' *Pflüger's Archiv für die gesammte Physiologie des Menschen und der Thiere*, **67**, 299–344.

Brown, T.G. (1911) 'The intrinsic factors in the act of progression in the mammal.' *Proceedings of the Royal Society of London. Series B: Biological Sciences*, **B84**, 308–319.

Burke, D., Ashby, P. (1972) 'Are spinal "presynaptic" inhibitory mechanisms suppressed in spasticity?' *Journal of the Neurological Sciences*, **15**, 321–326.

Capaday, C., Stein, R.B. (1986) 'Amplitude modulation of the soleus H-reflex in the human during walking and standing.' *Journal of Neuroscience*, **6**, 1308–1313.

Carr, L.J., Harrison, L.M., Evans, A.L., Stephens, J.A. (1993) 'Patterns of central motor reorganization in hemiplegic cerebral palsy.' *Brain*, **116**, 1223–1247.

Cazalets, J.R., Sqalli-Houssaini, Y., Clarac, F. (1992) 'Activation of the central pattern generators for locomotion by serotonin and excitatory amino acids in neonatal rat.' *Journal of Physiology*, **455**, 187–204.

Crenna, P. Frigo, C. (1984) 'Evidence of phase-dependent nociceptive reflexes during locomotion in man.' *Experimental Neurology*, **85**, 336–345.

de Vries, J.I.P., Visser, G.H.A., Prechtl, H.F.R. (1984) 'Fetal motility in the first half of pregnancy.' *In:* Prechtl, H.F.R. (Ed.) *Continuity of Neural Functions from Prenatal to Postnatal Life. Clinics in Developmental Medicine No. 94.* London: Spastics International Medical Publications, pp. 46–64.

Dietz, V. Berger, W. (1983) 'Normal and impaired regulation of muscle stiffness in gait: a new hypothesis about muscle hypertonia.' *Experimental Neurology*, **79**, 680–687.

—— —— (1984) 'Interlimb coordination of posture in patients with spastic paresis. Impaired function of spinal reflexes.' *Brain*, **107**, 965–978.

—— Ketelsen, U-P., Berger, W., Quintern, J. (1986) 'Motor unit involvement in spastic paresis. Relationship between leg muscle activation and histochemistry.' *Journal of the Neurological Sciences*, **75**, 89 103

—— Quintern, J., Sillem, M. (1987) 'Stumbling reactions in man: significance of proprioceptive and preprogrammed mechanisms.' *Journal of Physiology*, **386**, 149–163.

—— Discher, M., Faist, M., Trippel, M. (1990a) 'Amplitude modulation of the human quadriceps tendon jerk reflex during gait.' *Experimental Brain Research*, **82**, 211–213.

—— Faist, M., Pierrot-Deseilligny, E. (1990b) 'Amplitude modulation of the quadriceps H-reflex in the human during the early stance phase of gait.' *Experimental Brain Research*, **79**, 221–224.

—— Trippel, M., Berger, W. (1991) 'Reflex activity and muscle tone during elbow movements in patients with spastic paresis.' *Annals of Neurology*, **30**, 767–779.

—— Colombo, G., Jensen, L. (1994a) 'Locomotor activity in spinal man.' *Lancet*, **344**, 1260–1263.

—— Zijlstra, W., Duysens, J. (1994b) 'Human neuronal interlimb coordination during spilt-belt locomotion.' *Experimental Brain Research*, **101**, 513–520.

—— Colombo, G., Jensen, L. Baumgartner, L. (1995) 'Locomotor capacity of spinal cord in paraplegic patients.' *Annals of Neurology*, **37**, 574–582.

Drew, T. (1991) 'Visuomotor coordination in locomotion.' *Current Opinion in Neurobiology*, **1**, 652–657.

Duysens, J., Loeb, G.E. (1980) 'Modulation of ipsi- and contralateral reflex responses in unrestrained walking cats.' *Journal of Neurophysiology*, **44**, 1024–1037.

—— Pearson, K.G. (1980) 'Inhibition of flexor burst generation by loading ankle extensor muscles in walking cats.' *Brain Research*, **187**, 321–332.

—— Trippel, M., Horstmann, G.A., Dietz, V. (1990) 'Gating and reversal of reflexes in ankle muscles during human walking.' *Experimental Brain Research*, **82**, 351–358.

Edström, L. (1970) 'Selective changes in the sizes of red and white muscle fibres in upper motor lesions and Parkinsonism.' *Journal of the Neurological Sciences*, **11**, 537–550.

Eidelberg, E., Walden, J.G., Nguyen, L.H. (1981) 'Locomotor control in macaque monkeys.' *Brain*, **104**, 647–663.

Faist, M., Mazevet, D., Dietz, V., Pierrot-Deseilligny, E. (1994) 'A quantitative assessment of presynaptic inhibition of Ia afferents in spastics: differences in hemiplegics and paraplegics.' *Brain*, **117**, 1449–1455.

Forssberg, H. (1979a) 'Stumbling corrective reaction: a phase-dependent compensatory reaction during loco-motion.' *Journal of Neurophysiology*, **42**, 936–953.

—— (1979b) 'On integrative motor functions in the cat's spinal cord.' *Acta Physiologica Scandinavica*, Suppl. 474.

—— (1985) 'Ontogeny of human locomotor control. I. Infant stepping, supported locomotion and transition to independent locomotion.' *Experimental Brain Research*, **57**, 480–493.

—— Grillner, S. (1973) 'The locomotion of the acute spinal cat injected with clonidine i.v.' *Brain Research*, **50**, 184–186.

—— —— Rossignol, S. (1977) 'Phasic gain control of reflexes from the dorsum of the paw during spinal locomotion.' *Brain Research*, **132**, 121–139.

—— —— Halbertsma, J. (1980a) 'The locomotion of the low spinal cat. I. Coordination within a hindlimb.' *Acta Physiologica Scandinavica*, **108**, 269–281.

—— —— —— Rossignol, S. (1980b) 'The locomotion of the low spinal cat. II. Interlimb coordination.' *Acta Physiologica Scandinavica*, **108**, 283–295.

Fung, J., Stewart, J.E., Barbeau, H. (1990) 'The combined effects of clonidine and cyproheptadine with inter-active training on the modulation of locomotion in spinal cord injured subjects.' *Journal of the Neuro-logical Sciences*, **100**, 85–93.

Garcia-Rill, E. (1986) 'The basal ganglia and the locomotor regions.' *Brain Research*, **396**, 47–63.

—— Skinner, R.D. Fitzgerald, J.A. (1983) 'Control of locomotion using localized injections of GABA agonists and antagonists into the mesencephalic locomotor region (MLR).' *Neuroscience Abstracts*, **9**, 357.

Georgopoulos, A.P. (1991) 'Higher order motor control.' *Annual Review of Neuroscience*, **14**, 361–377.

Gollhofer, A., Schmidtbleicher, D., Dietz, V. (1984) 'Regulation of muscle stiffness in human locomotion.' *International Journal of Sports Medicine*, **5**, 19–22.

Grillner, S., Rossignol, S. (1978) 'On the initiation of the swing phase of locomotion in chronic spinal cats.' *Brain Research*, **146**, 269–277.

—— Zangger, P. (1979) 'On the central generation of locomotion in the low spinal cat.' *Experimental Brain Research*, **34**, 241–261.

—— Deliagina, T., Ekeberg, Ö., El Manira, A., Hill, R.H., Lansner, A., Orlovsky, G.N., Wallén, P. (1995) 'Neural networks that co-ordinate locomotion and body orientation in lamprey.' *Trends in Neurosciences*, **18**, 270–279.

Gurfinkel, V.S., Levik, Y.S., Popov, K. E. Smetanin, B.N. (1988) 'Body scheme in the control of postural activity.' *In:* Gurfinkel, V.S., Joffe, M.E., Massion, J. Roll, J.P. (Eds.) *Stance and Motion. Facts and Concepts.* New York: Plenum, pp. 185–193.

Hering, H.E. (1897) 'Ueber Bewegungsstörungen nach centripetaler Lähmung.' *Archiv für experimentelle Pathologie und Pharmakologie*, **38**, 266–283.

Hore, J., Vilis, T. (1985) 'A cellebellar-dependent efference copy mechanism for generating appropriate muscle responses to limb perturbations.' *In:* Bloedel, J.R., Dichgans, J., Precht, W. (Eds.) *Proceedings in Life Science. Cerebellar Functions.* Heidelberg: Springer, pp. 1–23.

Hufschmidt, A., Mauritz, K-H. (1985) 'Chronic transformation of muscle in spasticity: a peripheral contribution to increased tone.' *Journal of Neurology, Neurosurgery and Psychiatry*, **48**, 676–685.

Hultborn, H., Petersen, N., Brownstone, R., Nielsen, J. (1993) 'Evidence of fictive spinal locomotion in the marmoset (*Callitreix jacchus*).' *Society of Neuroscience Abstracts*, **19**, 539.

Ibrahim, I.K., Berger, W., Trippel, M., Dietz, V. (1993) 'Stretch-induced electromyographic activity and torque in spastic elbow muscles. Differential modulation of reflex activity in passive and active motor tasks.' *Brain*, **116**, 971–989.

Ito, M. (1982) 'The CNS as a multivariable control system.' *Brain Behaviour Science*, **5**, 552–553.

Jones, D.L., Mogenson, G.J. (1980) 'Nucleus accumbens to globus pallidus GABA projection: electrophysi-ological and iontophoretic investigations.' *Brain Research*, **188**, 93–105.

Kazennikov, O.V., Shik, M.L., Iakovleva, G.V. (1985) 'Synaptic responses of propriospinal neurons to stimulation of the stepping strip in the cat dorsolateral funiculus.' *Neurofiziologiia*, **17**, 270–278.

Lance, J.W. (1980) 'Spasticity: Disordered motor control.' *In:* Feldman, R.G., Young, R.R., Koella, W.P. (Eds.) *Symposium Synopsis.* Chicago: Year Book, pp. 485–495.

Lawrence, D.G., Kuypers, H.G.J.M. (1968) 'The functional organization of the motor system in the monkey. I. The effects of bilateral pyramidal lesions.' *Brain*, **91**, 1–14.

Lee, W.A., Boughton, A., Rymer, W.Z. (1987) 'Absence of stretch reflex gain enhancement in voluntarily activated spastic muscle.' *Experimental Neurology*, **98**, 317–335.

Leonard, C.T., Hirschfeld, H., Forssberg, H. (1991a) 'The development of independent walking in children with cerebral palsy.' *Developmental Medicine and Child Neurology*, **33**, 567–577.

—— —— Moritani, T., Forssberg, H. (1991b) 'Myotatic reflex development in normal children and children with cerebral palsy.' *Experimental Neurology*, **111**, 379–382.

Lovejoy, C.O. (1988) 'Evolution of human walking.' *Science*, **259**, 118–125

Lundberg, A., Malmgren, K., Schomburg, E.D. (1987) 'Reflex pathways from group II muscle afferents. 3. Secondary spindle afferents and the FRA: a new hypothesis.' *Experimental Brain Research*, **65**, 294–306.

Mendell, L.M. (1984) 'Modifiability of spinal synapses.' *Physiological Reviews*, **64**, 260–324.

Mori, S., Matsuyama, K., Takakusaki, K., Kanaya, T. (1988) 'The behavior of lateral vestibular neurons during walk, trot and gallop in acute precollicular decerebrate cats.' *In:* Pompeiano, O. Allum, J.H.J. (Eds.) *Vestibulospinal Control of Posture and Locomotion. Progress in Brain Research Vol. 76.* New York: Elsevier, pp. 211–220.

Myklebust, B.M., Gottlieb, G.L., Agarwal, G.C. (1986) 'Stretch reflexes of the normal infant.' *Developmental Medicine and Child Neurology*, **28**, 440–449.

Nacimiento, W., Mautes, A., Töpper, R., Oestreicher, A.B., Gispen, W.H., Nacimiento, A.C., Noth, J., Kreutzberg, G.W. (1993) 'B-50 (GAP-43) in the spinal cord caudal to hemisection: indication for lack of intraspinal sprouting in dorsal root axons.' *Journal of Neuroscience Research*, **35**, 603–617.

Okamoto, T., Goto, Y. (1982) 'Electromyographic study of normal infant and child gait.' *Journal of the Liberal Arts Department, Kansai Medical University*, **9**, 72–100.

Oppenheim, R.W. (1981) 'Ontogenetic adaptations and retrogressive processes in the development of the nervous system and behaviour: a neuroembryological perspective.' *In:* Connolly, K.J., Prechtl, H.F.R. (Eds.) *Maturation and Development: Biological and Psychological Perspectives. Clinics in Developmental Medicine No. 77/78.* London: Spastics International Medical Publications, pp. 73–109.

Orlovsky, G.N. (1969) 'Electrical activity in brainstem and descending paths in guided locomotion.' *Sechenov Physiological Journal*, **55**, 437–444.

Peiper, A. (1963) *Cerebral Function in Infancy and Childhood.* New York: Consultants Bureau.

Powers, R.K., Campbell, D.L. Rymer, W.Z. (1989) 'Stretch reflex dynamics in spastic elbow flexor muscles'. *Annals of Neurology*, **25**, 32–42.

Pozzo, T., Berthoz, A., Lefort, L., Vitte, E. (1991) 'Head stabilization during various locomotor tasks in humans. II. Patients with bilateral peripheral vestibular deficits.' *Experimental Brain Research*, **85**, 208–217.

Prechtl, H.F.R. (1984) 'Continuity and change in early neural development.' *In:* Prechtl, H.F.R. (Ed.) *Continuity of Neural Functions from Prenatal to Postnatal Life. Clinics in Developmental Medicine No. 94* London: Spastics International Medical Publications, pp. 1–15.

Prochazka, A., Sontag, K., Wand, P. (1978) 'Motor reactions to perturbations of gait: proprioceptive and somesthetic involvement.' *Neuroscience Letters*, **7**, 35–39.

Rosenfalck, A., Andreassen, S. (1980) 'Impaired regulation of force and firing pattern of single motor units in patients with spasticity.' *Journal of Neurology, Neurosurgery and Psychiatry*, **43**, 907–916.

Rossignol, S., Barbeau, H. (1993) 'Pharmacology of locomotion: an account of studies in spinal cats and spinal cord injured subjects.' *Journal of the American Paraplegia Society*, **16**, 190–196.

Saunders, J.B.deC.M., Inman, V.T., Eberhart, H.D. (1953) 'The major determinants in normal and pathological gait.' *Journal of Bone and Joint Surgery*, **35A**, 543–558.

Selverston A.I., Moulins, M. (1987) *The Crustacean Stomatogastric System.* Berlin: Springer Verlag.

Shik, M.L., Yagodnitsyn, A.S. (1977) 'The pontobulbar "locomotion strip".' *Neirofiziologiia*, **9**, 95–97.

—— Severin, F.V. Orlovsky, G.N. (1966) 'Control of walking and running by means of electrical stimulation of the mid-brain.' *Biophysics*, **11**, 756–765.

Sillar, K. (1991) 'Spinal pattern generation and sensory gating mechanisms.' *Current Opinion in Neurobiology*, **1**, 583–589.

Sinkjaer, T., Toft, E., Larsen, K., Andreassen, S., Hansen, H.J. (1993) 'Non-reflex and reflex mediated ankle joint stiffness in multiple sclerosis patients with spasticity.' *Muscle and Nerve*, **16**, 69–76.

Steeves, J.D., Jordan, L.M. (1980) 'Localization of a descending pathway in the spinal cord which is necessary for controlled treadmill locomotion.' *Neuroscience Letters*, **20**, 283–288.

Sutherland, D.H., Olshen, R., Cooper, L., Woo, S.L-Y. (1980) 'The development of mature gait.' *Journal of Bone and Joint Surgery*, **62A**, 336–353.

Thelen, E., Cooke, D.W. (1987) 'Relationship between newborn stepping and later walking: a new interpretation.' *Developmental Medicine and Child Neurology*, **29**, 380–393.

—— Skala, K., Kelso, J. (1987a) 'The dynamic nature of early coordination: evidence from bilateral leg movements in young infants.' *Developmental Psychobiology*, **23**, 179–186.

—— Ulrich, B.D., Niles, D. (1987b) 'Bilateral coordination in human infants: stepping on a split-belt treadmill.' *Journal of Experimental Psychology: Human Perception and Performance*, **13**, 405–410.

Thilmann, A.F., Fellows, S.J. Garms, E. (1990) 'Pathological stretch reflexes on the "good" side of hemiparetic patients.' *Journal of Neurology, Neurosurgery and Psychiatry*, **53**, 208–214.

—— —— —— (1991) 'The mechanism of spastic muscle hypertonus. Variation in reflex gain over the time course of spasticity.' *Brain*, **114**, 233–244.

White, T.D. (1980) 'Evolutionary implications of pliocene hominid footprints.' *Science*, **208**, 175–176.

von Holst, E. Mittelstaedt, H. (1950) 'Das Reafferenzprinzip (Wechselwirkungen zwischen Zentralnervensystem und Peripherie).' *Naturwissenschaften*, **37**, 464–476.

Yang, J.F., Stein, R.B. (1990) 'Phase-dependent reflex reversal in human leg muscles during walking.' *Journal of Neurophysiology*, **63**, 1109–1117.

Young, J.L., Mayer, R.F. (1982) 'Physiological alterations of motor units in hemiplegia.' *Journal of the Neurological Sciences*, **54**, 401–412.

Zelazo, P.R. (1983) 'The development of walking: new findings and old assumptions.' *Journal of Motor Behavior*, **15**, 99–137.

5

THE LOCOMOTOR DEVELOPMENT OF CHILDREN WITH CEREBRAL PALSY

David Scrutton and Peter Rosenbaum

There is a wealth of cross-sectional data about normal locomotor development. In general terms the milestones are well known and are useful in well baby clinics to highlight deviations from the norm. However, individual variations in the timing and especially the sequence of events are great and consequently the milestones must be used with caution in evaluating an individual. These variations probably make such cross-sectional data more useful to toy manufacturers than to the clinician (What size are most children needing a pusher-walker?); but unfortunately, we have so little information to call upon that these milestone data are still in common usage as the principal indicator of potential problems. The child's tone and postural preferences together with the family's typical pattern of locomotor development may be ignored, yet it is these factors which are often more useful indicators of whether the child is maintaining *appropriate* locomotor development. The concept of milestones also tends to overshadow the characteristics of movement, which, in the event of there being some pathology, are usually more pathognomonic than simple achievement. In other words, the quantitative information provided by milestones is in itself insufficient without qualitative descriptions of a child's pattern of development. What follows is a brief outline of several of the principal factors to be considered when assessing a child's motor development.

Sequence and timing

Some clinicians still consider that the order in which children achieve locomotor milestones is dictated by the need to learn one skill (*e.g.* crawling) before another (*e.g.* walking) because the earlier skill provides something of value essential to the quality of the ensuing one. This, they claim, can lead to children being prevented from advancing to a higher level of locomotor achievement because they cannot do (or do sufficiently well) an earlier skill. Anyone having experience of children with disability will know that this is a mistaken belief, but it is probably Robson (1970) who has done most to make us aware of the varying sequences of normal development and so make such rigid notions untenable. A child who gets to standing and walking while still showing difficulty with an earlier achieved milestone may not walk well, but that is a reflection of an *underlying* problem of coordination, not with the failure to perfect the first milestone *per se*.

The sequence of locomotor development of a child without disability appears to be governed by several factors including the following.
• *The child's family pattern.* Although the majority of infants follow a prone developmental

sequence which, combined with normal tone, favours a sit/crawl/pull to stand sequence (often described as the correct locomotor development path), a sizeable proportion, perhaps 15%, do not. Depending on a number of factors they may shuffle (in a sitting position) instead of crawling, or omit the stage of floor-bound locomotion altogether, and they are early walkers. Very few (usually floppy infants) roll or creep as their predominant means of prewalking locomotion. These characteristics appear to be largely influenced by genetic factors (Robson 1970). Between-heel sitting is also usually familial.

• *The body's physical proportions.* Although, in the main, locomotor progress awaits the maturation of central control processes for certain abilities, some of these occur or are prevented from occurring simply because the physical proportions of the infant's body encourage or preclude them. For example, head lifting in supine is impossible until the rest of the body has the mass and lever arm length to counterbalance it. Thus head control is always a poor indicator of future locomotor progress in children with microcephaly, who excel at this skill.

• *Mechanical principles.* Any purposeful physical system has three components: a control mechanism, a power source and a structure. Considerations of locomotor development have usually focused largely on the development of the control system; but to move any mechanism efficiently requires that it is moved as its articulations, lever lengths and dispositions of masses naturally allow. The obvious corollary to this is that if the system is changed in any way it may be unwise to attempt to get it to mimic normal movement, without appreciating that this is certain to be achieved only at the expense of efficiency, if at all.

• *Muscle tone.* Not all normally developing children have what might be considered normal muscle tone. Some are hypotonic and very few are hypertonic, but without the mass movement synergies (mass patterning) one would expect from a central disorder of movement. The tone normalizes gradually but while variations are present they exert an effect on locomotor progress. Floppy infants may lack pelvic and shoulder girdle stability and this delays certain skills. Jan *et al.* (1975) have noted the early hypotonia of congenitally blind infants, which is associated with delayed motor development.

• *Loss of certain primitive responses and the appearance of balance and protective responses.* During the first year of life the more primitive postural responses are gradually replaced by the more mature and sophisticated balance and protective responses. Whether the latter develop independently and override the former's dominance, or can emerge only as the dominance of the primitive responses diminishes is uncertain. However, children who have the muscle tone and strength to allow any postural and movement ability never show the absence of primitive responses without the appearance of either the balance or protective responses. The central motor system itself can present a posturally unresponsive state only by atonia or extreme hypertonia, *e.g.* opisthotonus (see Paine 1964; Milani-Comparetti and Gidoni 1967a,b; Caputo *et al.* 1984, 1985; Thelen 1984; Cooke and Thelen 1987; Thelen and Cooke 1987).

• *Personality and intellect.* Some infants continuously explore, others are happy with the toy they have rather than the one just out of reach. In children without a disability this is an aspect of their personality; for the child with generalized developmental delay a reduction in exploration can be a reflection of their intellectual capacity. Either way such uninquisitive behaviour can influence the motor development of these children, in the first

example transiently but in the second profoundly. Many severely developmentally delayed children without a disorder of movement and having well developed balance (base retaining) responses* lack protective (base changing) responses and are very resistant to using them.
• *Environment.* Milani-Comparetti (personal communication, 1965) noted the absence of protective responses in a group of children at an orphanage who had been kept in their cots all day. They rapidly developed protective responses when placed in an environment where the responses were advantageous.

All these factors are influential with the child who has cerebral palsy (CP), although in the more severe forms muscle tone, primitive responses, balance and protective responses, and perhaps the child's intellectual and personality characteristics assume disproportionate influence. However, these factors do not work in isolation, rather they interact with each other and with the infant's environment influencing how movements develop. When selecting the intervention required for a child with CP, these are factors which may be as important as the type and distribution of the motor disorder (for example, see Robson and Mac Keith 1971). These three categories, pathology, natural variability and environment, cannot easily be separated and should be considered interactive rather than mutually exclusive.

Gross locomotor development can be viewed at its simplest as the story of learning how to cope with a higher centre of gravity and a narrower base in increasingly complex dynamic situations. Anything affecting these factors may influence the rate, path and ultimate limits of locomotor development.

Quality of movement

Physiotherapists in particular put much store by the quality of a movement and complain that developmental scales lack any consideration of this important feature. How a movement is performed can be as important in the long term as the bare achievement of a skill (Boyce *et al.* 1991). Quality is by no means easy to define but the following features are important.
• *Choice.* For a movement to have good quality it must match the circumstances precisely. To do this the child needs a multitude of possibilities available. Any limitation of choice will force the selection of a suboptimal movement even though it may achieve the movement's primary purpose.
• *Social appropriateness.* This is an important constraint on choice. How one eats at a picnic is usually different from the manner adopted at a dinner table. For many disabled people no such choice exists.
• *Functional efficiency.* An action has to be more than just achievable, that is reproducible, to be of use in daily life. In many circumstances, for example picking up a glass and drinking, it has to be effective first time because failure may mean tipping the glass over or spilling the contents. The threat of failure alone may stop the attempt. Such a restricted skill cannot really be considered an ability at all because it is of little or no use to the individual.

*There are two fundamentally opposed ways in which the body can respond to regain postural stability. Either the line of gravity is brought back within the existing base, or the base is changed so as to be under the (perhaps shifting) centre of gravity. The first reaction, here called a balance reaction, is unexploratory; the second, called the protective reaction, allows locomotion and hence exploration.

• *Physiological efficiency.* The energy used to achieve a desired goal is an important factor and most people with locomotor disability are less efficient than non-disabled persons. This means that they use more energy and get tired more quickly, so that the time over which an action, such as walking, can be sustained is limited. One aspect of this concerns the effort sometimes made to teach children with CP, usually those with spastic diplegia, to mimic the normal gait cycle and in particular the pendular swing of the lower leg. Knee flexor hypertonus makes this impossible for them, just as being in water does for us. In water we wade using a gait very similar to that of some people with spastic diplegia. They are walking with their most efficient gait; it may have disadvantages (socially, functionally, developmentally) but to change it, without surgery, could only lead to a further reduction in their mechanical efficiency.

• *Developmental efficiency.* The body appears to move in the easiest manner it can to achieve a goal; but what is efficient at one stage may lead to a reduction in efficiency at a later stage. Some repeated movements inevitably lead to secondary pathology which may increase the overall disability. For example, encouraging a young child with a mild spastic diplegia to walk about with 20° hip and knee flexion allows independence and exploration and permits more socially appropriate interaction with peers. However, over the next few years the disadvantages can be any or all of: fixed hip flexion deformity, short hamstrings, posterior knee capsule contracture, patella alta (high knee cap), loss of knee and hip extensor power in inner range, and lumbar lordosis with an exaggeration of all anteroposterior spinal curvatures.

• *Gracefulness.* Normal movement is graceful, coordinated, smooth and purposeful, such that even minor impediments can be quickly spotted. When taken to the limits of movement confidence, everyone's movements lose these attributes. Society expects that actions will be smooth and confidently executed and any marked deviation is hard for us to accept. Much of the conflict between the different schools of physical therapy concerns the relative importance attached to either the normality of appearance or the functional effectiveness of movement. When the aim of treatment is to achieve the nearest copy of normal movement, it acts as a block to functional independence as the child may be discouraged from practising aberrant movement. Up to a point in particular circumstances this may be excusable, but as a basis for treatment it is flawed because there is no way that the therapist can know in advance how close to normality a particular child can come. So there is no goal which, when it is achieved, signals the end of treatment, nor a scale by which one result can be judged better than another: it depends on the aim of the intervention. Function, however, provides its own measures: Can the person do it? Under what circumstances? And in what time frame? Also, the importance of a particular function to an individual ensures that priorities are set for treatment aims and the effort which is reasonable and sustainable to both patient and therapist. Making a judgement about how near a movement is to normality is quite different from assessing how near it is to that child's likely most effective function.

Cerebral palsy

Hemiplegia

Infants with congenital hemiplegia differ in their pattern of locomotor development but only in ways which can easily be predicted. The majority of infants with hemiplegia will wish to crawl and this may be difficult for them, primarily because of lack of support by one arm. Pelvic stability may not be efficient, and crawling can often be more of a prone shuffle. Sitting is more typically side-sitting, allowing arm support with the unaffected arm, trunk side flexion to the affected side and internal rotation of the hip on that side. If they are natural shufflers rather than crawlers they usually shuffle in the same asymmetric sitting posture. When getting into a standing position more effort is made by the unaffected leg which also bears more of the weight in supported standing. Given the circumstances none of this is surprising.

The appearance of motor milestones in children with hemiplegia need not be delayed and might commonly be described as late-normal; more mildly affected infants frequently show no delay at all. Any major delay in gross skills in a child with a presumed hemiplegia should lead one to look for another explanation; not infrequently such children have an asymmetric diplegia or a more generalized developmental delay.

Bilateral disorders
It will be apparent to those who have watched even a small number of children with bilateral CP that to discuss their motor development would be as difficult as it would be pointless. Although there are a few clinically useful groupings, children are truly different and will follow a sequence and timing unique to themselves. However, there are some points which need consideration.
• *Anatomical distribution of the disorder.* Bilateral CP nearly always involves four limbs and the trunk, but in some cases there is an almost complete absence of disorder of the upper trunk and upper limbs. There are also a small number of children who have true triplegia, usually sparing one upper limb. In the main, however, the involvement falls into three groups, with or without left/right asymmetry: equal involvement of upper and lower limbs (legs affected similarly to arms, L=A: usually called tetra- or quadriplegia); lower limbs more affected than upper limbs (L>A: diplegia); and a far smaller number whose upper limbs are clearly more involved than their lower limbs (L<A). This latter group are usually classified as having tetra/quadriplegia, but in association with microcephaly and pseudobulbar palsy are also classified as double hemiplegia. As was seen in the South-east England cohort (see below), a few children can be difficult to classify because if, for example, all four limbs are involved but one upper limb excessively so, then L>A, L=A or L<A ceases to have a useful meaning.

In general the diplegic group, often referred to as spastic diplegic irrespective of whether they have pyramidal or extrapyramidal hypertonus, have much the better locomotor prognosis because of better balance ability and the advantage of better upper limb function for reliable support.
• *Primitive responses.* The opportunity to attain any vertical posture is not precluded by retention of, for example, the asymmetric tonic neck reflex (ATNR), symmetric tonic neck response (STNR) or Moro response. However, it is much less likely, and function within these unsupported postures may remain difficult to the point of being hardly useful. A few children can overcome one, even dominant, primitive response. One of us remembers a child with a severe involuntary movement disorder who walked independently by using head turning

to initiate reciprocal leg flexion and extension. These and other retained primitive responses, particularly when they are so consistent as to be considered reflexes, may not be the cause of poor locomotor development. It is more likely that they are markers for the severity of CNS dysfunction.

The loss of these responses, which are usually gone by 5–6 months, is definitely an advantage for further motor development (Paine 1964, Bleck 1975, Badell-Ribera 1985, Watt *et al.* 1989, Campos da Paz *et al.* 1994, Trahan *et al.* 1994).

• *Balance and protective responses.* Spasticity, as opposed to other types of hypertonia, tends to preclude the effective use of protective responses. Dystonic (extrapyramidal) hypertonia does not and this is a major advantage with regard to locomotor development because it allows much greater security in any upright position.

• *Reciprocation.* Some children find that controlled reciprocal movements are difficult or impossible, particularly when they are under any stress. Hence bunny-hopping rather than a reciprocal crawl will nearly always be preferred when excited or hurrying. Children with hypertonic diplegia fall into two groups. First, those—usually spastic—who would rather not use a reciprocal movement of the legs for walking, but lock them into semiflexion and use a pseudoreciprocation by alternately rotating the pelvis around the vertical axis. And second, those—usually dystonic—who naturally reciprocate; they have no difficulty in attaining full extension of the hips and knees and usually walk with knee hyperextension during the stance phase. These children can easily crawl reciprocally unless they are excited.

• *Between-heel sitting.* 'W-sitting' is a position which has achieved almost mythical status. It is frequently castigated as the cause of femoral neck anteversion and so is banned by many therapists and orthopaedic surgeons. However, one has only to attempt this position oneself to realize that it is a posture no-one would adopt unless they were already comfortably able to do so, *i.e.* the child already has femoral neck anteversion. It does have a number of advantages. It gives a wide base with the centre of gravity in the middle of the base so that both hands are free for play. It aligns the pelvis to promote a good spinal posture and so allows better head control and hand function. It is also a position which easily translates to crawling or getting to a standing position. Its drawbacks are: it may help retain femoral neck anteversion, it can force the foot/ankle into equinus, and it can promote external tibial torsion. However, how real these assumed effects are is not known.

A further point concerns the worry that femoral neck anteversion is related to gait. If the child is unlikely to achieve more than household walking, one should consider whether between-heel sitting is anything but an advantage. Moreover, the structure of the hip joint is such that internal and external rotation in flexion (for sitting) bears little relationship to these movements in extension (for walking).

Thus, apart from the overt CP, a number of other factors may directly affect these children's locomotor development. CP is not a single disease entity nor even the sequela of one pathology, it is the outcome of many pathological events which can occur at any developmental stage, pre-, peri- or postnatally. This is only a little less true when the disorder is more clearly defined, as for instance diplegia, quadriplegia, etc. CP is a disorder of movement, but it is not necessarily a disorder only of movement. The causal event(s) may have involved other

TABLE 5.1
Children with bilateral cerebral palsy from the 1989 and 1990 cohorts of the South-east England study

Year	Live births in region	Number with bilateral CP	Rate/1000 live births	Sex Male	Female	Deaths
1989	51,073	90	1.76	59	31	5
1990	52,086	85	1.63	43	42	3
Total	103,159	175	1.69	102	73	8*

*Two further children died after age 4 years.

CNS functions, which are often more subtle and less easily classified but which may significantly affect the child's locomotor performance. By focusing exclusively on the motor aspects of a child's disability it is easy to neglect other impairments, for example sensory function or skeletal deformities that contribute to the overall functional limitations.

South-east England study

Subjects

The children in this cohort were collected primarily for a study of the natural history of hip dysplasia in children with bilateral CP. The geographical area chosen is that covered by the South East Thames Regional Health Authority, with a population of 3.6 million and approximately 51,000 live births per annum. The children described here are from the first two years of the study (1989, 1990), in which period there were 103,159 live births (Table 5.1). Since hip dysplasia is not a feature of hemiplegia, children referred with hemiplegia were examined only to ensure that those with bilateral, but markedly asymmetric, disorders were not lost to the study. The children with hemiplegia were then excluded. Children who acquired their disorder after the age of 18 months are included in the hip study, but are classified as having late acquired CP and do not appear in the data presented here.

Data from the eight children who died before they achieved any recorded milestones were excluded. Two other children died after the age of 4 years and their data are included in what follows.

From the cohort reported on here 217 children were examined at home; of these, 42 did not match the study criteria. Data were not obtained for all children: eight died before the age of 4 years; permission to take part was refused for three; and 16 joined but it proved impossible to collect data from them. This left 148 children from whom data on locomotor development to age 4 years have been collected.

Measures

The motor milestones are defined in Table 5.2. These data were not collected solely to monitor gross locomotor function, but also because the functions may relate to hip development. These measures are easily monitored and were agreed upon prior to the study in discussions with the 100 or more physiotherapists treating the children locally. One measure, getting to sitting position and sitting independently, was included as a guide to the severity of the motor disorder.

TABLE 5.2
The locomotor milestones and the abbreviations used throughout the text

Name in text	Measure	Comments
To Sit	Getting to sitting position and sitting on the floor; from supine or prone into any sitting position and maintaining it for 15 seconds without propping with arms	This is a non-hip-related measure of general motor ability
Crawl	Crawling on hands/elbows and knees—reciprocal or bunny hop—used as a means of locomotion daily	A hip-use-related measure of weight bearing and hip movement
Chair to Stand	Getting to standing position against furniture from sitting on a chair	This was included because many of the children were likely to be having a Conductive Education based programme
Floor to Stand	Getting to standing against furniture from any lying position on the floor	
Cruise	Cruise along furniture/wall—even if placed in standing—for two steps sideways in either (not necessarily both) directions	Not asking for the ability to get to stand because this is a hip-related measure. Once achieved, parents will usually encourage their child to do this even though the child cannot attain the position
Stand Balanced	Stand—even if placed—without any aid or help to balance for 15 seconds. May use ankle–foot orthosess, knee orthoses or special footwear	This is a balance and base measure, rather than a movement ability measure
To Stand Alone	Get to standing without support and stand for 15 seconds. May use ankle–foot orthoses and special footwear	This is a movements, base and balance measure
Walk with Aid	Walking with a (hand held) walking aid, but no personal help, for ten steps	A measure of movement ability eliminating balance; but also upper limb function
Walk Alone	Walking independently for ten steps. May use ankle–foot orthoses or special footwear	A movement and balance measure
Use Walk/Coast	Walking with or without a walking aid or orthoses, as the usual means of locomotion indoors	This milestone may appear a more advanced skill than 'walk alone', but it is a hip-use-related milestone which some children attain by intermittent cruising combined with only a few steps to the next support. This is referred to as 'coasting' in the text

INITIAL EXAMINATION

Before being accepted into the study the children were seen in their homes or at a local clinic by the researcher. After informed consent was obtained from the parents, the children were examined and a number of specific items recorded. For the purposes of this chapter the presence or absence of ATNR and pseudobulbar palsy, and the distribution between the limbs of relative severity of disability, are the most relevant. The mean age of initial examination was 21 months with a standard deviation of 10 months. No child was examined before the age of 1 year, to allow the motor disorder to 'stabilize'. By 33 months of age 90% had been examined. However, when corrected for gestational age, 19% were at 12 months or less.

DATA COLLECTION
Data were collected at intervals of six months by questionnaire completed by the child's physiotherapist with the help of the parents/carers. Very few children were referred late and consequently few questionnaire returns relied on memory or case notes.

RECORDING OF AGE
For simplicity all ages were collected as from birth, but then corrected for gestational age. Thus the terms 'achieved' and 'not achieved' mean by 4 years, after correction for gestational age.

Results
The results relate to the 148 children (90 male, 58 female) for whom records are available up to the age of 48 months. Of these, 48 (32%) failed to achieve any recorded locomotor milestone. There were no significant sex differences for any of the milestones. The number of children not achieving a particular milestone and the percentage of subjects so failing are shown in Table 5.3. One hundred children (68%) achieved at least one skill (Table 5.4).

INDIVIDUAL MILESTONES
• *To Sit.* This is operationally defined as getting into a sitting position and sitting without support for 15 seconds. Of the 92 children who achieved this milestone, all but nine achieved Cruise, but 35 failed to achieve Walk Alone by 4 years. When initially examined 11% of the 92 children produced an ATNR as opposed to 61% of the 56 children who failed To Sit. Only 31% had a pseudobulbar palsy as opposed to 77% of those who failed To Sit.

Table 5.5 and Figure 5.1 show how the age of attaining the To Sit milestone relates to further locomotor progress. Thus, of those up to the 25th centile (11 months) all achieved Cruise but two did not achieve Walk Alone; whereas of those up to the 90th centile (30 months) four did not achieve Cruise and 28 did not achieve Walk Alone. Of the 83 children who achieved both To Sit and Cruise, 20 (24%) achieved Cruise first. Fifty-six children (38%) did not achieve To Sit by the age of 4 years.
• *Cruise.* Sixty-four children (43%) did not achieve this milestone by 4 years. Of these, nine achieved To Sit, three achieved Crawl, nine achieved Chair to Stand, five achieved Floor to Stand, and four achieved Walk with Aid. All of those achieving Cruise (n=84) achieved To Sit except one child who achieved Cruise at 22 months, Crawl at 47 months, Chair to Stand at 20 months, Floor to Stand at 27 months and Walk with Aid at 24 months.
• *Walk with Aid.* Not every child who walked alone needed to have a prior period using a walking aid, and it might clarify the bare figures in Tables 5.3 and 5.4 to state that of the 57 children who walked alone by 4 years, 13 never used a walking aid and 44 did. There are also another 26 children who use a walking aid but cannot yet walk alone.

TABLE 5.3
**Number of children in study (N = 148) unable
to achieve each milestone by 48 months**

Milestone	Number of children	%
To Sit	56	38
Crawl	65	44
Chair to Stand	57	39
Floor to Stand	60	41
Cruise	64	43
Stand Balanced	81	55
To Stand Alone	96	65
Walk Alone	91	61
Use Walk/Coast	86	58
Walk with Aid*	65	48

*N = 135 only (13 walked alone without needing
a walking aid).

TABLE 5.4
Children achieving each milestone by 48 months

Milestone	Number of children	Age of achieving milestone (months) Median	Range
To Sit	92	16	5–46
Crawl	83	17	6–47
Chair to Stand	91	20	7–45
Floor to Stand	88	21	6–48
Cruise	84	20	8–48
Stand Balanced	67	24	10–48
To Stand Alone	52	25	11–48
Walk with Aid	70	22	12–48
Walk Alone	57	28	14–48
Use Walk/Coast	62	26	14–48

ASYMMETRIC TONIC NECK REFLEX

From Table 5.6 and Figures 5.2 and 5.3 it can be seen that the retention of an ATNR as a reflex long after it would normally have disappeared does not preclude any milestone being attained, but it is associated with a greatly reduced likelihood of this, confirming it as a marker for a more severe disorder.

A pseudobulbar palsy is also a marker for a more severe locomotor disorder, although obviously not in such a direct fashion, *viz.* congenital suprabulbar paresis (Worster-Drought 1956).

UPPER/LOWER LIMB DISTRIBUTION OF DISORDER

As expected, those with a diplegic distribution (legs more involved than the arms) do much better than those with equal involvement of upper and lower limbs (quadriplegia) who, apart from other difficulties, usually have a primary balance problem. The balance difficulties

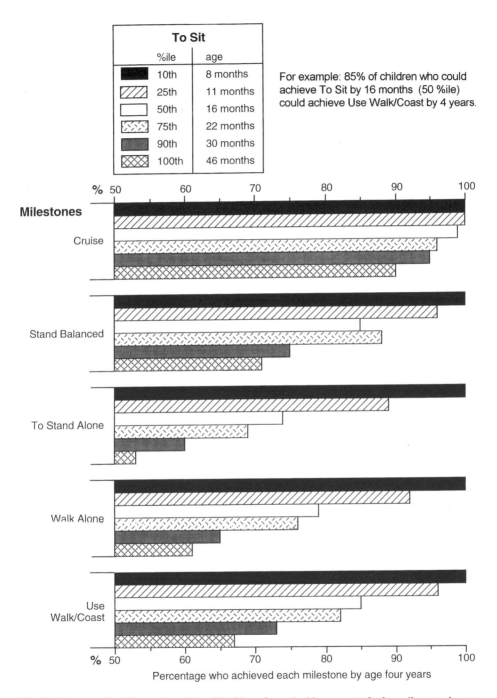

Fig. 5.1. How the 92 children who achieved To Sit performed with respect to further milestones by age 4 years. For example, 85% of children who could achieve To Sit by 16 months (50th centile) could achieve Use Walk/Coast by 4 years. (See also Table 5.5.)

111

TABLE 5.5

Numbers of subjects achieving To Sit and Sit Unsupported, with centile ages, and subsequent milestone achievements for each centile group for Cruise, Stand Balanced, To Stand Alone, Walk Alone and Use Walk/Coast*

To Sit and Sit Unsupported			Cruise			Stand Balanced			To Stand Alone			Walk Alone			Use Walk/Coast		
			Failing skill	Milestone achieved		Failing skill	Milestone achieved		Failing skill	Milestone achieved		Failing skill	Milestone achieved		Failing skill	Milestone achieved	
n	Centile	Age (months)	n	90% by (months)	All by (months)	n	90% by (months)	All by (months)	n	90% by (months)	All by (months)	n	90% by (months)	All by (months)	n	90% by (months)	All by (months)
8	10	8	0	—	22	0	—	26	0	—	28	0	—	33	0	—	32
24	25	11	0	—	33	1	—	48	3	—	48	2	42	48	1	45	48
47	50	16	1	28	36	7	43	48	12	40	48	10	41	48	7	44	48
67	75	22	1	30	48	12	43	48	21	36	48	16	41	48	12	44	48
81	90	30	4	39	48	20	39	48	32	36	48	28	41	48	22	44	48
90**	100	46	9	39	48	26	44	48	40	45	48	35	42	48	30	46	48

*One child achieved Cruise without To Sit; another child achieved Stand Balanced without To Sit.
**92 children achieved To Sit but the ages are unknown for 2.

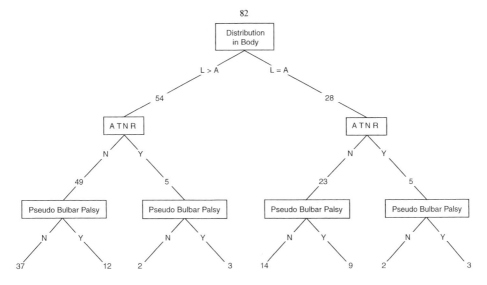

Fig. 5.2. Number of children achieving To Sit by 4 years, and the effect of distribution in the body, ATNR and pseudobulbar palsy.

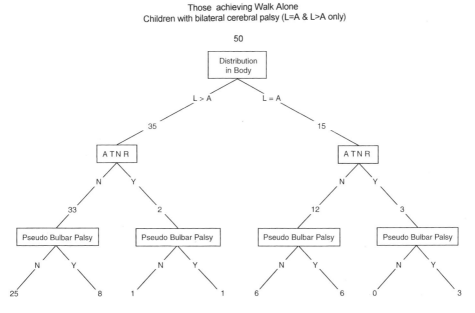

Fig. 5.3. Number of children achieving Walk Alone by 4 years, and the effect of the distribution in the body, ATNR and pseudobulbar palsy.

TABLE 5.6
Percentage of children achieving each milestone in each category (see text)

| Milestone | ATNR[1] | | Bulbar palsy | | Distribution in body[2] | |
	Absent (n = 104)	Present (n = 44)	Absent (n = 71)	Present (n = 77)	Legs = Arms (n = 76)	Legs>Arms (n = 59)
To Sit	79	23	83	39	37	92
Crawl	72	18	75	35	30	86
Chair to Stand	79	21	79	42	38	90
Floor to Stand	77	18	81	37	34	88
Cruise	73	18	75	37	30	86
Stand Balanced	58	16	60	30	25	68
To Stand Alone	48	5	47 **	23	18	54
Walk with Aid	66	23	71	32	28	80
Walk Alone	50	11	49 **	27	20	59
Use Walk/Coast	55	11	58	24	21	63

On χ^2, all differences significant at $p<0.001$ except, ** $p<0.01$.
[1]ATNR as tested at initial (entry) examination (see text).
[2]Ten children were classified Legs<Arms; three children were unclassifiable.

for those with diplegia are the result of a poor base. This can be seen (Table 5.6) in the contrast between the achievement percentages for all hand support milestones and those milestones for which the feet form the only base. In the main more severe involvement of the legs (L>A) is a marker for a less generalized disorder but this relationship may be an indirect one, for only six of the 59 children in this (diplegic) category had an ATNR. It should also be emphasized that children were classified on the basis of a single examination and 19% of these examinations took place when the infants were less than 1 year, corrected for gestational age. All the children will be re-examined after they have reached 5 years.

Ontario study

Few studies are available of the patterns of longitudinal motor development of children with CP. In fact the data reported in this chapter represent rare examples of systematic studies of changes in motor development in children with CP. A small body of information has accumulated which describes some prognostic factors relating to the later acquisition of specific motor skills in this population (Crothers and Paine 1959, Beals 1966, Molnar and Gordon 1976, Sutherland *et al.* 1980, Bleck 1987, Watt *et al.* 1989, Campos da Paz *et al.* 1994). However, these studies are not consistent in methods, populations or findings, and much uncertainty remains regarding the natural history of motor development and outcomes of children with CP.

In a series of studies carried out in Ontario, Canada over the past ten years, data have been collected on the motor development of a population of children with CP. These data were collected systematically, in a standardized manner, with a valid and reliable instrument specifically designed to assess gross motor function in this population. The Gross Motor Function Measure (GMFM) (Russell *et al.* 1989, 1993) is an 88-item criterion-referenced observational measure of gross motor activities in children. The items cover the spectrum of motor functions that preschool children would ordinarily readily accomplish by the age of 4 or 5: lying, rolling, sitting, standing and walking/running/jumping. The GMFM was created to measure quantitative change in motor function in children with CP, and has been validated as an evaluative instrument capable of detecting clinically important changes in motor function in children with CP over a six month period (Russell *et al.* 1989, Guyatt *et al.* 1992). The measure is now being widely used as a clinical outcome measure in intervention studies (Bjornson *et al.* 1990; Bower and McLellan 1992, 1994; Parker *et al.* 1993; Evans *et al.* 1994; McLaughlin *et al.* 1994).

In the course of creating and validating the GMFM, and later the Gross Motor Performance Measure (GMPM) (Boyce *et al.* 1995, Gowland *et al.* 1995), data were collected on the gross motor function of over 300 children ranging in age from 1 month to 19 years. These included 63 normally developing preschool children, and 215 children with CP. The latter group had been prospectively classified clinically as having mild (n=53), moderate (n=99), or severe (n=63) CP, although no standardization of this classification was used, nor was any attempt made to assess the reliability with which classifications were made. Children in this study were drawn from a population believed to be representative of children with CP in Ontario. They were in fact a convenience sample of children receiving therapy services in two of southern Ontario's ambulatory specialized treatment programmes. These two services were typical of those in which the great majority of therapy support for children with disabilities is provided. These programmes provide a variety of conventional treatment and service activities for children with a wide range of physical/functional disabilities. Children receive the programme practised in the administrative region in which they live.

The parents of children in the case records of the two centres were approached for permission to enroll their children in the study. The children were not a randomly chosen sample; rather, an effort was made to select children representing a broad spectrum of age and clinical severity of CP. It was expected that younger children would, in general, show more change in motor function than older children. Thus, although the children ranged in age from less than 12 months to mid-adolescence, approximately 70% were aged 7 or below. A strategy was devised to ensure that the recruitment included children across the spectrum of severity of motor disability (Russell *et al.* 1989, Boyce *et al.* 1995).

Approximately 80% of the children had some form of spastic CP, with the remainder showing evidence of other forms of motor impairment. Of those with spastic syndromes, roughly 82% had bilateral CP and the rest presented with hemisyndromes. In the results that follow, children are grouped only by the clinical classification of severity used by each therapist. The data are not presented separately by type of motor disability, though the 30 children with hemisyndromes were all classified as mild. The findings presented here are thought to be representative of children with CP in Canada at the present time. However, it is important to appreciate that the data are not drawn from an epidemiologically sampled population.

The GMFM was developed as a change-detecting measure, and is meant to be used serially to assess the extent of change in motor function over time. Because it seemed likely that the GMFM scores would also discriminate children by age and severity, we decided to plot first assessments of each child against age, by severity grouping. Although the data

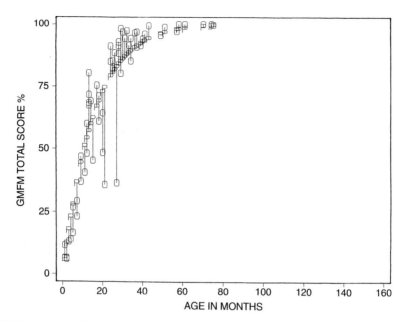

Fig. 5.4. The pattern of gross motor development of normal preschool children (n=63), by age, as assessed by the Gross Motor Function Measure. 'O' represents actual scores of individual children; 'P' plots the mean growth curve derived by the formula GMFM = $\theta(1-e^{-\lambda t})$. See text for details.

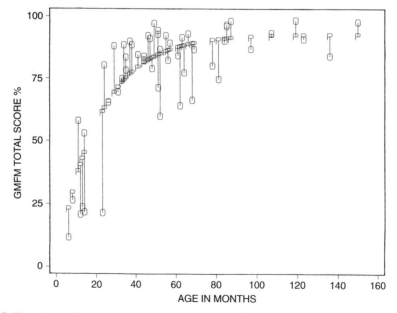

Fig. 5.5. The pattern of gross locomotor development of children with mild cerebral palsy (n=53), by age, as assessed by the Gross Motor Function Measure. 'O' represents actual scores of individual children; 'P' plots the mean growth curve derived by the formula GMFM = $\theta(1-e^{-\lambda t})$. See text for details.

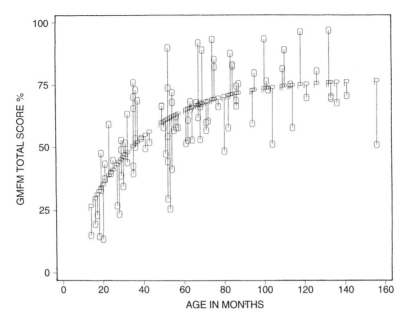

Fig. 5.6. The pattern of gross motor development of children with moderate cerebral palsy (n=99), by age, as assessed by the Gross Motor Function Measure. 'O' represents actual scores of individual children; 'P' plots the mean growth curve derived by the formula GMFM = $\theta(1-e^{-\lambda t})$. See text for details.

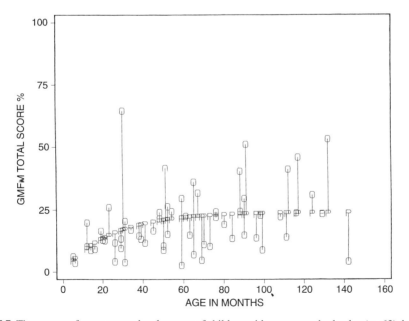

Fig. 5.7. The pattern of gross motor development of children with severe cerebral palsy (n=63), by age, as assessed by the Gross Motor Function Measure. 'O' represents actual scores of individual children; 'P' plots the mean growth curve derived by the formula GMFM = $\theta(1-e^{-\lambda t})$. See text for details.

TABLE 5.7
Statistical parameters describing Figures 5.4–5.7

Severity	n	θ (SE)	λ (SE)
Normal	63	100.00 (0.0)	0.064 (0.003)
Mild	53	92.23 (3.28)	0.047 (0.006)
Moderate	99	76.9 (3.44)	0.029 (0.003)
Severe	63	23.6 (2.99)	0.041 (0.016)

are cross-sectional, we believed that it might be possible to discern patterns of motor development that would provide clues concerning both the rate of change and the eventual motor achievements of children with CP.

The motor growth curves of the normally developing preschool children and of the children with mild, moderate and severe CP are shown in Figures 5.4–5.7. Note that the GMFM score is a percentage, based on how much a child accomplishes (partial or complete success on each item) as a proportion of the total possible on the scale. In this scoring system no adjustment is made for age or severity of motor disability. It is readily apparent to the eye that these curves differ in both slope and the value of the asymptote. Despite the variation above and below each best-fit line, there are significant differences in the ultimate asymptotic values of these four curves.

The curves were created using the mathematical formula $GMFM = \theta(1-e^{-\lambda t})$, in which the major independent variables are: θ, the value of the asymptote; λ, the rate of change in the curve as it rises from 0; and t, the time over which the change occurs. Table 5.7 gives the numerical values for these parameters for each of the curves. The different λ values describe numerically the variations in rate of acquisition of motor skills among the four groups of children. It can be seen that in general the most rapid rise in GMFM scores, reflecting the most rapid change in motor development, occurs in the preschool years and in children with the least disability.

It may be helpful to place the λ values into a clinical context. A 10-year-old with CP who achieves a GMFM total score of 92 would be independently ambulatory, with an awkward gait on uneven surfaces or inclines, and show some difficulty with run and jump. A child of 10 with a GMFM total score of 77 would at best walk on an even surface with the aid of mobility device, climb stairs using a rail, but require wheeled mobility to travel any distance or to travel over uneven ground. Total GMFM scores below 25 in a 10-year-old imply, at best, supported sitting, without any capacity for independent mobility, except perhaps through the use of powered mobility aids.

Several cautions about these data should be emphasized. First, the severity classification is unstandardized and was applied by a large number of physiotherapists who used individual judgements to place each child in this three-level scale. It is therefore likely that some proportion of children belong in a level above or below the one in which they were placed. Second, the data displayed in Figures 5.4–5.7 represent a cross-sectional aggregation of GMFM information from different children. Anthropometric curves are usually created by amalgamating individual longitudinal data sets acquired by following large numbers of subjects prospectively to collect information on within-subject growth. These data are then combined and enable investigators to discern both mean growth patterns and between-subject variations. In this way it is possible to obtain means and variances for the population, something that is not available in the data presented here. Third, the curves describe only gross motor function, without any additional information about potential confounders of motor development in children with CP. For example, the curves do not take account of variations in the intelligence, general health and sensory function of the children nor in therapeutic support. Thus these curves represent at best a crude display of the motor progress of children with CP, by severity, across the childhood years.

Discussion

CP is a major cause of physical disability and motor impairment in children (Stanley and Alberman 1984). However, the natural history of the locomotor development of this population is still poorly understood and has not been systematically described and documented. This is surprising given the number of rehabilitation professionals engaged in the management of these children, the variety of interventions that have been advocated and the high cost of lifelong care. Moreover, several interventions including drug therapy, orthopaedic surgery and neurosurgery are invasive, have potentially adverse effects, and place very considerable demands on the child, the family and health care resources. In the absence of objective data on the natural course of motor development in children with CP, it is difficult to evaluate the extent to which specific interventions improve motor function beyond what might be expected as a consequence of natural growth and development.

Few reports in the literature offer either the systematic perspective of the English data presented here, or the severity-based cross-sectional picture of locomotor development illustrated in the Ontario data. Both studies contribute new information and understanding about locomotor progress in children with CP, and both have limitations that are important to recognize. From a consideration of these two projects some directions for future investigation are evident.

One of the strengths of the South-east England study is that it is a prospective, population-based enquiry. Thus no selection biases appear to be operating that might give a misleading picture of locomotor development in children with CP. The children were ascertained when young, all were examined by the same therapist on entry to the study, and data were collected at a closely specified age (48 months, corrected for gestational age). The children are being followed up using a protocol-based procedure. However, several considerations should be borne in mind. The study was designed to explore the natural history of hip dysplasia rather than chart locomotor development in the population. Hence the data are not as specific or detailed as one might wish regarding locomotor development. A related point concerns the measurement of motor milestones. These data were recorded by a large number of therapists but we have no information on inter-observer agreement or reliability. The

119

data therefore are probably less reliable than might be obtained had they been collected by a smaller number of highly trained research staff using an instrument specifically designed to assess locomotor development.

The Ontario research differs both in terms of how the data were collected and what they demonstrate. In the Ontario study data were collected by trained observers (Russell *et al.* 1994), using a standardized criterion-referenced measure of known reliability and validity. Efforts were made to assess locomotor function across both age and severity dimensions, in order to sample the range of children with CP seen and treated in children's rehabilitation programmes. The clinical assessment of severity applied prospectively to each child made it possible to use this factor in analysis of the data, though it is important to appreciate that assessment of severity was not standardized.

However, the report on the Ontario work presented here is cross-sectional and derives from a single observation, although the data were treated in a manner similar to longitudinal data on height, weight or head circumference. While these growth curves are suggestive of characteristic patterns of locomotor development in children with CP, they should be treated as pilot data indicating what might be useful in describing motor development in this population. A second limitation is the lack of standardization of the severity classification. Thus, while it is possible to discern clearly different patterns of motor development among the three subgroups of children with CP, there is inevitably a good deal of noise in the data.

A fuller understanding of the locomotor development of children with CP will be possible only with carefully structured prospective studies that combine, among other factors, elements of the English and Canadian work. Such a study is currently being planned in Ontario. The Ontario project is designed to create motor growth curves analogous to those used to describe the physical growth of children. This will be achieved by serial assessments of children with CP aged 12 months to 12 years, whose motor progress will be charted in a systematic manner for a minimum of three years. Locomotor function will be assessed regularly, using the GMFM. A clinical classification of severity of motor disability will be applied prospectively, using the Gross Motor Function Classification System recently created by Palisano and co-workers at the Neurodevelopmental Clinical Research Unit, McMaster University, Hamilton, Ontario (Palisano *et al.*, in press). This descriptive five-level system focuses on self-initiated movement, and particularly examines sitting (truncal control) and mobility. In addition to severity and motor function information, standardized data will be collected on covariable factors that might influence motor outcomes, including cognitive ability, sensory impairments, behavioural and personality factors, family and sociodemographic variables, and type and amount of treatment.

The expected outcome of this study is a series of growth curves that plot patterns of motor development for children with CP according to age and severity of disability. We believe that these curves will be widely applicable to an understanding of motor development in children with CP, controlling for 'severity' and for co-morbidities. They will contribute important new information for the study and understanding of the conditions collectively called 'cerebral palsy'. These curves will also provide a backdrop against which to compare both standard and innovative interventions designed to improve motor outcome in children with CP. Equally important, we believe, will be the potential to use these 'natural history' observations in our ongoing clinical work; in discussions with parents about locomotor prognosis; and to target interventions relevant to each child's motor capabilities and expected functional outcome.

What do the data from these investigations tell us about approaches to understanding motor function in children with CP? The English study demonstrates the possibility of determining an early and fairly precise prognosis for locomotor function for children with CP. This clearly will help improve the specification of treatment aims and the targeting of treatment. The Ontario study complements these observations by adding the dimension of the severity of disability and by using an objective clinical measure of motor function applicable to all children with CP. Together these studies point a way forward, toward the collection of standardized prospective observations of children with CP, which will improve our understanding of the needs of both individual children and populations of children with disordered motor development.

ACKNOWLEDGEMENTS

The South-east England study has relied on the cooperation of paediatricians to refer their patients and the children's physiotherapists to provide the six-monthly developmental data. The main (hip) study is being carried out in partnership with Gillian Baird, who has provided paediatric advice throughout. David Scrutton would like to thank them all. The study is supported by research grants from Mencap City Foundation and Scope (formerly The Spastics Society).

The Ontario work represents the collaboration of a number of researchers. Peter Rosenbaum wishes to recognize the contributions of Dianne Russell, Bob Palisano, Stephen Walter, Barb Galuppi and Ellen Wood, all of whom are co-investigators in the research projects outlined here. This work has been supported by grants from the Easter Seal Research Institute, Health Canada and the Medical Research Council of Canada.

REFERENCES

Badell-Ribera, A. (1985) 'Cerebral palsy: postural–locomotor prognosis in spastic diplegia.' *Archives of Physical Medicine and Rehabilitation*, **66**, 614–619.

Beals, R. K. (1966) 'Spastic paraplegia and diplegia. An evaluation of non-surgical and surgical factors influencing the prognosis for ambulation.' *Journal of Bone and Joint Surgery*, **48A**, 827–846.

Bjornson, K., McLaughlin, J., Graubert, C., Roberts, T., Hays, R., Hoffinger, S. (1990) 'Gross motor function post selective dorsal rhizotomy: a pilot study.' *Pediatric Physical Therapy*, **2**, 214.

Bleck, E. E. (1975) 'Locomotor prognosis in cerebral palsy.' *Developmental Medicine and Child Neurology*, **17**, 18–25.

—— (1987) *Orthopaedic Management in Cerebral Palsy. Clinics in Developmental Medicine No. 99/100.* London: Mac Keith Press.

Bower, E., McLellan, D.L. (1992) 'Effect of increased exposure to physiotherapy on skill acquisition of children with cerebral palsy.' *Developmental Medicine and Child Neurology*, **34**, 25–39.

—— —— (1994) 'Assessing motor-skill acquisition in four centres for the treatment of children with cerebral palsy.' *Developmental Medicine and Child Neurology*, **36**, 902–909.

Boyce, W.F., Gowland, C., Rosenbaum, P.L., Lane, M., Plews, N., Goldsmith, C.H., Russell, D.J., Wright, V., Zdrobov, S. (1991) 'Measuring quality of movement in cerebral palsy: a review of instruments.' *Physical Therapy*, **71**, 813–819.

—— —— —— —— —— —— —— Potter, S., Harding, D. (1995) 'The Gross Motor Performance Measure: validity and responsiveness of a measure of quality of movement.' *Physical Therapy*, **75**, 603–613.

Campos da Paz, A., Burnett S.M., Braga, L.W. (1994) 'Walking prognosis in cerebral palsy: a 22-year retrospective analysis.' *Developmental Medicine and Child Neurology*, **36**, 130–134.

Capute, A.J., Palmer, F.B., Shapiro, B.K., Wachtel, R.C., Ross, A., Accardo, P.J. (1984) 'Primitive reflex profile: a quantitation of primitive reflexes in infancy.' *Developmental Medicine and Child Neurology*, **26**, 375–383.

—— Shapiro, B.K., Palmer, F.B., Ross, A., Wachtel, R.C. (1985) 'Normal gross locomotor development: the influences of race, sex and socio-economic status.' *Developmental Medicine and Child Neurology*, **27**, 635–643.

Cooke, D.W., Thelen, E. (1987) 'Newborn stepping: a review of puzzling infant co-ordination.' *Developmental Medicine and Child Neurology*, **29**, 399–404. *(Annotation.)*

Crothers, B., Paine, R.S. (1959) *The Natural History of Cerebral Palsy.* Cambridge: Harvard University Press. (Reprinted 1988 as *Classics in Developmental Medicine No. 2.* London: Mac Keith Press.)

Evans, C., Gowland, C., Rosenbaum, P., Willan, A., Russell, D., Weber, D., Plews, N. (1994) 'The effectiveness of orthoses for children with cerebral palsy.' *Developmental Medicine and Child Neurology*, **36** (Suppl. 70), 26–27. *(Abstract.)*

Gowland, C., Boyce,W.F., Wright, V., Russell, D.J., Goldsmith, C.H., Rosenbaum, P.L. (1995) 'Reliability of the Gross Motor Performance Measure.' *Physical Therapy*, **75**, 597–602.

Guyatt, G.H., Kirshner, B., Jaeschke, R. (1992) 'Measuring health status: what are the necessary measurement properties.' *Journal of Clinical Epidemiology*, **45**, 1341–1345.

Jan, J.E., Robinson, G.C., Scott, E, Kinnis, C (1975) 'Hypotonia in the blind child.' *Developmental Medicine and Child Neurology*, **17**, 35–40.

McLaughlin, J.F., Bjornson, K.F., Astley, S.J., Hays, R.M., Hoffinger, S.A., Armantrout, E.A., Roberts,T.S. (1994) 'The role of selective dorsal rhizotomy in cerebral palsy: critical evaluation of a prospective clinical series.' *Developmental Medicine and Child Neurology*, **36**, 755–769.

Milani-Comparetti, A, Gidoni, E.A. (1967a) 'Pattern analysis of motor development and its disorders.' *Developmental Medicine and Child Neurology*, **9**, 625–630.

—— —— (1967b) 'Routine developmental examination in normal and retarded children.' *Developmental Medicine and Child Neurology*, **9**, 631–638.

Molnar, G.E.,Gordon, S.U. (1976) 'Cerebral palsy: predictive value of selected clinical signs for early prognostication of motor function.' *Archives of Physical Medicine and Rehabilitation*, **57**, 153–158.

Paine, R.S. (1964) 'The evolution of infantile postural reflexes in the presence of chronic brain syndromes.' *Developmental Medicine and Child Neurology*, **6**, 345–361.

Palisano, R., Rosenbaum, P., Walter, S., Russell, D., Wood, E., Galuppi, B. (in press) 'Development and validation of a Gross Motor Function Classification System for children with cerebral palsy.' *Developmental Medicine and Child Neurology*.

Parker, D.F., Carriere, L., Hebestreit, H., Salsberg, A., Bar-Or, O. (1993) 'Muscle performance and gross motor function of children with spastic cerebral palsy.' *Developmental Medicine and Child Neurology*, **35**, 17–23.

Robson, P. (1970) 'Shuffling, hitching, scooting or sliding: some observations in 30 otherwise normal children.' *Developmental Medicine and Child Neurology*, **12**, 608–617.

—— Mac Keith, R.C. (1971) 'Shufflers with spastic diplegic cerebral palsy: a confusing clinical picture.' *Developmental Medicine and Child Neurology*, **13**, 651–659.

Russell, D.J., Rosenbaum, P.L., Cadman, D.T., Gowland, C., Hardy, S., Jarvis, S. (1989) 'The Gross Motor Function Measure: a means to evaluate the effects of physical therapy.' *Developmental Medicine and Child Neurology*, **31**, 341–352.

—— Gowland, C., Hardy, S., Lane, M., Plews, N., McGavin, H., Cadman, D., Jarvis, S. (1993) *The Gross Motor Function Measure Manual.* (Available from D. Russell, Bldg. 74, Chedoke-McMaster Hospitals, Hamilton, Ontario, Canada L8N 3Z5.)

—— —— Lane, M., Gowland, C., Goldsmith, C.H., Boyce, W.F., Plews, N. (1994) 'Training users in the Gross Motor Function Measure: methodological and practical issues.' *Physical Therapy*, **74**, 630–636.

Stanley, F., Alberman, E. (Eds.) (1984) *The Epidemiology of the Cerebral Palsies. Clinics in Developmental Medicine No.87.* London: Spastics International Medical Publications.

Sutherland, D.H., Olshen, R., Cooper, L., Woo, S.L-Y. (1980) 'The development of mature gait.' *Journal of Bone and Joint Surgery*, **62A**, 336–353.

Thelen, E. (1984) 'Learning to walk: ecological demands and phylogenetic constraints'. *In:* Lipsitt, L.P., Rovee-Collier, C. (Eds.) *Advances in Infancy Research, Vol. 3.* Norwood, NJ: Ablex, pp. 213–250.

—— Cooke, D.W. (1987) 'Relationship between newborn stepping and later walking: a new interpretation.' *Developmental Medicine and Child Neurology*, **29**, 380–393.

Trahan, J., Marcoux, S. (1994) 'Factors associated with the inability of children with cerebral palsy to walk at six years: a retrospective study.' *Developmental Medicine and Child Neurology*, **36**, 787–795.

Watt, J.M., Robertson, C.M.T., Grace, M.G.A. (1989) 'Early prognosis for ambulation of neonatal intensive care survivors with cerebral palsy.' *Developmental Medicine and Child Neurology*, **31**, 766–773.

Worster-Drought, C. (1956) 'Congenital suprabulbar paresis.' *Journal of Laryngology and Otology*, **70**, 453–463.

6
INTERACTION OF MUSCLE MATURATION WITH MOVEMENT AND POSTURE

Jean-Pierre Lin

Any given posture or movement depends on a continuous interaction of peripheral and central mechanisms. The physical properties of the limb segments narrowly define the range and economy of action, so that motor control begins with the anatomical arrangements of the limb segments and the physical properties of the muscles as the peripheral elements of the motor system. These in turn interact with simple and complex reflexes, postures and voluntary motor activation to produce controlled posture or movement. The endless repertoire of skilled actions which develop or are learned, is undoubtedly based on a constant evolutionary honing of these peripheral and central elements.

The development of motor control from the newborn period to adulthood is achieved against the parallel somatic growth of the body and hence increases in limb inertia which impose further demands on motor physiology. As will be seen, inertia can be controlled by posture, which modifies limb length and prevents unwanted oscillations. Movement at speed presents great challenges to the motor system in terms of the energy consumption and force output required to overcome inertia while at the same time maintaining the accuracy and smoothness of movements. The delicate alternating movements of which adults are capable are markedly different from the motor output in newborn infants which begins with obligate postures, complex reflexes and mass movements that can be provoked by nonspecific stimuli: the classical example being the startle response. However, the exact mechanisms which underpin this emergent control are poorly understood.

The study of motor development has predominantly focused on the maturation of central nervous system elements such as the brain, spinal cord and peripheral nerves. Certain functions such as walking undoubtedly unfold according to a developmental plan and require no conscious learning, in contrast to, for example, a dance routine or using a pencil, both of which are learned culture-dependent actions and not innate features of human motor development. The basic reciprocating mechanisms for walking are likely to be laid out at spinal level, sharing much in common with more primitive vertebrate movements (Grillner *et al.* 1986). Nevertheless, even standing and walking change considerably with age, indicating that changing cortical inputs modify either the basic spinal patterns or the selection of a repertoire of spinal patterns. The tendency to co-contraction and flexion synergies in infancy changes in the second year of life to that of a phasic interplay of muscles and the production of joint assymmetries which are necessary for a mature gait, a feature which fails to emerge in the child with cerebral palsy (Leonard *et al.* 1991). Further examples of the mismatch between muscle activation patterns and the physical demands of standing are provided by Nashner's tilt platform experiments (Nashner *et al.* 1983, Nashner 1985). In these noninvasive experiments, subjects attempted to remain standing on a platform which was made to tilt unexpectedly. Healthy controls reacted to such perturbations by activating their muscles in a distal-to-proximal fashion serving to stabilize the muscles and joints closest to the moving surface first. By contrast, subjects with damage to the central nervous system tended to activate muscles in a proximal-to-distal sequence which in effect produced an unstable motor strategy through a failure to control the joints closest to the weight-bearing surface, allowing the distal segments to flail in an unstable manner relative to the supporting surface. Such a reversal of motor patterning with brain damage indicates the importance of motor sequencing for normal motor control (see Chapter 3). These findings illustrate how injury to the central nervous system may produce disordered motor control, but do not explain the role of muscles and their receptors in normal motor development and in disordered states.

This chapter deals mainly with peripheral influences on motor control. It will illustrate, mainly by reference to studies at the ankle joint, how apparently complex central phenomena can be influenced by relatively simple peripheral events, and will explore the significance of these influences for our understanding of motor development and disordered motor control. The control of alternating movements will be described in terms of physical constraints, followed by a description of how the motor system is organized peripherally to meet these constraints. The concept of the functional joint range and optimum motoneuron output will be shown to play a crucial role in motor control. These findings provide a further scientific framework for the understanding of motor control and its development as well as indicating how a variety of peripherally directed treatments might affect it.

The physics of motion and anatomical–inertial control

All movements of the body are built up from the rotatory motion of limbs about joints, whether these are slow and smooth or brisk and jerky. All movements involve overcoming inertia which is the property of all physical objects to resist a change in their state of rest or motion (Newton's First Law). Overcoming inertia requires force, which is the product of mass and acceleration ($F = ma$), and at their simplest level, all movements require a continuous matching of the forces developed by muscles with the inertial characteristics of the limbs. Although the mass of the body is invariable (ignoring the fluctuations in insensible losses), and the mass of the limb segments remains constant, the physiological rearrangement of the limb segments in relation to each other can profoundly affect the speed of rotatory movements by altering the inertial characteristics of the system. Clapping hands as fast as you can with outstretched arms while movement is restricted to the shoulder joints is more difficult and more tiring than clapping from the wrist, owing to the increased inertia of the outstretched arms compared with the hands alone. The inertia of a limb can be shown to increase with the fifth power of the limb length, so that a doubling of limb length results in a 32-fold increase in the inertia (Walsh and Wright 1987). Relatively small peripheral changes can thus exert an enormous influence on motor speed, a good example being the spin of the ballet dancer or ice skater. Inertia is acceleration-dependent. For oscillating

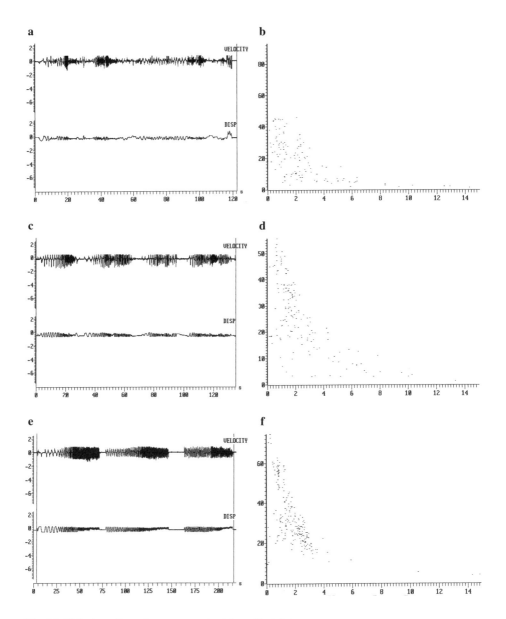

Fig. 6.1. Voluntary alternating movements at the ankle joint.

    (a, c, e) The displacement crosses the 0° position (neutral) at large amplitudes with slow frequencies and at low amplitude with high frequencies of oscillation for subjects aged 3, 6 and 36 years respectively. Note that the joint angle stays close to neutral (0°) as the frequency of oscillation increases.

    (b, d, f) As the frequency of voluntary oscillation increases, so the amplitude of displacement at the ankle joint diminishes. The amplitude is inversely related to the square of the frequency (equation 2, see text), irrespective of age. Horizontal divisions = 5 seconds. Vertical divisions: 1 unit = 33.25°, and 0 = neutral joint angle or right angle position of the foot with the shaft of the tibia. Negative values indicate plantarflexion, positive values indicate dorsiflexion.

126

motion, the limb repeatedly changes direction, accelerating from a position of rest at each turning point; the frequency of voluntary alternating movements at a joint is therefore governed in absolute terms by the ability to overcome inertia, that is to say, the ability to modulate the force exerted by muscles.

What are the physical laws governing alternating movements? For any oscillating system, the acceleration varies with the square of the frequency as given by the equation:

$$\text{Acceleration} = (2\pi f)^2 A \sin 2\pi f t \qquad \text{(equation 1)},$$

where f = frequency of oscillation, A = amplitude of oscillation, and t = time. A doubling in frequency therefore requires a four-fold increase, and a trebling of the frequency a nine-fold increase in the acceleration necessary to move the limb. Ultimately there are limits to the accelerations which muscles can generate, which in turn limits the forces which they can develop.

One way in which the frequency of oscillations can be increased is by diminishing the amplitude of oscillation. This is because the amplitude of oscillation of any system (including a limb about a joint) varies inversely with the square of the frequency of oscillation, as can be seen by rearranging equation 1 so that for any given fixed maximum acceleration, the frequency of oscillation can only increase if the amplitude of movement is reduced:

$$A = \text{Acceleration}/(2\pi f)^2 \sin 2\pi f t \qquad \text{(equation 2)}.$$

The relationship between amplitude and frequency of oscillation is illustrated in Figure 6.1 which shows isotonic alternating movements at the ankle joint at increasing frequencies (plots a, c and e) for subjects aged 3, 6 and 36 years respectively. The corresponding plots of the relation between amplitude of motion and frequency for the same subjects are shown in plots b, d and f. Irrespective of age, as the frequency of voluntary oscillations increases, the amplitude diminishes.

Contractile properties of muscle and the functional joint range

Simple, physical, non-neural constraints have been shown to regulate motion. How have these physical constraints shaped the body's motor strategies? Altering the posture of the limb can be shown to influence the frequency of oscillation, which introduces the concept of the functional joint range. In isotonic alternating plantarflexion and dorsiflexion of the hindfoot at the ankle joint, slow oscillations can encompass the whole of the joint range, but the fastest oscillations, which require the greatest accelerations (equation 1), occur about the joint angle which corresponds to the right angle of the foot with the shaft of the tibia (Figs. 6.1, 6.2), i.e. they occur about the mid-range of the muscle's length. Such rapid oscillations are impossible at the extremes of the joint angle range for several very good reasons, which are revealed by the following series of simple experiments that demonstrate further, peripheral motor constraints on motion.

Effect of joint angle on motoneuron excitability, muscle twitch force and twitch time

The following demonstrations may at first appear far removed from the common experience of voluntary movements, but they serve to illustrate mechanisms regulating movement intrinsic to muscles and their spinal motoneuron connections. The basic experimental design evolved from measurements of calf muscle twitches following a tap to the Achilles tendon

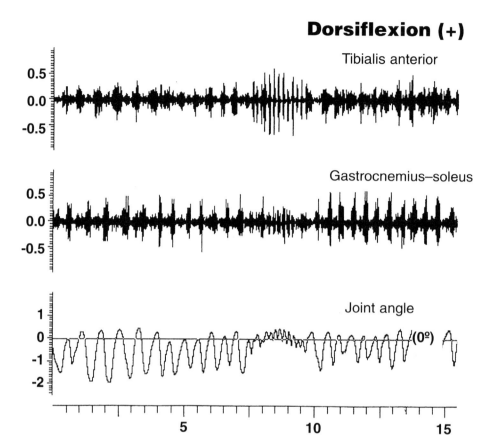

Fig. 6.2. Voluntary alternating movements at the ankle joint, the triphasic response and functional joint range. (Reproduced by permission from Lin *et al.* 1996.)

Low amplitude surface EMG discharges are recorded from the tibialis anterior and gastrocnemius–soleus muscles during alternating movements and are seen to interplay in a 'triphasic pattern' (see Jeannerod 1988 for further discussion). For slow, large amplitude movements, the EMG discharges occur in broad, sustained bursts of low amplitude. At the fastest oscillations close to neutral, the discharges become larger and are very brief (phasic). Neutral appears to be the optimum joint angle for the fastest movements at the ankle. Horizontal divisions = 0.5 s. Vertical divisions: 1 unit = 33.25°, and 0 = neutral joint angle or right angle position of the foot with the shaft of the tibia. Negative values indicate plantarflexion, positive values indicate dorsiflexion.

to elicit a monosynaptic ankle jerk (stretch reflex). Details of these experiments have, in part, been published elsewhere (Walsh *et al.* 1993; Lin *et al.* 1994, 1996a).

The influence of gravity is abolished by lying the subject on their side. The knee-joint is flexed to 90° to eliminate the gastrocnemius muscle influence which acts across both the ankle and knee-joints. Surface electrodes are placed over the midline of the calf muscle at the maximum calf diameter and close to the insertion of the muscles with the Achilles tendon. The ball of the foot rests in contact with a 20 kg load cell which is embedded in a

a.

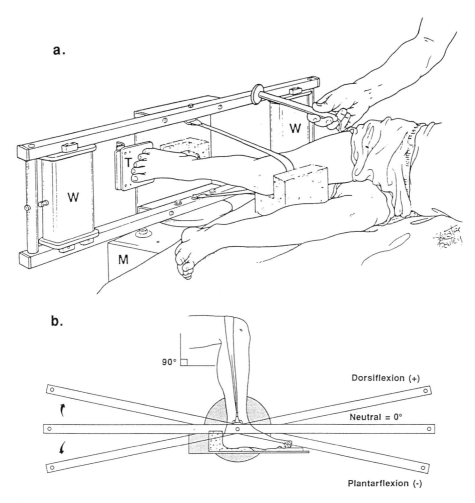

b.

90°

Dorsiflexion (+)

Neutral = 0°

Plantarflexion (-)

Fig. 6.3. High inertia ankle jerk method for eliciting soleus muscle twitches in children and adults. (Reproduced by permission from Walsh 1992.)

    (a) Artist's impression of the apparatus: note heavily-weighted ends of the beam (W), the force plate (T) and torque motor (M). The soleus muscle twitch is reflexly elicited with an Achilles tendon tap.

    (b) View from above showing the position of the knee joint and the axis of the beam and torque motor coaxial with the ankle joint. The ankle joint position and hence the soleus muscle length may be specified by varying the torque applied by the electric motor.

heavily-weighted beam which is coaxial to the ankle joint. The beam may be rotated by a printed electric motor (Fig. 6.3) which allows the ankle joint angle to be varied by preset increments. Measurements begin with the foot at the position of resting plantarflexion (arbitrarily designated as a negative joint angle) and with each increment into dorsiflexion, the soleus muscle is lengthened and the tension in the muscle increases, reaching a maximum at full dorsiflexion (designated a positive joint angle). A typical recording shows the

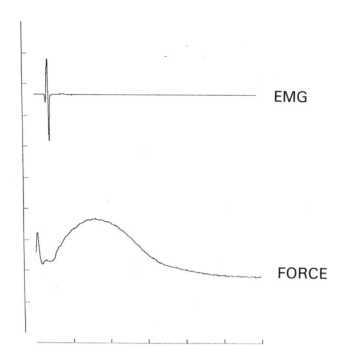

Fig. 6.4. The ankle jerk soleus reflex EMG and whole muscle mechanogram.

    The tendon tap artefact seen on the force trace causes a reflex depolarization of the spinal alpha-motoneurons followed by a synchronous soleus muscle depolarization lasting 14.4 ms (EMG trace) some 12–35 ms later, depending on the length of the leg. The muscular contraction (force trace) follows the EMG discharge and lasts 278 ms. The traces represent four consecutive trigger-averaged taps allowing the muscle to settle between taps. Horizontal divisions = 100 ms. Vertical divisions: EMG trace = 1 mV; force trace = 6.4 N. Joint angle neutral (*i.e.* sole of foot at 90° to shaft of tibia). 31-year-old male, right leg.

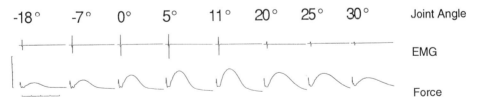

Fig. 6.5. Change in ankle jerk soleus reflex EMG and force with soleus muscle length (data from healthy 31-year-old male, right leg.)

    The ankle jerk has been elicited at resting plantarflexion (−18°) and at subsequent positions through to 30° of dorsiflexion. (i) The EMG amplitude increases to reach a maximum between 0° and 5° and declines with further dorsiflexion. (ii) The twitch force increases with each dorsiflexing increment to reach a maximum at 11° and declines with further dorsiflexion. (iii) The twitch time increases with each dorsiflexing increment to reach a maximum in full dorsiflexion at 30°. Each point represents the average of four consecutive tendon taps. Horizontal divisions = 100 ms. Vertical bar: EMG trace = 2 mV; FORCE trace = 12.8 N.

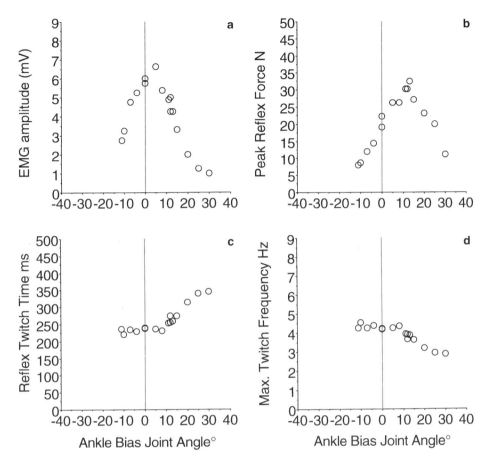

Fig. 6.6. Graphic plot of change in soleus reflex EMG, twitch force and twitch frequency against joint angle. Data taken from Figure 6.5.

(*a*) Soleus reflex EMG amplitude (mV); (*b*) soleus reflex peak force (N); (*c*) soleus reflex twitch time (ms); (*d*) soleus reflex twitch frequency (Hz). Neutral angle = 0°. Each point is the average of four consecutive tendon taps. Note influence of increasing soleus muscle length on all three parameters. The twitch frequency falls from 4 Hz at –11° of plantarflexion to 2.75 Hz at 30° of dorsiflexion.

tendon tap artefact on the force trace, followed some 12–25 ms later (depending on age), by a brief biphasic EMG discharge corresponding to the electrical activation of the soleus muscle by the spinal motoneurons, and finally the mechanical twitch represented by a slowly rising and falling force (Fig 6.4). When this reflex is elicited at steadily increasing increments of dorsiflexion from the resting angle, through neutral, to maximum dorsiflexion, three phenomena are evident (Fig 6.5):

(1) The reflex EMG reaches a peak close to neutral and diminishes markedly in amplitude with further dorsiflexion, suggesting that muscle length modulates the motoneuron pool by initially facilitating and then inhibiting the reflex discharge.

131

(2) The peak twitch force generated by the tendon tap steadily rises, reaching a peak at 5–10° of dorsiflexion, and then it too declines markedly with further dorsiflexion, implying that the optimum joint angle (or muscle length) for reflex force generation lies close to the mid-range of the muscle length, the fully shortened and maximally lengthened muscle being reflexly weak. This is because fewer motoneurons participate in force generation at the extremes of the joint angle (see below).

(3) The twitch time steadily increases with each increment of dorsiflexion, almost doubling with maximum dorsiflexion: a muscle which has been lengthened takes longer to relax.

These three important findings are graphically represented in Figure 6.6.

Motoneuron excitability, muscle contractility and the voluntary functional joint range

The simple experiments described above demonstrate the influence of the joint angle, and hence muscle length, on reflex excitability, twitch force and twitch time, and the findings accord well with the observations on the functional joint range at the ankle illustrated in Figures 6.1 and 6.2. Rapid alternating movements at the ankle are most easily performed close to neutral, becoming slower in either full equinus or full dorsiflexion. To what extent does the joint angle determine the electrical output from the motoneurons and the mechanical output of the muscles?

In maximum equinus, the spinal motoneuron pool is poorly excitable if not refractory to stimulation and thus the twitch force generated is weak, partly because fewer motor units can be recruited but also because the muscle, being fully shortened, is at a mechanical disadvantage. It is therefore difficult to generate large muscular accelerations close to full plantarflexion, so that although the muscle twitch time is brief, only slow movements are possible in equinus because of the feeble accelerations and hence feeble force generation at this angle. In equinus the motor system at the calf is at a neuromechanical disadvantage, even though the brief twitch times should theoretically favour rapid movements.

Close to neutral, the mid-range of the muscle's length, the spinal motoneurons are readily recruited, and consequently the twitch force is large and capable of generating the large muscular accelerations necessary for rapid alternating movement.

Close to maximum dorsiflexion, the motoneurons become refractory to stimulation, so fewer motor units are recruited with comparable stimuli. The muscle, which is fully elongated, has an excessively slow twitch time making rapid movements difficult because of a neurotemporal disadvantage. The neutral joint angle thus coincides with the position of maximum neuro-mechanico-temporal advantage of the motor system.

When directly electrically stimulated along the tibial nerve, the muscle is capable of generating large forces (Fig. 6.7). This direct electrical stimulation of the muscle bypasses the muscle spindle and the spinal alpha-motoneurons, and under these conditions the mechanical output from the muscle continues to increase with increasing muscle length beyond neutral, concordant with the findings of Sale *et al.* (1982). This contrasts with the twitch forces induced by reflex contractions of the muscles which clearly diminish with increasing dorsiflexion. The spinal motoneurons appear to override the muscle's natural tendency to match increasing length with increasing force generation. Muscle stretch therefore influences the output from either the muscle spindle or the alpha-motoneurons. Experiments

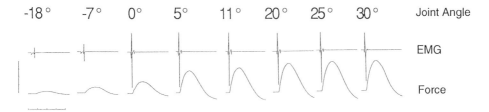

| -18° | -7° | 0° | 5° | 11° | 20° | 25° | 30° | Joint Angle |

Fig. 6.7. Changes in directly stimulated soleus muscle twitch force with increasing muscle length.

Same subject as for Figures 6.5 and 6.6. The soleus muscle is directly electrically stimulated along the tibial nerve in the popliteal fossa at the same joint angles as for Figure 6.5. The stimulus artefact is visible as a small downward deflection on the EMG trace. At −11° and −6° of flexion the electrical stimulus artefact is followed by an H-reflex EMG discharge some 35 ms later with relatively weak twitch forces. With dorsiflexion at the ankle, a very large discharge occurs within a few milliseconds of the electrical stimulus to produce a direct depolarization of the muscle, the M response, which bypasses the muscle spindle and spinal alpha-motoneurons. The M response remains relatively constant with incremental dorsiflexion to 30°. However, the soleus twitch force and twitch time both increase serially with each increment of dorsiflexion. By contrast, the H-reflex amplitude diminishes with each stretch increment beyond 0°. This demonstrates spinal alpha-motoneuron modulation by muscle stretch and the concept of the optimum neuromuscular joint angle. Each trace represents the average of four consecutive stimuli. Horizontal bar = 100 ms. Vertical bar: EMG trace = 2 mV; FORCE trace = 12.8 N.

on the influence of joint angle on the H-reflex (Hoffmann reflex, an electrically stimulated ankle jerk) demonstrate that it is the spinal alpha-motoneurons which become refractory with increasing applied muscle stretch (Burke and Lance 1973, Burke 1983). The H-reflex is obtained by electrically stimulating the afferent sensory fibres, bypassing the muscle spindle. The motoneuron output could be modulated by muscle length and/or tension. However, according to Houk and Henneman (1967), muscle-tension-sensing Golgi tendon organs are stimulated during active muscle contractions but are relatively quiescent during passive changes in muscle length. Al-Falahe *et al.* (1990) were also able to confirm with microneurographic techniques that during movements of moderate speed, human tendon organs behave as monitors of the amount of muscle contraction whereas muscle spindles behave as stretch receptors. So it appears most likely that muscle length alone acts as the main peripheral modulator of motoneuron output.

Clearly the joint angle, which represents muscle length, has a profound influence on the neurophysiology of neuromechanical coupling and hence motion at the ankle joint. Voluntary and involuntary control of motion at the ankle presumably makes constant use of this interaction between muscle and the spinal motoneurons. Such control is achieved by alterations to muscle length (or bias angle) which sets the optimum joint angle for optimum muscle performance at any given joint for any given limb. The posture of the limb partly presets or determines the motor output, *i.e.* makes use of the peripheral neuromuscular constraints to modulate the desired action. One aspect of voluntary motor control is to select the appropriate joint angle for the task. During a continuously varying task, this changing joint angle contributes at a peripheral level, and at very short latencies to a continuous modulation of spinal motoneuron output. It has been demonstrated that the highest sustainable firing rates of human motoneurons innervating intrinsic muscles of the hand are significantly lower in the absence of feedback from the target muscle (Gandevia *et al.* 1990, Macefield *et al.* 1991).

These ankle experiments can be extended to other joints such as wrist or metacarpophalangeal (MCP) joints. For each case, there is a joint angle that favours the maximum speed of alternating movements that corresponds to the muscle length at which maximum accelerations, and hence forces, can be generated.

Cortical control of muscle force

The foregoing sections have shown how the changing posture of the limb as it moves through a given joint range continuously modulates motoneuron output. In addition, the brain plays a crucial role in selecting the motor units involved in any given motor task. Henneman *et al.* (1974) studied spinal motor unit firing in isometric tasks and demonstrated that a smooth increase in force output could be produced by a combination of first increasing the firing rate of motor units and secondly by recruiting more units from a given spinal motor unit pool. Isometric tasks thus begin with the recruitment of slow and relatively weak (small) motor units and as further force is required these fire more rapidly until still further forces can only be achieved by recruiting larger, more rapidly firing units. This graded recruitment of spinal motor units of steadily increasing size and firing frequency has come to be known as the Hennemann Size Principle (Jones and Round 1990). At a cortical level, Evarts (1968) demonstrated that corticomotoneuron firing rate is correlated with force generation. Further studies (Evarts *et al.* 1983) have shown that the populations of pyramidal tract neurons with the slowest firing frequencies also had the slowest conduction latencies, whereas fast firing pyramidal tract neurons had the fastest conduction latencies, indicating an anatomical basis to force generation at the cortical level. These and other relevant studies are examined in depth by Porter and Lemon (1993). The modulation of the size and firing frequency of cortical and spinal motoneurons clearly determines the production of smooth and sustained motor tasks.

Alternating movements and age: do muscles develop?

Alternating movements (or oscillations) can be measured at the ankle, wrist and MCP joints in children and adults (Fig. 6.8). The frequency of such voluntary oscillations roughly doubles between the ages of 3 and 11 years, irrespective of the joint under study, and remains relatively constant thereafter (Lin *et al.* 1996). Several factors could account for this speeding up.

(1) Central candidate structures for the increases in speed with age include:

(i) Cortical maturation of cortical motoneurons and connections. It is believed that unlearned, repetitive alternating movements in a single plane at one joint are generated in the primary motor strip of the precentral gyrus (see Porter and Lemon 1993 for detailed discussion), in contrast to more complex tasks requiring increasing levels of concentration such as the orderly successive opposition of the finger tips with the thumb [as in the dexterity test of Denckla (1973)] which appear to originate in the supplementary motor area as demonstrated by cerebral blood flow studies (Orgogozo and Larsen 1979, Roland *et al.* 1980).

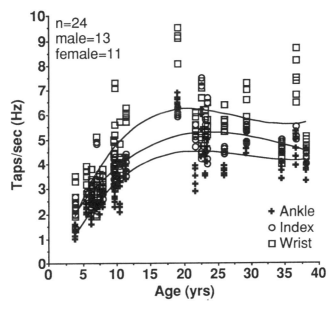

Fig. 6.8. Changes in voluntary isotonic alternating movements (tap frequency) at the ankle, metacarpophalangeal and wrist joints with age.

(a) Ankle tap frequency at the ankle joint. (b) Index finger tap frequency at the metacarpophalangeal joint. (c) Wrist tap frequency at the wrist joint. Data recorded in Hertz (taps/s). Note the doubling in tap frequency for each joint between 3 and 11 years of age.

The supplementary motor area has an important role in the initiation and control of non-repetitive complex movements, and Orgogozo and Larsen refer to it as a 'supramotor area' which is functionally of a higher hierarchical order than the primary rolandic areas. Activation of the supplementary motor area has been demonstrated noninvasively by functional magnetic resonance imaging in healthy adult controls (Santosh *et al.* 1995). Work on the cerebral localization of complex motor tasks demonstrates the complexity of the cerebral organization of movement, and a number of studies have shown that a variety of surgical lesions can impair alternating movements. Ablation of the medial part of the frontal lobe (which includes the supplementary motor area) in three patients resulted in a characteristic sequence of recovery: stage 1, a postoperative global akinesia which was most prominent contralaterally and associated with speech arrest; stage 2, a spontaneous motor recovery albeit with a marked reduction in spontaneous movements, facial expression and speech; and stage 3, a disturbance of alternating movements of the hands long after the other functions had recovered (Laplane *et al.* 1977). In another study, stimulation of the 'frontal speech area' during the course of epilepsy surgery investigations resulted in combinations of speech arrest, writing arrest or impaired rapid alternating movements of the tongue, fingers and toes (Lesser *et al.* 1984). These authors used chronic subdural electrode stimulation techniques to demonstrate that rapid finger and tongue movements could be interrupted by stimulation over quite wide areas of the posterior aspects of the third frontal gyrus. It is

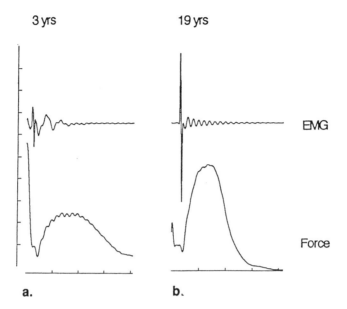

Fig. 6.9. Influence of age on soleus muscle reflex twitch time.

(a) Boy aged 3 years. *(b)* Male aged 19 years. Note that while peak force is achieved within 110 ms for both ages, the child's relaxation time is almost twice as long as that of the adult. Each trace represents four consecutive tap averages. Horizontal divisions = 100 ms. Vertical bar: EMG trace = 1 mV; FORCE trace = 6.4 N.

reasonable to suppose that in healthy development, there is a maturation of neurons and their connections involved in motor tasks. Likewise, it is possible to demonstrate that as a child's walking matures from infancy, co-contractions of muscle groups which produce stiff and ungainly movements give way to a phasic interaction of EMG activity leading to joint asynchronies and smoother movements (Leonard *et al.* 1991). This maturation suggests an emerging motor engram (both spinal and cortical) for walking and other movements. Notwithstanding central nervous maturation, the details of which will need further elucidation, before any slowness or clumsiness of movements in any given child are ascribed to disordered cortical processes it is worth pausing to consider other factors. In this context, the observations of Denckla (1973) demonstrating a speeding up of sequential finger movements with age in children has been attributed almost entirely to the maturation of central structures, although a peripheral contribution to this maturation is described below.

(ii) Central conduction from the corticomotoneuron to the spinal motoneuron reaches a maximum speed at 18 months of age (Eyre *et al.* 1991) and is thus unlikely to be responsible for the increasing speed of alternating movements between 3 and 11 years of age.

(2) Peripheral candidate structures for the increases in speed with age include:

(i) Peripheral nerve conduction velocity, which more than doubles from birth to adulthood from 28.5 to 82 m/s; however, despite this, the latency (conduction time) along the nerves increases because of their increase in length so that the latency of the H-reflex increases

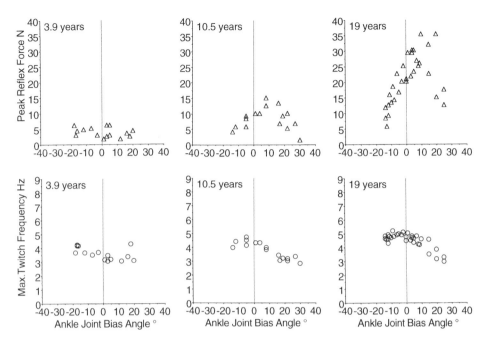

Fig. 6.10. Changes with age in soleus peak twitch force and twitch frequency plotted against joint angle.
Data plots for males aged 3.9, 10.5 and 19 years respectively. (Each point represents an average of four consecutive taps.) The peak twitch force and twitch frequency vary with muscle length (joint angle) for all subjects. When compared at the neutral angle (0°) the effects of age are clearly evident for all parameters. Twitch force rises from about 2.5–4.9 N at age 3 years to 29.4–39.2 N in adulthood. Likewise the twitch frequency rises from 3 Hz at age 3–4 years to 5 Hz at age 19 years.

from 15 to 28 ms between birth and adulthood (Mayer and Mosser 1973). Such an increase in nerve conduction latency would have a tendency to slow down the speed of alternating movements with age, and be at variance with the observed speeding up.

(ii) Muscles themselves could provide the rate-limiting step. Figure 6.9 shows the typical soleus twitch profiles for a boy aged 3 and a 19-year-old adult at neutral joint angle. The child's twitch profile is slower than the adult's. The changes with age of reflex EMG, twitch force and soleus twitch frequency (the reciprocal of the soleus twitch time) are illustrated in Figure 6.10 for male subjects aged 3.9, 10.5 and 19 years. The soleus twitch force clearly increases with age. Likewise, the isometric soleus twitch frequency at neutral increases from 3 Hz at 3 years to 4.5 Hz at 10.5 years and 5 Hz at 19 years. Similar changes with age are measurable in females, the soleus twitch frequency at neutral increasing from 2.5 Hz at 3 years to just over 4 Hz in the early twenties. Scott *et al.* (1985) found it difficult to fatigue the tibialis anterior muscles of healthy children, implying that children exhibit slower, non-fatigueable, type 1 muscle phenotypes with an oxidative metabolism. Brooke and Engel (1969) showed that muscle fibre diameter increases with age so that sex differences begin to emerge round about 10 years of age. There is some histochemical evidence to support

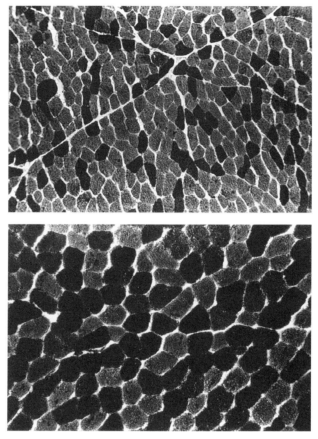

Fig. 6.11. Changes in quadriceps myosin ATPase isoforms with age.
    (a) Child aged 8 years with small diameter, rounded, loosely packed muscle fibres with predominantly slow twitch (pale, type 1) fibres. *(b)* Adult aged 18 years with tightly packed, polygonal fibres with 51% fast twitch (dark, type II) fibres. Incubated at pH 10.4; ×80 magnification. (Reproduced by permission from Lexell *et al.* 1992.)

the notion of muscular maturation with age, although the two most recent histological studies offer conflicting data. Maturation from a slow to a fast phenotype was demonstrated by Lexell *et al.* (1992) in a study involving 22 muscle biopsy subjects aged 5–36 years who had died accidentally. A slow muscle phenotype of the vastus lateralis muscle was clearly evident in the children (Fig. 6.11). Elder and Kakulas (1993) demonstrated in 19 newborn infants and 35 children that while the tibialis anterior muscle half-relaxation time speeds up between 5 and 16 months of age, that of the posterior calf muscles slows over a similar period. Nevertheless, some infants demonstrated persistence of slow muscle phenotypes, and in a parallel study of 43 subjects aged from 22 weeks gestation to 28 years there was a greater preponderance of slow (type 1) muscle phenotypes in children than in adults in samples of triceps brachii, vastus lateralis, biceps brachii and tibialis anterior muscles.

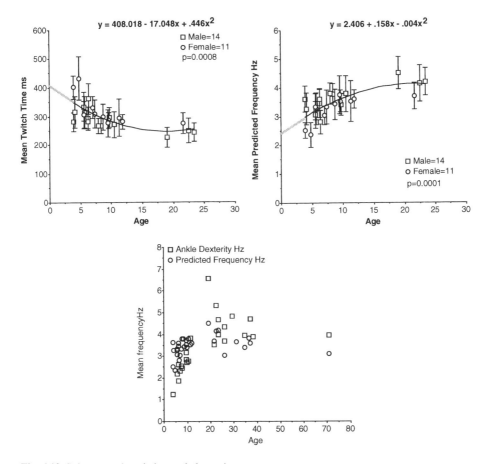

Fig. 6.12. Soleus muscle twitches and alternating movements.
(a) Change in soleus twitch time with age for 25 subjects: ten male and 11 female aged 11 years or under, and four adults. (b) The inverse of the soleus twitch time gives the 'predicted frequency', *i.e.* the number of twitches per second [same subjects as in (a)]. (c) Superimposed mean voluntary ankle dexterity (25 cases) and predicted soleus twitch frequencies (31 cases): age range 3.9–70 years.

Some of the mechanisms by which the twitch profile might speed up with age have been studied (Margareth *et al.* 1980, Zubrzycka-Gaarn and Sarzala 1980) and may relate to the ontogeny of the sarcoplasmic reticulum enzyme biochemistry which regulates calcium re-uptake and hence muscle relaxation. It is not known what factors may influence such muscle maturation, although a variety of internal and external stimuli are known to affect the myosin-ATPase expression in muscle.

At least three principle mechanisms for the observed increases in motor speed in the first decade of life can be identified. The first of these is the undoubted increase in force generation crucial for overcoming inertia and hence the production of faster movements with age. Second, faster relaxation times logically should facilitate the production of faster

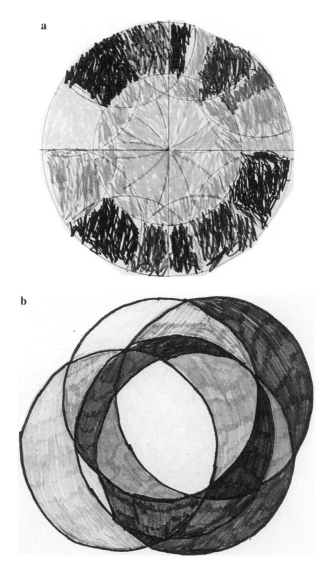

Fig. 6.13. Development of drawing skills. The ability to rapidly colour in may reflect the changes in motor control described in this chapter.

(a) 4-year-old boy shading: the coarse (slow) strokes of large amplitude are unable to fill the geometric shape adequately. (b) 7-year-old boy: fine, closely packed (fast), short strokes of colouring which completely fill in the shape, leaving few bare patches. This change in shading (colouring) skills with age may reflect the greater ease of performing rapid alternating movements with increasing age in the first decade and may depend on three factors. (1) Muscle maturation such as an increase in the contractile force and faster relaxation times of muscles. (2) Children learn that they can go faster by reducing the amplitude of the strokes, *i.e.* they experimentally 'discover' that the amplitude of movement is inversely related to the square of the frequency of movement. (3) The older child finds that there is an optimum joint angle at which such movements can be executed: this corresponds to the optimum neuromuscular angle.

140

alternating movements by allowing more muscle twitches per second, as illustrated in Figure 6.12 which shows: (a) the changes in soleus twitch times with age, (b) the predicted soleus frequency (or inverse soleus twitch time), and (c) the relationship between predicted soleus frequency and actual voluntary alternating movements at the ankle in adults and children. Third, there may be a learning curve for the performance of rapid tasks involving experience of the functional joint range and optimal joint angle as described below.

What is the practical significance of these observations for child development? Evidence for motor maturation can also be seen in pictures, for instance colouring in shapes, a task which requires alternating movements at the wrist and forearm. The 4-year-old makes broad, coarse (slow) strokes (Fig. 6.13a), whereas the 7-year-old uses short, close-knit (rapid) strokes which provide a denser, more even covering of the paper (Fig. 6.13b). In their everyday lives, childrens' movements show an adaptation to the physical and neuro-muscular constraints described above. It is hypothesized that the older child optimizes the neuromuscular output by appropriate postural adjustments which include making small-amplitude strokes which in turn allow a higher frequency of alternating movements. It is also likely that the older child's rapid strokes are being performed close to the functional mid-range of the muscle at which the maximum forces can be generated, whereas the younger child, by making large-amplitude strokes, will produce slower movements and is working quite literally at a physical disadvantage.

Despite these compelling arguments for a peripheral control of motor function by means of short-loop spinal modulation presented here and by others (Hagbarth *et al.* 1975, Al Falahe *et al.* 1990, Gandevia *et al.* 1990, Macefield *et al.* 1991), there are isolated case reports of voluntary alternating movements occuring in the presence of complete deaffer-entation in man (Rothwell *et al.* 1982) and in primates (Polit and Bizzi 1979). The extent to which such movements can be modulated remains unclear. Also, these findings were obtained in adults who presumably had experienced normal sensory feedback as children (or young primates) so that the situation in these cases is that of a loss of a sensory modality rather than development from birth without sensory feedback. These interesting questions are dealt with in some depth by Jeannerod (1988).

Conclusions

Dexterity may be governed by the maturation of peripheral and central structures in which selected postures maximize motoneuron recruitment and force output. The principles of physics dictate that for a fixed force generation, the frequency of oscillation is inversely proportional to the amplitude of movement. The concept of the physiological joint range has been explored in detail to show that the motoneuron pool is difficult to recruit at the extremes of the joint range, maximum recruitment occurring close to the middle of the physio-logical joint range. The production of the fastest alternating voluntary movements occurs close to this physiological mid-range and must, by definition, be of low amplitude. Despite the increases in limb length and consequent 32-fold increase in limb moment of inertia between the ages of 3 years and adulthood, such alternating movements almost double in frequency between 3 and 10 years of age. This speeding up cannot be adequately explained in terms of the shortening of the central conduction time, from cortex to spinal cord, since maturity has already been achieved by the age of 18 months. The peripheral nerve conduction time actually increases with age, despite the fact that the conduction velocity increases, because of the lengthening of the nerves as the limbs grow. Physiological and histochemical evidence exists to support the hypothesis that the muscles mature to produce fast-twitch muscles within the first decade by a combination of increased speed of contraction and, above all, relaxation. Muscles also increase in strength with age and this permits the generation of greater acceleration and deceleration. The excitability of the spinal motoneuron pool, muscle mechanical output and twitch profile are exquisitely sensitive to the joint angle, which is dictated by muscle length to produce a given posture. Such postures (muscle lengths) serve to select, specify or facilitate a given motor output. The growing child may learn by trial and error to use the joint angle (posture) which optimizes motoneuron recruitment and force output and hence produces the fastest movements. By specifying such postures during the course of voluntary tasks, the cortex is in effect selecting a position of optimum neuromuscular output.

These peripheral factors are constantly modulated to produce the final motor pattern for control, and they appear to undergo a process of maturation as the child grows. This concept of muscle maturation accords well with the demonstrable plasticity of the muscle twitch phenotype which can be altered by a variety of external and internal mechanical and electrical stimuli, both natural and artificial (Buller *et al.* 1960, Salmons and Sréter 1976, Pette 1980). After injury to the central nervous system, weakness and immobility together with abnormal passive and dynamic postures are likely to alter movements and affect speed and force by imposing a dysfunctional joint range within which neither force of contraction nor speed can be generated. The impact of central lesions is in effect to render the spinal motoneurons refractory to recruitment because of weak or reduced descending corticospinal inputs and the inhibitory effects of the dysfunctional posture. It is hypothesized that in pathological hind-foot equinus, dexterity is reduced according to these dual inhibitory influences (personal data, unpublished). The influence of congenital damage to the central nervous system and therapeutic manipulations of muscle length, both in the long and short term, on the neuromuscular system and in particular on muscle twitch times and reflex excitability, sheds further light on the pathophysiology of phenomena such as clonus and could help us not only to understand the natural history of certain motor disabilities, but also to tailor better approaches to neurological rehabilitation based on physiological principles.

ACKNOWLEDGEMENTS

This work was made possible by an Edinburgh University Faculty of Medicine George Guthrie Research Fellowship held by the author from 1991–1994 and was carried out at the Royal Hospital for Sick Children, Edinburgh. The author is indebted to the children and adults who participated in the studies; to Dr Keith Brown for clinical insights; to Dr Geoffrey Walsh for sharing his long experience in studying human motor physiology and with whose collaboration most of these studies were executed; and finally to Dr Mayank Dutia for invaluable technical assistance in the use of computer technology.

REFERENCES

Al-Falahe, N.A., Nagaoka, M., Vallbo, Å.B. (1990) 'Response profiles of human muscle afferents during active finger movements.' *Brain*, **113**, 325–346.

Brooke, M.H., Engel, W.K. (1969) 'The histographic analysis of human muscle biopsies with regard to fiber types. 4. Children's biopsies.' *Neurology*, **19**, 591–605.

Buller, A.J., Eccles, J.C., Eccles, R.M. (1960) 'Interactions between motoneurones and muscles in respect of the characteristic speeds of their responses.' *Journal of Physiology*, **150**, 417–439.

Burke, D. (1983) 'Critical examination of the case for or against fusimotor involvement in disorders of muscle tone.' *In:* Desmedt, J.E. (Ed.) *Motor Control Mechanisms in Health and Disease. Advances in Neurology, Vol. 39.* New York: Raven Press, pp. 133–150.

—— Lance, J.W. (1973) 'Studies of the reflex effects of primary and secondary spindle endings in spasticity.' *In:* Desmedt, J.E. (Ed.) *New Developments in Electromyography and Clinical Neurophysiology. Vol. 3.* Basel: Karger, pp. 475–495.

Denckla, M.B. (1973) 'Development of speed in repetitive and successive finger-movements in normal children.' *Developmental Medicine and Child Neurology*, **15**, 635–645.

Elder, G.C.B., Kakulas, B.A. (1993) 'Histochemical and contractile property changes during human muscle development.' *Muscle and Nerve*, **16**, 1246–1253.

Evarts, E.V. (1968) 'Relation of pyramidal tract activity to force exerted during voluntary movement.' *Journal of Neurophysiology*, **31**, 14–27.

Eyre, J.A., Miller, S, Ramesh, V. (1991) 'Constancy of central conduction delays during development in man: investigation of motor and somatosensory pathways.' *Journal of Physiology*, **434**, 441–452.

Gandevia, S.C., Macefield, G., Burke, D., McKenzie, D.K. (1990) 'Voluntary activation of human motor axons in the absence of muscle afferent feedback. The control of the deafferented hand.' *Brain*, **113**, 1563–1581.

Grillner, S., Broden, L., Sigvardt, K., Dale, N. (1986) 'On the spinal network generating locomotion in the lamprey: transmitters, membrane properties and circuitry.' *In:* Grillner, S., Stein, P., Stuart, P., Forssberg, H., Herman, R. (Eds.) *Neurobiology of Vertebrate Locomotion. Wenner–Gren International Symposium Series, No. 45.* London: MacMillan, pp. 335–352.

Hagbarth, K-E., Wallin, G., Löfstedt, L. (1975) 'Muscle spindle activity in man during voluntary fast alternating movements.' *Journal of Neurology, Neurosurgery, and Psychiatry*, **38**, 625–635.

Henneman, E., Clamann, H.P., Gillies, J.D., Skinner, R.D. (1974) 'Rank order of motoneurons within a pool: law of combination.' *Journal of Neurophysiology*, **37**, 1338–1349.

Houk, J., Henneman, E. (1967) 'Responses of Golgi tendon organs to active contractions of the soleus muscle of the cat.' *Journal of Neurophysiology*, **30**, 466–481.

Jeannerod, M. (1988) *The Neural and Behavioural Organization of Goal-Directed Movements. Oxford Psychology Series No. 15.* Oxford: Oxford University Press.

Jones, D.A., Round, J.M. (1990) *Skeletal Muscle in Health and Disease.* Manchester: Manchester University Press.

Laplane, D., Talairach, J., Meininger, V., Bancaud, J., Orgogozo, J.M. (1977) 'Clinical consequences of corticectomies involving the supplementary motor area in man.' *Journal of the Neurological Sciences*, **34**, 301–314.

Leonard, C.T., Hirschfeld, H., Forssberg, H. (1991) 'The development of independent walking in children with cerebral palsy.' *Developmental Medicine and Child Neurology*, **33**, 567–577.

Lesser, R.P., Lueders, H., Dinner, D.S., Hahn, J., Cohen, L. (1984) 'The location of speech and writing functions in the frontal language area. Results of extraoperative cortical stimulation.' *Brain*, **107**, 275–291.

Lexell, J., Sjöström, M., Norlund, A-S., Taylor, C.C. (1992) 'Growth and development of human muscle: a quantitative morphological study of whole vastus lateralis from childhood to adult age.' *Muscle and Nerve*, **15**, 404–409.

Lin, J-P., Brown, J.K. (1991) 'Peripheral and central mechanisms of hindfoot equinus in childhood hemiplegia.' *Developmental Medicine and Child Neurology*, **34**, 949–965.

—— —— Walsh, E.G. (1994) 'Physiological maturation of muscles in childhood.' *Lancet*, **343**, 1386–1389.

—— —— —— (1996) 'The maturation of motor dexterity: or why Johnny can't go any faster.' *Developmental Medicine and Child Neurology*, **38**, 244–254.

Macefield, G., Gandevia, S.C., Bigland-Ritchie, B., Gorman, R., Burke, D. (1991) 'The discharge rate of human motor neurones innervating ankle dorsiflexors in the absence of muscle afferent feedback.' *Journal of Physiology*, **438**, 219P.

Margareth, A., Salviati, G., Dalla Libera, L., Betto, R., Biral, D., Salvatori, S. (1980) 'Transition in membrane macromolecular composition and in myosin isoenzymes during development of fast-twitch and slow-twitch muscles.' *In:* Pette, D. (Ed.) *Plasticity of Muscle.* Berlin: Walter de Gruyter, pp. 193–208.

Mayer, R.F., Mosser, R.S. (1973) 'Maturation of human reflexes: studies of electrically evoked reflexes in newborns, infants and children.' *In:* Desmedt, J.E. (Ed.) *New Developments in Electromyography and Clinical Neurophysiology. Vol. 3.* Basel: Karger, pp. 294–307.

Nashner, L.M. (1985) 'A functional approach to understanding spasticity.' *In:* Struppler, A., Weindl, A. (Eds.) *Electromyography and Evoked Potentials.* Berlin: Springer, pp. 22–29.

—— Shumway-Cook, A., Marin, O. (1983) 'Stance posture control in select groups of children with cerebral palsy: deficits in sensory organization and muscular coordination.' *Experimental Brain Research*, **49**, 393–409.

Orgogozo, J.M., Larsen, B. (1979) 'Activation of the supplementary motor area during voluntary movement in man suggests it works as a supramotor area.' *Science*, **206**, 847–850.

Pette, D. (Ed.) (1980) *Plasticity of Muscle.* Berlin: Walter de Gruyter.

Polit, A., Bizzi, E. (1979) 'Characteristics of motor programs underlying arm movements in monkeys.' *Journal of Neurophysiology*, **42**, 183–194.

Porter, R., Lemon, R. (Eds.) (1993) *Corticospinal Function and Voluntary Movement.* Oxford: Clarendon Press.

Roland, P.E., Skinhøj, E., Lassen, N.A., Larsen, B. (1980) 'Different cortical areas in man in organization of voluntary movements in extrapersonal space.' *Journal of Neurophysiology*, **43**, 137–150.

Rothwell, J.C., Traub, M.M., Day, B.L., Obeso, J.A., Thomas, P.K., Marsden, C.D. (1982) 'Manual motor performance in a deafferented man' *Brain*, **105**, 515–542.

Sale, D., Quinlan, J., Marsh, E., McComas, A.J., Belanger, A.Y. (1982) 'Influence of joint position on ankle plantarflexion in humans.' *Journal of Applied Physiology*, **52**, 1632–1642.

Salmons, S., Sréter, F.A. (1976) 'Significance of impulse activity in the transformation of skeletal muscle muscle type.' *Nature*, **263**, 30–34.

Santosh, C., Rimmington, J.E., Best, J.K. (1995) 'Functional magnetic resonance imaging at 1T: motor cortex, supplementary motor area and visual cortex activation.' *British Journal of Radiology*, **68**, 369–374.

Scott, O.M., Vrbová, G., Hyde, S.A., Dubowitz, V. (1985) 'Effects of chronic low frequency electrical stimulation on normal human tibialis anterior muscle.' *Journal of Neurology, Neurosurgery, and Psychiatry*, **48**, 774–781

Walsh, E.G. (1992) *Muscles, Masses and Motion. Clinics in Developmental Medicine No. 125.* London: Mac Keith Press.

—— Wright, G.W. (1987) 'Inertia, resonant frequency, stiffness and kinetic energy of the human forearm.' *Quarterly Journal of Experimental Physiology*, **72**, 161–170.

—— —— Davies, A. , Lin, J-P., Thompson, J. (1993) 'A comparison of the mechanogram of the ankle jerk in men and women: observations using an adjustable dorsiflexing torque, high inertia mechanical filter and automatic readout system.' *Experimental Physiology*, **78**, 531–540.

Zubrzycka-Gaarn, E., Sarzala, M.G. (1980) 'Sarcoplasmic reticulum and sarcolemma during development.' *In:* Pette, D. (Ed.) *Plasticity of Muscle.* Berlin: Walter de Gruyter, pp. 209–223.

7
DEVELOPMENT AND FUNCTION OF CUTANEOMUSCULAR REFLEXES AND THEIR PATHOPHYSIOLOGY IN CEREBRAL PALSY

Andrew Lloyd Evans

It has been known for many years that cutaneous stimulation can elicit motor reflex responses which provide information about the functional integrity and developmental state of the central nervous system. Perhaps the best known of these is the plantar response (Babinski 1898). Modest electrical stimulation of the digits produces a reflex modulation of ongoing muscle activity recorded from the skin surface during steady voluntary contraction of the upper (Caccia *et al.* 1973) or lower limb muscles (Jenner and Stephens 1982), which is usually only visualized after signal averaging.

At the cellular level, during ongoing muscle activity, the pattern of discharge of a single motoneuron is determined by the summed effects of a large variety of synaptic inputs, including supraspinal and peripheral afferent influences via interneurons (Lundberg 1975). Peripheral afferent influences include information from cutaneous, muscle and joint receptors. Taking one of these inputs and altering it in a regular fashion while the other inputs remain relatively constant can be used to produce predictable changes in muscle activity. This provides an indirect method for studying the synaptic connections of motor units. Only changes time-locked to the stimulus are extracted from the naturally occurring spike train produced by the motoneuron (Stephens *et al.* 1976). This can be used to infer other contributions to the firing pattern, such as those from descending pathways. Recording cutaneomuscular reflexes (CMRs) therefore provides a noninvasive method of monitoring activity in spinal and transcortical pathways involved in the reflex control of muscle activity.

Conduction in peripheral and central pathways
A number of studies have documented developmental sequences in individual central and peripheral neural pathways.

Peripheral sensory conduction
Conduction velocity in peripheral nerves matures by early to mid-childhood. Desmedt *et al.* (1973) have reported that the conduction velocity of sensory fibres in the median and ulnar nerves reached adult values at 12–18 months of age. Eyre *et al.* (1991) used median nerve sensory evoked responses to determine age-related changes in peripheral sensory pathways in the upper limbs. Conduction delays became shorter in early life as conduction

velocity increased, but from the age of 5 years conduction velocity remained constant and conduction delays increased progressively in proportion to arm length. This was paralleled by a progressive reduction in threshold stimulus intensity for exciting peripheral sensory nerves, which reached a minimum at age 5 years and remained constant thereafter.

Peripheral motor conduction
Thomas and Lambert (1960) and Gamstorp (1963) found that motor fibre conduction velocities of nerves in the upper limb increased markedly from birth until 3-4 years. Two studies (Eyre *et al.* 1991, Müller *et al.* 1991) used magnetic stimulation to determine changes in conduction delays with age in peripheral motor pathways. Peripheral conduction times obtained after cervical motor root stimulation reach adult values by 3–5 years. Similar maturation is found in the lower limbs following stimulation of lumbar motor roots, adult values being reached by about 3 years (Müller *et al.* 1991). The threshold stimulus intensity for exciting peripheral motor nerves reduced progressively until 5 years and then remained constant. Other studies have shown the anatomical substrate underlying these changes in peripheral conduction. Myelination in spinal roots and peripheral nerves is complete by the age of 2 years. Axon diameters attain adult values by 2–5 years (Rexed 1944, Gutrecht and Dyck 1970). Nerve conduction in the preterm and term neonate has been reviewed by Khater-Boidin and Duron (1992).

Central sensory conduction
Desmedt *et al.* (1976) described the maturational sequence of cortical sensory evoked responses. They noted that the N1 component, which is developmentally the first to appear, reduced its duration with increasing age, and had not reached an adult configuration by the eighth year after birth. The development of spinal evoked responses has been documented in childhood by Cracco *et al.* (1979) and Kamimura *et al.* (1988). These groups found that intraspinal sensory conduction velocity increased until 5 years or later. Taylor and colleagues (Taylor and Fagan 1988, George and Taylor 1991) found that central conduction times measured using sensory evoked responses after median nerve stimulation progressively reduced and reached adult values by 6 to 8 years. Müller *et al.* (1994) found that afferent pathways reached adult values by 5–7 years. Similar values were found by Lauffer and Wenzel (1986). The maturation of the somatosensory system was most rapid during the first three weeks of life.

Others have found slightly differing results. Allison *et al.* (1983, 1984) using median nerve sensory evoked responses found a small nonsignificant reduction in central conduction time, but their study had a lack of data from children less than 4 years old. Eyre *et al.* (1991) used median nerve sensory evoked responses to measure how central somatosensory conduction changed during development. Conduction delays fell rapidly from birth to 2 years, thereafter remaining constant at adult values.

Central motor conduction
Studies in central motor conduction have also led to inconsistent conclusions.
Khater-Boidin *et al.* (1992), using electrical percutaneous stimulation of the brain and

146

spinal cord found that at birth, the conduction velocity of central motor fibres along the spinal cord was about 10 m/s, four or five times slower than the lowest values published for adult subjects.

Eyre *et al.* (1991) and Müller *et al.* (1991, 1994) used magnetic brain stimulation to determine changes in central motor conduction. Müller's group used magnetic stimulation with relaxed rather than active muscle. Clear responses in the upper extremity could be obtained only after the first year of life, and in the lower extremity they could not be obtained before the fourth year of life. Efferent pathway conduction reached adult values by the age of 10 years. There was no evidence for constant central conduction times.

Eyre's group used magnetic stimulation on a background of active muscle. They found a similar developmental time course compared with their study of sensory pathways. The most rapid reduction was in the first year of life. This rapid reduction reflects the progress of myelination and increase in axon diameter in the corticospinal pathway over this time period (Nathan and Smith 1955, Yakovlev and Lecours 1967). It was concluded that the maximum fibre diameters in central pathways increase with age in proportion to height, leading to constant central conduction delays.

The difference between the two studies using magnetic stimulation may result from a variety of levels of muscle contraction in the active muscle protocol, which is less easy to control than using a relaxed muscle protocol. This would give differing levels of pre-innervation, leading to significant latency shifts when measuring central conduction.

Summary of conduction studies

These studies suggest that peripheral sensory and motor conduction velocities mature by mid-childhood. Changes in peripheral conduction thereafter relate to linear growth. There is debate about whether central sensory and motor conduction velocities continue to increase with increasing linear growth, resulting in a relatively constant central conduction time, or whether central conduction time continues to decrease. Constancy of central conduction time may be important in the development of motor control by removing the potentially confusing factor of changing time patterns in neural transmission as a child grows. However, the bulk of the evidence is in favour of central conduction time continuing to decrease until late childhood. Whether central conduction is constant or not, changes in peripheral and central conduction with age are relevant to the study of maturation of reflex control of movement in children.

Reflexes in development

Reflex behaviour begins *in utero*, and responses to fine tactile stimuli may be elicited as early as 7.5 weeks gestation in the human fetus. At this time, facial stimulation produces reflex movement of the body (Fitzgerald and Windle 1942, Hooker 1958). As gestation continues, the repertoire of reflex behaviour increases, and the movements become progressively more sophisticated, with a cephalocaudal progression and better localization of responses. A number of functional reflex arcs develop and some can be related to anatomical investigations of fetal maturation (Hooker 1958). From about 10 weeks reflex responses of the upper limb to local stimuli can be elicited. Partial finger closure begins at about 11 weeks and the grasp reflex begins at about 18 weeks gestation (Hooker 1958).

Systematic studies have been undertaken of the extensive repertoire of neonatal reflex behaviours (André-Thomas *et al.* 1960, Amiel-Tison and Grenier 1980). Touwen (1976) has shown how reflexes such as the Moro, Babinski and stepping reflexes change over the first two years of life. These studies have led to the idea that primitive reflexes present at birth are either superseded by or incorporated into more sophisticated and higher levels of neural control. Twitchell (1970) found that the grasp reflex fractionated into responses of individual fingers between 16 and 40 weeks postnatal age. Exploratory grasping developed between 20 and 44 weeks, and thumb–finger opposition did not appear until the grasp reflex could be fractionated during the second half year of life. He considered each more complex form of voluntary grasping to be anticipated by a more complex reflex substrate. Infantile reflexes did not disappear, but evolved during maturation. Sherrington (1951) also referred to the progressive central modification of the reflex substrate of behaviour during development.

It is possible to use specific reflexes to study activity in specific pathways. Developmental changes in the H-reflex have been studied by Thomas and Lambert (1960), Mayer and Mosser (1969) and Vecchierini-Blineau and Guiheneuc (1981). They found that reflex excitability diminished over the first four years of life and considered this to be the result of supraspinal suppression. Berger *et al.* (1984, 1985) studied leg muscle EMG activity and stretch reflex responses both during normal gait and following perturbations during stance and gait in children aged between 6 months and 8 years. During normal gait up to the age of 4 years large short-latency reflex potentials were seen in the gastrocnemius as the forefoot reached the ground. Perturbations during stance produced short-latency reflex responses, more prominent in younger children. Perturbations during the stance phase of gait produced similar short-latency responses which disappeared at 5 years. These short-latency reflex potentials were followed by long-lasting longer latency responses which became shorter and more phasic with increasing age. These longer latency components were thought to follow an intraspinal path. Both short and longer latency responses showed developmental changes, presumably related to changes in descending modulation of the reflex pathways.

In the normal adult, tendon reflexes are confined to the muscle stimulated. A number of studies have shown that muscle responses to stretch may be much more widespread in early childhood. In the upper limb the biceps stretch reflex has a low threshold, and can even be elicited in relaxed muscle in children under 2 years old. The threshold increases over the first 6 years to mature values. Up to 4 years reflex responses also occur in a variety of other upper limb muscles, sometimes with amplitudes greater than the biceps response (O'Sullivan *et al.* 1991).

There have been similar findings in the lower limb (Myklebust *et al.* 1986, Myklebust 1990, Leonard *et al.* 1991). Achilles tendon taps produce responses in both agonist and antagonist muscle pairs or in more widespread muscle groups in infants. This reflex radiation becomes restricted over the first 6 years of life. The radiation of reflex response is thought to occur because of exuberant afferents from the stimulated muscles to alpha-motoneurons of other muscles. These projections might become more restricted with age.

The use of CMRs to study central nervous pathways

Short-latency responses

CMRs have been used as a tool with which to investigate the central nervous system since the turn of the century. Sherrington (1903, 1910) systematically studied the CMRs in the hind limbs of spinal and decerebrate cats and dogs. He concluded that variety in the reflex responses observed related to differences in intraspinal interconnections. Hagbarth (1952, 1960) also found that in the cat and in man CMRs varied depending on the site and type of stimulation employed. The timing of the earliest phase of the CMRs elicited in the foot was so short that Hagbarth considered this to be a spinally mediated reflex. This compares well with CMRs investigated in the foot by Jenner (1981) and Jenner and Stephens (1982). The onset of the earliest phases of other CMRs such as the abdominal reflex (Hagbarth and Kugelberg 1958) also occur at a latency compatible with a spinal pathway, although Hagbarth and Kugelberg comment that in this reflex cerebral outflow may influence spinal interneuronal transmission.

Long-latency responses

The existence of longer latency components in a variety of reflexes raises the question whether the reflex pathways are more extensive than merely intraspinal. CMRs may show more than one phase. The blink (Rushworth 1962), abdominal (Hagbarth and Kugelberg 1958), and plantar responses (Grimby 1963) have more than one phase.

Caccia *et al.* (1973) recorded rectified and averaged surface EMGs from the abductor pollicis brevis following stimulation of the digital nerves of the index finger. They failed to show an excitatory response at spinal latency, but did show two phases of inhibition each followed by an excitation. They considered the different latency responses to reflect differences in the conduction velocities of afferent fibres responsible for each phase, but did not consider the possibility of a transcortical or long loop reflex.

Using median nerve stimulation at the wrist and recording from the abductor pollicis brevis, Conrad and Aschoff (1977) showed a direct muscle response, a spinal reflex response and a third, longer latency, excitatory reflex response. The last response was more prominent in isotonic compared with isometric contractions. This reflex component could also be produced by cutaneous afferent stimulation and was diminished, delayed or absent in hemiplegic patients. The authors considered that this evidence supported the existence of a transcortical reflex pathway for the long-latency response, with muscle and cutaneous afferent inputs.

Pathways involved in the CMR

In normal adults, these CMRs are typically triphasic (Fig. 7.1). They consist of a short-latency increase in muscle electrical activity or excitatory component (E1), followed by a short-latency decrease or inhibitory component (I1) and then a second, more prominent, long-latency increase or excitatory component (E2). The mature adult configuration for intrinsic hand muscles shows an E2 component of greater amplitude than E1.

Measurement of sensory and motor conduction times suggests that the E1 and I1 components have latencies compatible with spinal pathways (Jenner 1981, Jenner and Stephens 1982). The afferent pathway for this component is probably via the fast conducting group

149

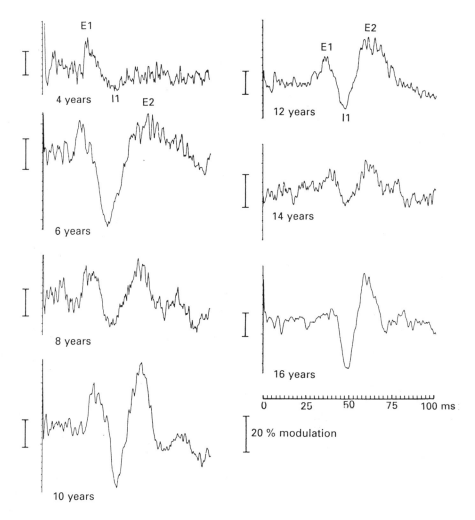

Fig. 7.1. Representative recordings obtained throughout childhood of the cutaneomuscular reflex response from the first dorsal interosseous muscle during a sustained index finger abduction. The short latency spinal components (E1 and I1) are present throughout. The longer latency E2 component is present in these examples from age 6. With increasing age, the E2 component becomes the more dominant of the excitatory components, greater in amplitude than E1. Each recording comprises 512 sweeps. Vertical calibration bar: 20% modulation of pre-stimulus background EMG.

II fibres which originate mainly from cutaneous receptors. The efferent limb of the reflex pathway is via the fast conducting alpha-motoneurons. Jenner (1981) found a central delay for E1 in the first dorsal interosseous muscle of 2.4–6.2 ms. Allowing 1 ms per synapse and perhaps 1 ms for central conduction through relatively slowly conducting spinal interneurons, only relatively few interneurons can be involved. Lesions of the motor cortex or internal capsule affecting the upper motoneuron result in an increase in amplitude of E1.

The I1 component may follow a spinal segmental inhibitory pathway receiving similar descending input to E1 as it is abolished by lesions that exaggerate E1. However, in hemiplegic cerebral palsy the I1 component may be found bilaterally when the non-hemiplegic side is stimulated, suggesting either reorganization or uncovering of spinal circuitry or, less likely, a supraspinal pathway (Carr *et al.* 1993). This is further discussed in Chapter 9.

E2 has many of the characteristics of a long loop, transcortical reflex. The timing of E2 related to sensory evoked responses supports the hypothesis that it follows a transcortical route (Jenner and Stephens 1982). In Jenner's study (1981) the E2 component was delayed, reduced in amplitude or abolished by localized lesions affecting the dorsal columns, sensorimotor cortex or descending motor pathways.

Changes in the CMR during development
There is maturation in the CMR from late gestation to late childhood which involves changes in both the latency and the configuration of the reflex. Maturational sequences for the CMR have been described for the forearm flexor and extensor muscles (Issler and Stephens 1983). Maturational changes in the lower limb have also been studied but will not be described here.

Issler and Stephens showed that CMRs in the finger flexor or extensor muscles of the forearm were monophasic and excitatory at birth, even visible on single EMG sweeps without the need for averaging. There was a powerful synchronous action potential at spinal latency only. The latency was high in preterm infants, falling to a minimum value early in the first year, and increased again from about 5 years to reach adult values in the teenage years. In the forearm extensor muscles the E1 component amplitude decreased and was followed by the appearance of I1 within the first year of life. The long-latency excitatory component of the reflex (E2) did not appear until the second year of life, at about 15 months. By the age of 2 years all the children in the study had three components to the response, but the point at which the adult configuration was reached was not clearly determined although a relatively mature response was seen at 5 years. Over the age range covered in this study, the response in the forearm flexors remained monophasic at spinal latency. It was concluded that E1 followed a simple spinal pathway by comparison with measurements of tendon jerk latency.

In a CMR study conducted at the University College and Middlesex School of Medicine, London (Evans *et al.* 1989, 1990), we made recordings from 127 normal children aged 3–18 years. In order to examine the relationship between stage of reflex motor development and manual dexterity, 67 subjects in the age range 4–11 years were selected for study on the basis of their ability to perform tests of rapid individual finger movements (Denckla 1973, Touwen 1979). Electrical stimuli of pulse width 100 µs were delivered from a constant current stimulator at 3 per second via ring electrodes placed either side of the proximal interphalangeal joint of the index finger. Perceptual threshold was determined, and stimuli at twice threshold for perception were then delivered for 2–3 minutes while the subject held a steady hand posture. Each subject performed three tasks: (1) an isometric abduction of the index finger against resistance; (2) a power grip (Napier 1956), for which the subject grasped a rigid cylinder of appropriate size; and (3) a ball grip (Griffiths 1943), for which

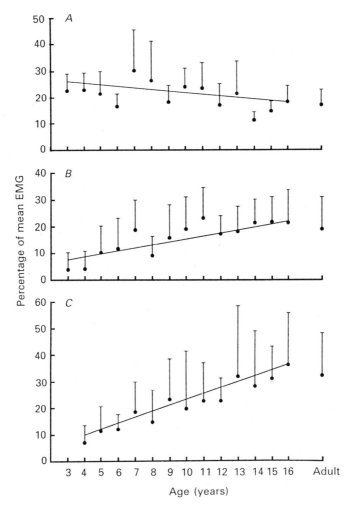

Fig. 7.2. Changes in the peak amplitude of the E1 component (A), the I1 component (B) and the E2 component (C) of the CMR recorded from first dorsal interosseous with increasing age. The ordinate shows the percentage modulation of mean rectified EMG level. The mean value and standard deviation of peak amplitudes are shown for each age group studied. The adult data for comparison are from Evans *et al.* (1989) and the linear regression lines exclude these data.

the subject held a ball of appropriate size. Subjects were required to perform each task in such a manner that EMG remained at a constant level equivalent to 10–20% of the level obtained during a maximal isometric abduction of the index finger against resistance. Surface EMGs were recorded from the first dorsal interosseous muscle of the preferred hand. EMG signals were amplified, filtered, rectified and averaged, time locked to each stimulus, and recorded on tape for off-line analysis using a microcomputer averaging system. Usually it was necessary to average up to 500 sweeps in order to identify and measure the reflex components. Latency and peak amplitudes normalized with respect to background level of EMG were measured. Figure 7.1 shows representative examples of CMRs from the first dorsal interosseous muscle at different ages for abduction of the index finger. There were changes in both peak amplitude and latency of the three components.

CHANGES IN LATENCY

There was a progressive increase in the latency of the E1 component of about 1 ms per year of life from 3 to 14 years. Using arm length as an indicator of linear growth, an estimate of change in peripheral conduction velocity was obtained by dividing arm length by the E1 latency. These values did not change with age, in accord with other studies quoted above.

The latency of I1 increased by 0.8 ms per year of life, reaching adult values at 14 years, and the latency of E2 increased by 0.4 ms per year of life to late adolescence. An estimate of central conduction time was obtained by subtracting the E1 from the E2 latency and showed a reduction in central delay of 0.6 ms per year over the age range tested.

The apparent decline in central conduction has to be interpreted with some caution as it is difficult to know exactly where E2 component starts. The measured reduction in central delay could be the result of an increase in the size of the synaptic effect of the underlying reflex pathways involved in E2 curtailing the duration of the preceding inhibitory events, producing I1 rather than any change in conduction time *per se* along the different reflex pathways concerned.

CHANGES IN REFLEX COMPONENT AMPLITUDE

E1 showed a small but significant decrease with age (Fig. 7.2a). At the age of 4 years only three out of seven children showed an I1 component (Fig. 7.2b). From the age of 4 to 9 years there was a progressive increase in the proportion of children showing this component and from the age of 10 years all children had an I1, which also showed a progressive increase in amplitude with age.

In early childhood the E2 component was generally absent. No 3-year-old had one. This component was first seen at the age of 4 years during an abduction of the index finger. The appearance of the component was followed by an increase in amplitude until the adult configuration of the reflex was obtained in the mid-teenage years (Fig. 7.2c). From the age of 12 years onwards, all the subjects had an E2 component.

In early childhood very few children showed a dominant E2. That is, if an E2 component was present, it was usually smaller than E1. Through childhood there was a progressive increase in the proportion of children who showed a dominant E2. By the age of 13–15 years a similar proportion of subjects showed a dominant E2 component when compared with adults (Evans *et al.* 1989).

The development of the motor control apparatus to produce the finest independent finger movements, such as those requiring the independent action of the intrinsic hand muscles, seems to require a prolonged period of development. The amplitude changes in all three components may reflect increasing activity in supraspinal pathways during maturation. This may involve anatomical development of pathways and connections and/or increasing use of pre-existent pathways.

153

There is considerable evidence both from animals and from man that the long descending motor tracts have a prolonged period of development. In the hamster, development of the pyramidal tract, in terms of growth into the spinal cord, penetration of the spinal grey and myelination, is entirely postnatal and takes a relatively prolonged time course (Reh and Kalil 1981, 1982). Although these pathways can function before myelination, forepaw movements in young animals are slower and less well coordinated than in the adult. The development of fine coordinated movements of the extremities may depend upon the myelination of the pyramidal tract and its ability to carry high frequency action potentials (Reh and Kalil 1982). In the rabbit, pyramidal tract development, in terms of increasing fibre diameter and myelination, continues until adulthood (Franson and Hildebrand 1975). These changes are associated with a decrease in conduction time (Conway *et al.* 1969).

The majority of direct corticomotoneuronal connections in the adult rhesus monkey are established postnatally (see Chapter 8). Studies on the development of the human brain and spinal cord between infancy and adulthood are uncommon. Those on the development of the pyramidal tract are all based on light microscopic studies, which may not give an accurate indication of myelination (Wozniak and O'Rahilly 1982). Larroche (1966) found that myelination of the pyramidal tract began in the third trimester of gestation, but the bulk of pyramidal tract myelination was postnatal. Yakovlev and Lecours (1967) suggested that pyramidal tract myelination began postnatally and continued into the third year of life, although their study included few child brains.

THE ABILITY TO PERFORM RAPID FINGER MOVEMENTS AND THE CONFIGURATION OF THE CMR

The speed of performance of the repetitive and sequential finger movements increased with age. From age 4 to 9 years this increase in speed was pronounced, and there was little change after this time. The size of E2 recorded during index finger abduction also increased with age. The E2 component is thought to involve activity in pathways including the corticospinal tract, which is involved in fine motor control. A relationship between ability to perform rapid finger movements and E2 amplitude might therefore be expected. However, no simple relationship between E2 amplitude and ability to perform accurate and rapid finger movements emerged. Those subjects lacking an E2 when recorded during index finger abduction were likely to perform poorly in tests of rapid finger movement. However, a larger than average E2 component was not associated with a better than average ability to perform these tests. No clear relationship emerged, presumably because many neural circuits are required for control of finger movement and only some of these are involved in generating the CMR. Müller and Hömberg (1992), using magnetic brain stimulation to measure conduction times in the fastest efferent motor pathways, found that central motor conduction could be related to speed of performance on repetitive movements.

The normal development of manipulative motor behaviours has received detailed observational study (Griffiths 1970; Denckla 1973, 1974; Sheridan 1975; Illingworth 1980; Ziviani 1983). These studies have shown continued acquisition of fine motor skills up to the age of 8–10 years and beyond. Our own study showed that changes can take place in reflex behaviour over the same long period. These changes in reflex circuitry may therefore play a part in the maturation of fine motor control during childhood.

Effects of task on the CMR during normal development

The components of the CMR showed different configurations when recorded during hand grips as compared with during abduction of the index finger. Typically during a grip E1 was larger than when recorded during an index finger abduction, and both the I1 and E2 were reduced. The increase in size of the E1 during grips was particularly pronounced in the younger children and prompts comparison with the grasp reflex seen in the newborn infant. The increase of the E1 and reduction of the I1 component during a grip may result from a reduction in descending pathway activity which is excitatory to inhibitory interneurons. It is possible that the pyramidal tract is more active during relatively independent use of the fingers than during whole hand grips. The similarity of the changes in the E2 component at all the ages studied suggests that similar mechanisms for these changes exist at all ages.

Physiological relevance of reflex modulation

Cutaneous afferent input is likely to play an important part in the control of movement. For whole hand grips involving the cooperation of a number of muscles in a rather crude movement this feedback might not require to be routed via the cortex but would perhaps be more usefully and efficiently routed via the spinal cord. For more sophisticated fine and exploratory finger movements it might be necessary for sensory feedback to be routed via the cortex, at least to some extent.

The CMRs recorded during whole hand grips showed a larger excitatory spinal E1 component, a smaller inhibitory spinal I1 component, and a much smaller or absent transcortical E2 component than those recorded during more isolated finger movements. CMRs recorded during relatively isolated finger movements showed much larger transcortical E2 components. This suggests that for relatively crude movements such as grips, sensory input tends to act at a spinal level, whereas for relatively isolated finger movements sensory input acts more at a cortical level in the reflex control of finger movement. This could be of great practical relevance as cutaneous input reinforcing a crude movement such as a grip would leave the cortex free for more important processing activities, whereas for novel exploratory or complex movements of the digits sensory feedback via the cortex would be of considerable practical use.

Cells in the motor cortex involved in producing movements of the distal extremities are influenced by cutaneous and other types of afferent input from the related part of the limb. A tight input–output circuitry has been demonstrated for sensory input to some motor cortex cells. Sensory input from the hand can modulate activity in pyramidal tract neurons. This modulation seems to be more pronounced for precision grips involving few fingers, with greater pyramidal tract neuronal activity compared with that recorded during whole hand grips (see Chapter 8).

Abnormalities of the CMR in cerebral palsy

CMR recordings were made in 21 subjects with spastic cerebral palsy (CP) with upper limb involvement (15 'pure', 6 mixed spastic/dyskinetic) aged 4–17 years (Evans *et al.* 1991). For each child where possible the reflex was recorded from each hand during a power grip (39 recordings) and during as close an approximation to an isometric isolated abduction or

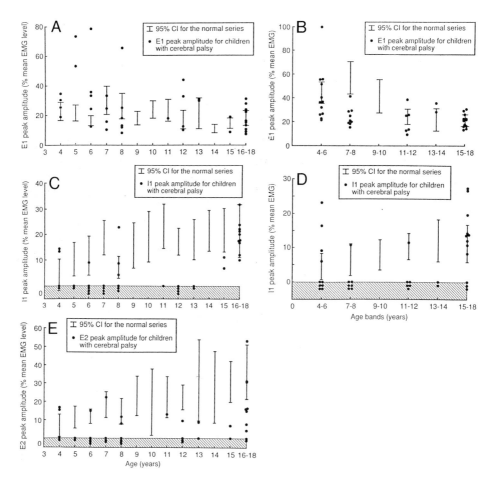

Fig. 7.3. The amplitude, expressed as percentage modulation of background EMG, of the three components of the CMR recorded from children with spastic CP. Data, presented as individual points, are compared with 95% confidence intervals obtained from normal children. Hatched areas denote absence of the component. (A) E1 amplitude recorded during a voluntary sustained relatively isolated movement of the index finger. (B) E1 recorded during a power grip. (C) I1 recorded during a voluntary sustained relatively isolated movement of the index finger. (D) I1 recorded during power grip. (E) E2 recorded during a voluntary sustained relatively isolated movement of the index finger.

flexion of the index finger that the child could perform (40 recordings). The ability of each child to perform finger movements was also assessed. Since some of the children with CP were substantially smaller for their age than normal children, comparison of reflex delays was carried out following adjustment for the size of the subject.

Comparison of estimated peripheral conduction velocities for the children with CP with the data from the normal children revealed that 24/40 were within the normal range, but 13/40 were below. CP results from a brain lesion, or lesions, acquired early in life and therefore would not be expected to have any direct effect on peripheral conduction velocities. However, there are often secondary effects related to nutrition and growth, and it is also known that trauma to peripheral nerves frequently occurs in individuals with central nervous lesions resulting in a reduction of peripheral conduction velocities.

E2 was present in 18/40 recordings; 8/18 of the adjusted latencies were within the normal range and 2/18 above, but 8/18 were below. This reduction could result from a delay or deficit in central myelination which has been described by Johnson *et al.* (1983, 1987) using magnetic resonance imaging in children with CP.

Figure 7.3a shows the E1 amplitudes when the CMRs were recorded during relatively isolated finger movements. These are expressed as percentage modulations of the mean EMG level and are compared with the 95% confidence intervals obtained from the normal series. During such a movement, the CMRs of all the children with CP had an E1 component. In these children this reflex component was significantly larger in 15/40 recordings compared with the normal series and was significantly smaller in 11/40. When recorded during a power grip, the E1 amplitude was greater for 27 of the 39 limbs in which recordings were obtained than when recorded during a relatively isolated finger movement (Fig. 7.3b). In only one instance was the E1 component very much larger in comparison with the normal series.

Figure 7.3c shows the I1 peak amplitudes recorded from children with CP compared with the 95% confidence intervals for the normal series at various ages. 22/40 showed a smaller than expected I1 component and 14/40 were within normal limits. When the task was changed from a relatively isolated finger movement to a power grip in the normal series, the I1 component was significantly smaller or absent at all ages studied. This result was also seen in the children with CP (Fig. 7.3d).

When the CMR was recorded during a relatively isolated finger movement, E2 was present less often than would be expected in normal children (Fig. 7.3e). Moreover, if an E2 component were present, it was seldom larger than the E1 component.

In the normal series of children, when the reflex was recorded during a power grip the E2 component was significantly smaller or absent at all ages studied than when recorded during a relatively isolated movement of the index finger. However, in all 18 reflexes recorded in children with CP, this component was absent or smaller when recorded during a power grip.

All the children with CP were slower performing the tests of finger movement than the normal children. There was no clear relationship between the presence or size of E2 recorded during a relatively isolated finger movement and the ability to perform repetitive or sequential finger movements.

Recordings made from adults with recently acquired central motor lesions have shown that the E1 component of the CMR tends to be increased in amplitude whereas the E2 component is reduced in size or absent. This suggests a reduction in descending modulation of the spinal components of the reflex and a reduction in corticospinal activity, upon which the longer latency (E2) component is dependent. It might be expected that the E1 component of the CMR recorded from children with spastic CP with evidence of pyramidal dysfunction would be exaggerated and the E2 component attenuated. In a grasp, the E1 might be even further exaggerated. However, exaggerated E1 components were not seen. In only one child was the size of the E1 component recorded during a power grip well outside the 95% confidence intervals obtained for the normal children. In some instances, the E1 component recorded during a relatively isolated finger movement was larger than expected. Some children experienced great difficulty when required to abduct or flex the index finger with little involvement of the remaining fingers. In these instances, the first dorsal interosseous muscle would not have been used in relative isolation, and this task may not have differed markedly from the power grip.

It is known from animal studies that a lesion acquired during the early neonatal period can produce quite different effects from one that is acquired during adulthood. The changes in CMR configuration seen in children with CP suggest that early damage to the central nervous system in man also results in different effects when compared to damage occurring in maturity. This might occur for a number of reasons, including rearrangement of central motor connections which might be more feasible in children than in adults. This is explored further in Chapter 9.

The previously described maturational changes in the configuration of the CMR may have a role in the development of motor skills during childhood. Such maturational changes appear to be less well developed in children with CP since E2 was not present in all children above the age of 12 years and was the dominant component less frequently than in normal children. The E2 component is dependent on the integrity of the dorsal columns, sensorimotor cortex and pyramidal tract. It is therefore not surprising that this component was found to be smaller than normal, since all the children in our study had some degree of pyramidal dysfunction. Pyramidal activity is known to be essential for the execution of fine manipulative skills (Lawrence and Hopkins 1976), many of which require the participation of the first dorsal interosseous muscle. Children with CP tend to have poorly developed manipulative ability, presumably in part due to a lesion of the motor cortex or pyramidal tract which is reflected by the relative immaturity of the CMR.

REFERENCES

Allison, T., Wood, C.C., Goff, W.R. (1983) 'Brainstem auditory, pattern-reversal visual, and short-latency somatosensory evoked potentials: latencies in relation to age, sex and brain and body size.' *Electroencephalography and Clinical Neurophysiology*, **55**, 619–636.
—— Hume, A.L., Wood, C.C., Goff, W.R. (1984) 'Developmental and aging changes in somatosensory, auditory and visual evoked potentials.' *Electroencephalography and Clinical Neurophysiology*, **58**, 14–24.
Amiel-Tison, C., Grenier, A. (1980) *Evaluation Neurologique du Nouveau-né et du Nourisson*. Paris: Masson.
André-Thomas, Chesni, Y., Saint-Anne Dargassies, S. (1960) *The Neurological Examination of the Infant. Little Club Clinics in Developmental Medicine No. 1.* London: Medical Advisory Committee of the National Spastics Society.
Babinski, J.F.F. (1898) 'On the phenomenon of the toes and its semeiotic value.' *English translation in:* Wilkins, R.H., Brody, I.A. (1967) 'Neurological Classics II: Babinski's Sign.' *Archives of Neurology*, **17**, 441–446.
Berger, W. Altenmüller. E. Dietz, V. (1984) 'Normal and impaired development of children's gait.' *Human Neurobiology*, **3**, 163–170.
—— Quintern, J., Dietz, V. (1985) 'Stance and gait perturbations in children: developmental aspects of compensatory mechanisms.' *Electroencephalography and Clinical Neurophysiology*, **61**, 385–395.
Caccia, M.R., McComas, A.J., Upton, A.R.M., Blogg, T. (1973) 'Cutaneous reflexes in small muscles of the hand.' *Journal of Neurology, Neurosurgery and Psychiatry*, **36**, 960–977.

Carr, L.J., Harrison, L.M., Evans, A.L., Stephens, J.A. (1993) 'Patterns of central motor reorganization in hemiplegic cerebral palsy.' *Brain*, **116**, 1223–1247.

Conrad, B., Aschoff, J.C. (1977) 'Effects of voluntary isometric and isotonic activity on late transcortical reflex components in normal subjects and hemiparetic patients.' *Electroencephalography and Clinical Neurophysiology*, **42**, 107–116.

Conway, C.J., Wright, F.S., Bradley, W.E. (1969) 'Electrophysiological maturation of the pyramidal tract in the post-natal rabbit.' *Electroencephalography and Clinical Neurophysiology*, **26**, 565–577.

Cracco, J.B., Cracco, R.Q., Stolove, R. (1979) 'Spinal evoked potential in man: a maturational study.' *Electro-encephalography and Clinical Neurophysiology*, **46**, 58–64.

Denckla, M.B. (1973) 'Development of speed in repetitive and successive finger-movements in normal children.' *Developmental Medicine and Child Neurology*, **15**, 635–645.

—— (1974) 'Development of motor co-ordination in normal children.' *Developmental Medicine and Child Neurology*, **16**, 729–741.

Desmedt, J.E., Noel, P., Debecker, J., Nameche, J. (1973) 'Maturation of afferent conduction velocity as studied by sensory nerve potentials and by cerebral evoked potentials.' *In:* Desmedt, J.E. (Ed.) *New Developments in Electromyography and Clinical Neurophysiology. Vol. 2.* Basel: Karger, pp. 52–63.

—— Brunko, E., Debecker, J. (1976) 'Maturation of the somatosensory evoked potentials in normal infants and children, with special reference to the early N_1 component.' *Electroencephalography and Clinical Neurophysiology*, **40**, 43–58.

Evans, A.L., Harrison, L.M., Stephens, J.A. (1989) 'Task-dependent changes in cutaneous reflexes recorded from various muscles controlling finger movement in man.' *Journal of Physiology*, **418**, 1–12.

—— —— —— (1990) 'Maturation of the cutaneomuscular reflex recorded from the first dorsal interosseous muscle in man.' *Journal of Physiology*, **428**, 425–440.

—— —— —— (1991) 'Cutaneomuscular reflexes recorded from the first dorsal interosseous muscle of children with cerebral palsy.' *Developmental Medicine and Child Neurology*, **33**, 541–551.

Eyre, J.A., Miller, S. (1992) 'Assessment of motor pathways.' *In:* Eyre, J.A. (Ed.) *The Neurophysiological Examination of the Newborn Infant. Clinics in Developmental Medicine No. 120.* London: Mac Keith Press, pp. 124–154.

—— —— Ramesh, V. (1991) 'Constancy of central conduction delays during development in man: investigation of motor and somatosensory pathways.' *Journal of Physiology*, **434**, 441–452.

Fitzgerald, J.E., Windle, W.F. (1942) 'Some observations on early human fetal movements.' *Journal of Comparative Neurology*, **76**, 159–167.

Franson, P., Hildebrand, C. (1975) 'Postnatal growth of nerve fibres in the pyramidal tract of the rabbit.' *Neurobiology*, **5**, 8–22.

Gamstorp, I. (1963) 'Normal conduction velocity of ulnar, median and peroneal nerves in infancy, childhood and adolescence.' *Acta Paediatrica Scandinavica*, Suppl. 146, 68–76.

George, S.R., Taylor, M.J. (1991) 'Somatosensory evoked potentials in neonates and infants: developmental and normative data.' *Electroencephalography and Clinical Neurophysiology*, **80**, 94–102.

Griffiths, H.E., (1943) 'Treatment of the injured workman.' *Lancet*, 1, 729–733,

Griffiths, R. (1970) *The Abilities of Young Children: A Comprehensive System of Mental Measurement for the First Eight years of Life.* London: Child Development Research Centre.

Grimby, L. (1963) 'Normal plantar response: integration of flexor and extensor reflex components.' *Journal of Neurology, Neurosurgery and Psychiatry*, **26**, 39–50.

Gutrecht, J.A., Dyck, P.J. (1970) 'Quantitative teased-fiber and histologic studies of human sural nerve during postnatal development.' *Journal of Comparative Neurology*, **138**, 117–130.

Hagbarth, K.E. (1952) 'Excitatory and inhibitory skin areas for flexor and extensor motoneurones.' *Acta Physiologica Scandinavica*, **26**, Suppl. 94, 7–58.

—— (1960) 'Spinal withdrawal reflexes in the human lower limbs.' *Journal of Neurology, Neurosurgery and Psychiatry*, **23**, 222–227.

—— Kugelberg, E. (1958) 'Plasticity of the human abdominal skin reflex.' *Brain*, **81**, 305–318.

Hooker, D. (1958) *Evidence of Prenatal Function of the Central Nervous System in Man. James Arthur Lecture on the Evolution of the Human Brain, 1957.* New York: American Museum of Natural History.

Illingworth, R.S. (1980) *The Development of the Infant and Young Child. Normal and Abnormal. 7th Edn.* London: Churchill Livingstone.

Issler, H., Stephens, J.A. (1983) 'The maturation of cutaneous reflexes studied in the upper limb in man.' *Journal of Physiology*, **335**, 643–654.

159

Jenner, J.R. (1981) 'Cutaneous reflexes in man studied in health and disease.' M.D. thesis, University of London.

—— Stephens, J.A. (1982) 'Cutaneous reflex responses and their central nervous pathways studied in man.' *Journal of Physiology*, **333**, 405–419.

Johnson, M.A., Pennock, J.M., Bydder, G.M., Steiner, R.E., Thomas, D.J., Hayward, R., Bryant, D.R.T., Payne, J.A., Levene, M.I., *et al.* (1983) 'Clinical NMR imaging of the brain in children: normal and neurologic disease.' *American Journal of Roentgenology*, **141**, 1005–1018.

—— —— Dubowitz, L.M.S., Thomas, D.J., Young, I.R. (1987) 'Serial MR imaging in neonatal cerebral injury.' *American Journal of Neuroradiology*, **8**, 83–92.

Kamimura, N., Shichida, K., Tomita, Y., Takashima, S., Takeshita, K. (1988) 'Spinal somatosensory evoked potentials in infants and children with spinal cord lesions.' *Brain and Development*, **10**, 355–359.

Khater-Boidin, J., Duron, B. (1992) 'Nerve conduction.' *In:* Eyre, J.A. (Ed.) *The Neurophysiological Examination of the Newborn Infant. Clinics in Developmental Medicine No. 120.* London: Mac Keith Press. pp. 155–167.

—— Joly, H., Duron, B. (1992) 'Développement postnatal des voies motrices centrales. Étude électrophysiologique.' *Neurophysiologie Clinique*, **22**, 207–224.

Larroche, J-C. (1966) 'The development of the central nervous system during intrauterine life.' *In:* Falkner, F. (Ed.) *Human Development.* Philadelphia: W.B. Saunders, pp. 257–276.

Lauffer, H., Wenzel, D. (1986) 'Maturation of central somatosensory conduction time in infancy and childhood.' *Neuropediatrics*, **17**, 72–74.

Lawrence, D.G., Hopkins, D.A. (1976) 'The development of motor control in the rhesus monkey: evidence concerning the role of corticomotoneuronal connections.' *Brain*, **99**, 235–254.

Leonard, C.T., Hirschfeld, H., Moritani, T., Forssberg, H. (1991) 'Myotatic reflex development in normal children and children with cerebral palsy.' *Experimental Neurology*, **111**, 379–382.

Lundberg, A. (1975) 'Control of spinal mechanisms from the brain.' *In:* Tower, D.B. (Ed.) *The Nervous System. Vol. 1: The Basic Neurosciences.* New York: Raven Press, pp. 253–265.

Mayer, R.F., Mosser, R.S. (1969) 'Excitability of motoneurons in infants.' *Neurology*, **19**, 932–945.

Müller, K., Hömberg, V. (1992) 'Development of speed of repetitive movements in children is determined by structural changes in corticospinal efferents.' *Neuroscience Letters*, **144**, 57–60.

—— —— Lenard, H-G. (1991) 'Magnetic stimulation of motor cortex and nerve roots in children. Maturation of cortico-motoneuronal projections.' *Electroencephalography and Clinical Neurophysiology*, **81**, 63–70.

—— Ebner, B., Hömberg, V. (1994) 'Maturation of fastest afferent and efferent central and peripheral pathways: no evidence for a constancy of central conduction delays.' *Neuroscience Letters*, **166**, 9–12.

Myklebust, B.M. (1990) 'A review of myotatic reflexes and the development of motor control and gait in infants and children: a special communication.' *Physical Therapy*, **70**, 188–203.

—— Gottlieb, G.L, Agarwal, G.C. (1986) 'Stretch reflexes of the normal infant.' *Developmental Medicine and Child Neurology*, **28**, 440–449.

Napier, J.R. (1956) 'The prehensile movements of the human hand.' *Journal of Bone and Joint Surgery*, **38B**, 902–913.

Nathan, P.W., Smith, M.C. (1955) 'Long descending tracts in man. 1. Review of present knowledge.' *Brain*, **78**, 248–303.

O'Sullivan, M.C, Eyre, J.A., Miller, S. (1991) 'Radiation of phasic stretch reflex in biceps brachii to muscles of the arm in man and its restriction during development.' *Journal of Physiology*, **439**, 529–543.

Reh, T., Kalil, K. (1981) 'Development of the pyramidal tract in the hamster. I. A light microscopic study.' *Journal of Comparative Neurology*, **200**, 55–67.

—— —— (1982) 'Development of the pyramidal tract in the hamster. II. An electron microscopic study.' *Journal of Comparative Neurology*, **205**, 77–88.

Rexed, B. (1944) 'Contributions to the knowledge of the post-natal development of the peripheral nervous system in man.' *Acta Psychiatrica et Neurologica*, Suppl. 33, 1–205.

Rushworth, G. (1962) 'Observations on blink reflexes.' *Journal of Neurology, Neurosurgery and Psychiatry*, **25**, 93–108.

Sheridan, M.D. (1975) *From Birth to Five Years.* Windsor: NFER–Nelson.

Sherrington, C.S. (1903) 'Qualitative difference of spinal reflex corresponding with qualitative difference of cutaneous stimulus.' *Journal of Physiology*, **30**, 39–46.

—— (1910) 'Flexion-reflex of the limb, crossed extension-reflex, and reflex stepping and standing.' *Journal of Physiology*, **40**, 28–121.

160

—— (1951) *Man on his Nature. 2nd Edn.* Cambridge University Press.

Stephens, J.A., Usherwood, T.P., Garnett, R. (1976) 'Technique for studying synaptic connections of single motoneurones in man.' *Nature*, **263**, 343–344.

Taylor, M.J., Fagan, E.R. (1988) 'SEPs to median nerve stimulation: normative data for paediatrics.' *Electro-encephalography and Clinical Neurophysiology*, **71**, 323–330.

Thomas, J.E., Lambert, E.H. (1960) 'Ulnar nerve conduction velocity and H-reflex in infants and children.' *Journal of Applied Physiology*, **15**, 1–9.

Touwen, B. (1976) *Neurological Development in Infancy. Clinics in Developmental Medicine No. 58.* London: Spastics International Medical Publications.

—— (1979) *Examination of the Child with Minor Neurological Dysfunction. 2nd Edn. Clinics in Developmental Medicine No. 71.* London: Spastics International Medical Publications.

Twitchell, T.E. (1970) 'Reflex mechanisms and the development of prehension.' *In:* Connolly, K. (Ed.) *Mechanisms of Motor Skill Development.* London: Academic Press, pp. 25–40.

Vecchierini-Blineau, M.F., Guiheneuc, P. (1981) 'Excitability of the monosynaptic reflex pathway in the child from birth to four years of age.' *Journal of Neurology, Neurosurgery and Psychiatry*, **44**, 309–314.

Woźniak, W., O'Rahilly, R. (1982) 'An electron microscopic study of myelination of pyramidal fibres at the level of the pyramidal decussation in the human fetus.' *Journal für Hirnforschung*, **23**, 331–342.

Yakovlev, P.I., Lecours, A-R. (1967) 'The myelogenetic cycles of regional maturation of the brain.' *In:* Minkowski, A. (Ed.) *Regional Development of the Brain in Early Life.* Oxford: Blackwell, pp. 3–70.

Ziviani, J. (1983) 'Qualitative changes in dynamic tripod grip between seven and 14 years of age.' *Developmental Medicine and Child Neurology*, **25**, 778–782.

161

8
SKILLED ACTION AND THE DEVELOPMENT OF THE CORTICOSPINAL TRACT IN PRIMATES

R.N. Lemon, J. Armand, E. Olivier and S.A. Edgley

It is obvious that a large number of different factors must interact to produce normal motor development. Clinical studies (see Chapter 9) show us that the major sensory and motor systems must develop normally in order to provide the basic neural infrastructure for motor learning and acquisition of motor skills. A simple example, relevant to hand function, is that tactile exploration of objects by the hand requires a coordinated motor system to scan the object and to allow interpretation of the sensory signals that arise as a result of the movement. The integrity of both the sensory and motor pathways is essential. Although higher-level parts of the CNS will be required to process this information for cognitive and motor development, such processing cannot occur without the normal development and function of relatively low-level sensorimotor systems.

It is therefore important to understand how such systems develop. The major sensory pathways mature earlier than the motor pathways. In this chapter we shall discuss the particular importance of studying the corticospinal system, because of its special relationship to the control of hand function. Early damage to this system usually has severe consequences for the child's hand function, and it is essential that we begin to understand the major events in the timetable of normal corticospinal development.

Corticomotoneuronal connections and skilled hand movement
When compared to lower mammals there have been two key developments in the organization of the cortical control system in primates. The first is the increasingly dominant role played by the motor cortex and corticospinal tract, and the second is the appearance of direct, corticomotoneuronal (CM) connections which provide a monosynaptic linkage between the motor cortex and the spinal motoneurons. These developments have allowed cortical control of the arm and hand for visuomotor control and tactile exploration.

"The development of corticomotoneuronal projections, in particular, allowed the motor hierarchy to bypass spinal segmental mechanisms, and to break up the rigid synergies of the spinal apparatus by direct access to the motoneurones, to the final common path itself. As we shall see, the corticomotoneuronal system appears to play an important part in the fractionation of muscle activity allowing for independent movement of the digits under voluntary control; such movements are an essential part of all skilled hand function." (Lemon 1993)

The fibres of the primate corticospinal tract originate from many different motor and sensory areas of the frontal and parietal lobes (Dum and Strick 1991, Porter and Lemon 1993).

This probably represents a distributed system, in which to some extent the different areas can operate in parallel, although there is ample evidence to suggest that the different motor areas of the frontal lobe also have specific and characteristic functions (Porter and Lemon 1993, Tanji 1994). The corticospinal fibres descend through the internal capsule and cerebral peduncle and then pass through the brainstem, as the pyramidal tract, to the spinal cord (Fig. 8.1). The fibres give off extensive collaterals to many structures, including the red nucleus, reticular formation, and pontine and dorsal column nuclei. Most fibres then cross over and descend as the lateral corticospinal tract, making widespread connections at all levels of the spinal cord (Kuypers 1981, Armand 1982, Nathan *et al.* 1990). The uncrossed fibres are generally recognized to be more concerned with the control of axial and girdle musculature (Kuypers 1981). Little is known about the development of these uncrossed fibres in the primate (Galea and Darian-Smith 1995).

Several lines of evidence suggest that CM connections provide the capacity for the performance of relatively independent finger movements. First, it is now well established that all CM connections are excitatory and that inhibition occurs via oligosynaptic mechanisms. The largest excitatory postsynaptic potentials (EPSPs) generated by stimulation of the motor cortex or pyramidal tract are found amongst the motoneurons supplying the most distal muscles, those acting upon the digits (Porter and Lemon 1993). This finding has recently been confirmed in man, using noninvasive transcranial magnetic stimulation of the motor cortex (Palmer and Ashby 1992).

Lesion studies performed on primates have shown that bilateral pyramidotomy abolished the capacity to make fine finger movements (Tower 1940, Lawrence and Kuypers 1968, Lawrence and Hopkins 1976). Contactual hand-orienting responses, which are the normal link between tactile input and grip, were also seriously affected. These effects were only seen with complete lesions; subtotal damage was usually accompanied by very good recovery. These observations are, of course, reinforced by the effects on upper limb function of capsular lesions in man, where weakness and poverty of movement are most strikingly observed in the hands. However, it should not be forgotten that the fibres of the pyramidal tract are only a tiny percentage of the total population of fibres within the internal capsule: no figures are available at present, but even at the level of the cerebral peduncle the proportion of fibres actually destined for the spinal cord is probably around only 10% (Porter and Lemon 1993), so the proportion within the capsule must be much lower.

A final line of evidence comes from the comparative anatomy of the corticospinal system. Although the hands of different primates may appear very similar in musculoskeletal structure and biomechanical properties, their motor capacities are very different (Phillips 1971). Comparison of the digital dexterity and corticospinal projections of different primates by Heffner and Masterton (1975, 1983) led them to conclude that there was a good correlation between the number of CM connections and the index of dexterity. Species with the highest index of dexterity, including the ability to perform a thumb–index opposition, have numerous CM connections, while those in which such connections are weak or absent are less dexterous (Bortoff and Strick 1993, Lemon 1993).

In the macaque monkey, the CM projection appears to be limited to the most dorsolateral parts of the motoneuronal cell groups of lamina IX, where the motoneurons supplying the

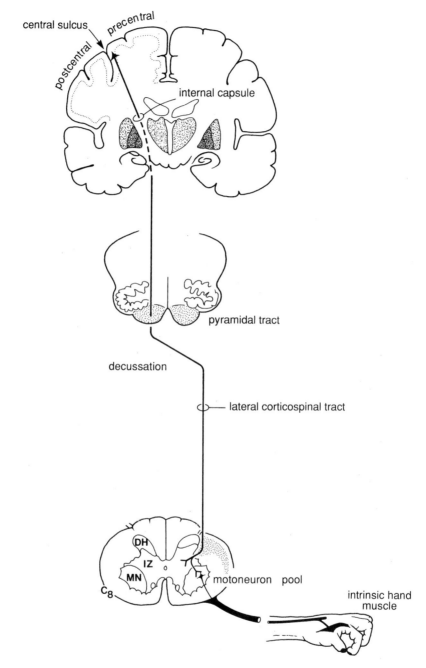

Fig. 8.1. The corticomotoneuronal system.

    The diagram shows that component of the corticospinal projection which arises from the precentral gyrus (primary motor cortex) and which primarily influences spinal interneurons (in the intermediate zone, IZ) and motoneurons (MN) via direct monosynaptic connections.

hand and finger muscles are located (Jenny and Inukai 1983). In man, the upper limb projections also involve motoneurons supplying the more proximal muscles groups (Kuypers 1981, Armand 1982).

Development of the corticospinal system

The development of the descending motor pathways, including the corticospinal tract, follows a well-defined sequence (Barkovich *et al.* 1992). In the initial stage corticospinal axons grow down the spinal cord. There is then a short 'waiting period' after which collaterals enter the grey matter and form synaptic contacts. Finally, the descending axons continue to grow and become myelinated.

Animal models of corticospinal development

Animal models are continuing to provide important insights into the processes which guide corticospinal development. However, before describing the results obtained from such models it is important to point out that some caution must be exercised in applying the results to human development. First, it is probable that the corticospinal tract carries out rather different functions in different species. Thus in lower mammals, such as the mouse and rat, which have provided most of what we know about molecular and cellular milestones in the developmental process, the corticospinal tract is relatively poorly developed, lacks any significant direct CM component, and is probably mostly concerned with the control of sensory input and some reflex functions (Porter and Lemon 1993). Second, the developmental timetable shows remarkable differences across species (Passingham 1985). In man and monkey, for example, corticospinal fibres have grown down the full extent of the spinal cord by birth, whereas in the rat, no fibres enter the spinal cord until just after birth. Although the macaque monkey is undoubtedly the best model we have, some differences between it and man have already emerged.

Exuberant corticospinal projections

A key feature of the developmental process in subprimates appears to be that an excessive number of axons and synapses are formed initially, and this excess is progressively eliminated at later stages. Thus, in the marsupial, carnivore and rodent, 'exuberant' corticospinal axons originate from cortical areas additional to those giving rise to the corticospinal projection in the adult (D'Amato and Hicks 1978; Reh and Kalil 1981; Schreyer and Jones 1982, 1988; Adams *et al.* 1983; Cabana and Martin 1984; Mihailoff *et al.* 1984; Kalil 1985; Stanfield and O'Leary 1985, Joosten *et al.* 1987). In addition, during the developmental period, the descending fibres make aberrant collaterals to supraspinal structures and to different parts of the spinal grey matter (Theriault and Tatton 1989, Alisky *et al.* 1992, Cabana and Martin 1985). For instance, in the cat, Alisky *et al.* (1992) observed that after a unilateral cortical injection of tracer in kittens of 4–5 weeks of age, there was a diffuse bilateral labelling in all parts of the grey matter. At 6–7 weeks after birth there was selective elimination of the transient ipsilateral projections to the dorsal horn and the dorsolateral part of the intermediate zone and the bilateral projections to the ventral horn leaving an adult-like pattern of termination.

A recent study by Galea and Darian-Smith (1995) indicates that there are also exuberant corticospinal fibres in the primate. They injected different types of fluorescent retrograde tracers into the spinal cord of young macaque monkeys. Their results showed that the patterns of corticospinal projections from the different cortical regions in the newborn and adult macaque were 'strikingly similar'. However, in the neonate they did find exuberant projections from cortical areas which skirted those giving rise to the projection in the adult. These areas included extensive regions of the cingulate gyrus, prefrontal cortex (area 12), lateral premotor cortex, peri-insular and intraparietal cortex. Galea and Darian-Smith also reported that large injections of tracer into the cervical dorsolateral funiculus labelled up to three times as many neurons in the neonate as in the adult. These authors favoured the idea that during the first 6–8 months of postnatal development, many of these neurons, which had descending projections to other subcortical targets, withdrew their corticospinal axon collaterals. Thus the total population of corticospinal neurons is steadily reduced during this period. By 5 months of age, exuberant cortical areas could no longer be detected by Biber *et al.* (1978).

As far as corticospinal projections are concerned, Armand *et al.* (1994, 1997) have found that corticospinal fibres from the motor cortex hand area project to the same regions of the spinal grey matter in neonatal and adult macaque monkeys, although with striking differences in the relative density of the projections to different parts of the grey matter (see below). No aberrant projections were detected. However, the contrast in the results from primates and non-primates may be due to the very considerable differences in the relative stage of development achieved by the different species at birth. The corticospinal system is so much more advanced in the neonatal primate; in man, for example, the fibres are thought to have reached sacral levels by a gestational age of 29 weeks (Humphrey 1960). Thus it is prob able that the early fetal stages of human corticospinal development are also exuberant in character, but that there has been a great deal of selection and elimination by birth. This is supported by the observation that such exuberance is most pronounced in prematurely born macaques (Galea and Darian-Smith 1995).

Development of primate corticomotoneuronal projections
Because the integrity of CM connections appears to be essential for skilled finger movements, it is important to understand the ontogeny of the projections of the corticospinal tract into the motoneuron nuclei innervating the hand and finger muscles. Kuypers (1962) was the first to study this question in macaques. He found that, at birth, corticospinal fibres had reached all levels of the spinal cord white matter. Corticospinal terminals were found in the spinal intermediate zone, but not in the motor nuclei. An important exception was the presence of a few terminals among the dorsal margins of the hand muscle motor nuclei at C8. Kuypers considered that an 'almost adult pattern' of terminal labelling, including much more extensive labelling in these hand motor nuclei, was present by 8 months of age.

This question has been reinvestigated recently by Armand *et al.* (1994, 1997), who used more modern and sensitive neuroanatomical tracing techniques. Large injections of the anterograde tracer WGA-HRP were made within the hand region of the primary motor cortex of macaque monkeys at different stages of development. After 72 hours, the animals were

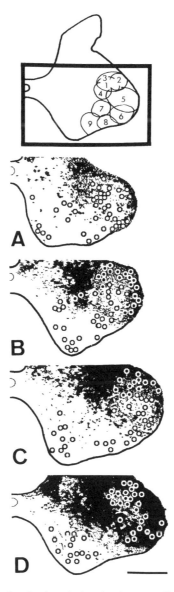

Fig. 8.2. Changes in corticospinal projections during development. Corticospinal anterograde labelling in the grey matter at the C8–Th1 junction in macaque monkeys of different ages: at 5 days (A), 2.5 months (B), 11 months (C), and in the adult (D). The inset in the top diagram (modified from Jenny and Inukai 1983) demarcates the region of grey matter represented below, and also shows the distribution of motor nuclei innervating nine selected hand and arm muscles: 1—first dorsal interosseous; 2—lateral lumbrical; 3—adductor pollicis; 4—abductor and flexor pollicis brevis; 5—flexor digitorum profundus and superficialis; 6—extensor digitorum communis, abductor and extensor pollicis longus; 7—flexor carpi ulnaris; 8—extensor carpi ulnaris; 9—triceps brachii. In A–D, the distribution of corticospinal terminal labelling is shown in black stipple. Circles indicate the locations of motoneurons. Calibration bar = 500 μm. (Reproduced by permission from Armand *et al.* 1994).

killed, frozen sections of the spinal cord were cut and histochemical procedures used to visualize the transported WGA-HRP. The densest projections resulting from these injections were found in the lower cervical spinal segments (C8–Th1).

In the adult monkey, terminal labelling was particularly heavy in the dorsolateral part of the intermediate zone and, although less dense, was also present throughout the dorsolateral group of motoneurons (Fig. 8.2D). There was no labelling of the ventral motoneurons, which supply axial and proximal arm muscles. This pattern confirmed earlier studies in the adult monkey (Kuypers 1981).

In a 5-day-old animal only weak labelling was observed (Fig. 8.2A), with very sparse projections to the dorsolateral motor nuclei. Fainter and more scattered labelling was also present in the centre of the motor nuclei, but no labelling was observed among the ventral motoneurons. At 2.5 months there was heavy labelling within the intermediate zone of the spinal grey, which formed a clear ring around the dorsolateral motor nuclei, and this dense labelling now extended into the most dorsal motoneurons (Fig. 8.2B); a more diffuse labelling was present among the other motor nuclei. At 11 months labelling was similar to that in the 2.5-month-old animal, with further penetration of corticospinal fibres into the lateral group of motoneurons (Fig. 8.2C). However, even at this age the labelling was still less extensive and less dense than in the adult (compare Figs. 8.2C and D).

Thus although small numbers of very fine corticospinal axon terminals do appear to reach the hand motor nuclei at birth, these projections are sparse even by comparison with the 2.5-month-old monkey. The general pattern is one of a protracted encroachment of the motor nuclei by the corticospinal fibres that takes at least a year. It is of interest that this postnatal expansion of projections is in distinct contrast to the retraction of aberrant corticospinal projections that characterizes other aspects of development, particularly in subprimate species (*cf.* Galea and Darian-Smith 1995).

Establishment of functional corticomotoneuronal connections in the primate
From a behavioural point of view it is much more important to know when corticospinal projections into the motor nuclei make synapses on target motoneurons and thereby establish functional corticomotoneuronal connections. But these changes are far more difficult to demonstrate. We do not yet know where on the extensive dendritic tree of the motoneurons the CM synapses are located, and, in any case, changes in corticospinal projections during development are paralleled by changes in the dendritic morphology of the target motoneurons (Goldstein *et al.* 1993, Dekkers *et al.* 1994). Thus analysis at the light microscopic level is unlikely to provide us with definitive information on functional connectivity. At the electron microscopic level, one study has demonstrated the existence, in the adult monkey, of CM connections (Ralston and Ralston 1985), but no information is yet available about the electron microscopic status of the developing CM connection.

A neurophysiological approach to this question has been to look at muscle responses to stimulation of the motor cortex using either invasive (Felix and Wiesendanger 1971) or noninvasive methods (Ludolph *et al.* 1987, Edgley *et al.* 1990, Flament *et al.* 1992). Because it can be used in man, there has been particular interest in the use of noninvasive transcranial magnetic stimulation (TMS) to investigate the development of the short-latency EMG responses that it evokes. The earliest component of these responses has been shown to be mediated by the CM system in both monkey (Edgley *et al.* 1990, Baker *et al.* 1994) and man (Baldissera and Cavallari 1993, Gracies *et al.* 1994).

In a longitudinal study of the effects of TMS on responses in infant macaques, Flament *et al.* (1992) applied TMS to young monkeys sedated with ketamine. No responses could be elicited in hand muscles until 4–5.5 months. These responses had much higher thresholds and longer latencies than in the adult. However, the low conduction velocities both centrally (see below) and peripherally make it difficult to determine whether or not these responses were monosynaptic in nature. Flament *et al.* pointed out that they could be mediated either by CM fibres (which are very slowly conducting for the first few months of life—Olivier *et al.* 1997) or by indirect pathways, possibly via corticorubrospinal or corticoreticulospinal pathways. These pathways appear to mature at an earlier stage than the corticospinal tract in all species studied (Langworthy 1933, Cabana and Martin 1984, Weidenheim *et al.* 1992, Kudo *et al.* 1993).

In the human neonate, it is not possible to obtain EMG responses to TMS in relaxed muscles, suggesting that the connections mediating these responses are rather weak (Koh and Eyre 1988, Müller *et al.* 1991). However, even in neonates, Eyre *et al.* (1991) found that TMS did elicit responses in actively contracted hand muscles. At birth, thresholds were high and latencies were long (around 32 ms, compared to 19 ms in adult subjects). These authors found a rapid decline in the latency of the evoked responses during the first two years after birth and then, from the age of 4 years, a progressive increase in total EMG response latencies. Once again, the lengthy central motor conduction time in neonates makes it difficult to assess whether or not the responses evoked by TMS are mediated monosynaptically. Further evidence against a significant corticospinal projection to the hand motor nuclei in man is provided by the work of Evans *et al.* (1990). They found that the long latency, presumably transcortical, E2 response that can be recorded in hand muscles in response to stimulation of the digital nerves is not present in newborn infants.

Thus we have as yet no conclusive evidence for functional CM connections in the newborn primate. In adult human subjects, the short latency of EMG responses to TMS has been taken as evidence of CM origin; in human neonates these responses are either absent or have very long latencies, and could be mediated by other pathways. In the newborn macaque monkey, EMG responses to TMS are not present. Interpretation of these results requires further study of the effect of TMS on the immature corticospinal system; no published data are yet available to show that it is activated by TMS.

Changes in the myelination and conduction velocity of corticospinal axons during development

In all species that have been studied, myelination of the corticospinal tract has been found to be a postnatal process (Reh and Kalil 1981, Schreyer and Jones 1982, Gribnau *et al.* 1986). Myelination does not appear to start until the axons have reached all levels of the spinal cord (Schreyer and Jones 1982). The first axons to be myelinated are the largest ones (Matthews and Duncan 1971, Reh and Kalil 1982). The wave of myelination and growth in axonal diameter produces a continuous increase in the conduction velocity of the whole tract (Oka *et al.* 1985; Armand *et al.* 1994; Olivier *et al.* 1994, 1997).

As has already been pointed out, in both monkey and man, corticospinal fibres reach all levels of the spinal cord before birth (Humphrey 1960, Kuypers 1962). In man, although the intracranial corticospinal fibres are probably myelinated before birth, there is no significant myelination of these fibres within the spinal cord at birth (Langworthy 1933, Yakovlev and Lecours 1967, Brody *et al.* 1987). However, other descending pathways are myelinating at this time (Weidenheim *et al.* 1992). Brody *et al.* (1987) found that myelination of the tract was still far from complete by the end of the second postnatal year. Half of the brains in their sample showed a mature pattern of myelination at the medullary pyramid by around 15 months; but a similar proportion did not achieve a mature pattern in the tract at the cervical level until 20 months of age.

The conduction velocity of corticospinal axons in the human neonatal spinal cord has been estimated to be about 10 m/s (Khater-Boidin and Duron 1991), compared to about 50–70 m/s in human adults. Investigations using TMS suggest that the maximum fibre diameter and conduction velocity of corticospinal axons could continue to increase until 14–16 years of age (Eyre *et al.* 1991, Olivier *et al.* 1997).

Olivier *et al.* (1997) measured the conduction velocity of the fastest corticospinal fibres in the same series of macaque monkeys that were used for the anatomical investigation. Their results showed that full myelination of corticospinal fibres in the spinal cord may not be complete until well into the second year of life. The fibres were stimulated by electrodes in the medullary pyramidal tract. Conduction velocity within the brain was determined from antidromic volleys recorded from the motor cortex (see Fig. 8.3A), while that of the corticospinal fibres within the cord was determined by recording the orthodromic volleys at different spinal levels.

Olivier *et al.* found large age-related changes in conduction velocity over both the cranial and spinal courses of the macaque corticospinal tract. Figure 8.3A shows the antidromic potential recorded from the motor cortex in an adult and in monkeys aged 11 and 2.5 months. This potential, the peak of which is arrowed in Figure 8.3, had onset latencies of 1.05, 1.13 and 2.32 ms, respectively. Since there are only minor increases in macaque brain size after 2–3 months of age (Holt *et al.* 1975), these latency changes must reflect an increase in conduction velocity of the fastest conducting pyramidal fibres over their cranial course. This change was particularly marked from 2.5 to 11 months.

Figure 8.3B shows the changes in conduction velocity estimated over the spinal course of the corticospinal tract. The conduction velocity of the fastest fibres increased from 7.8 m/s in the 5-day-old monkey, to 28.4 m/s in the 2.5-month-old monkey, and then to 54.8 m/s in the 11-month-old monkey. In the adult the conduction velocity was 72.6 m/s, ten times faster than in the newborn monkey. The time constant of the exponential fitted to the four data points plotted in Figure 8.3B is eight months, and predicts that an adult conduction velocity would not be reached until about 16 months of age. Further, while there was little or no difference in the antidromic latency between the 11-month-old and the adult, there was still a substantial difference in the spinal conduction velocity. Taken together these results were interpreted as confirming a rostrocaudal maturation of the corticospinal tract (Langworthy 1933, Brody *et al.* 1987).

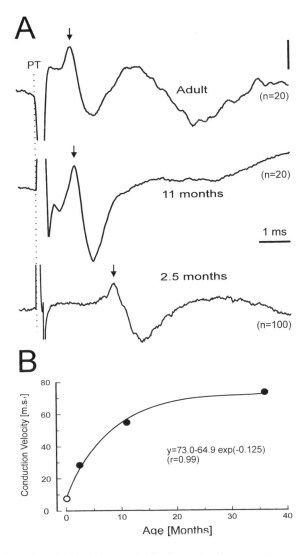

Fig. 8.3. Changes in corticospinal conduction velocity during development. (Reproduced by permission from Armand *et al.* 1994).

A. Antidromic volleys recorded from the exposed surface of the primary motor cortex to stimulation of the pyramidal tract (PT) in adult, 11- and 2.5-month-old monkeys, respectively. The dotted line indicates the onset of PT stimulation, and the positive peak of the antidromic response is arrowed in each case. Note that the response has a much longer latency in the 2.5-month-old as compared to the adult monkey, but there is little difference between the 11-month-old and adult cases. n = average number of sweeps. Calibration bar = 20 µV (adult and 11-month-old), 10 µV (2.5-month-old).

B. Relationship between age and conduction velocity of corticospinal axons in the spinal cord. In three monkeys (filled circles), this was estimated by the difference between the latencies of orthodromic volleys excited by PT stimulation and recorded at two spinal levels. In the 5-day-old monkey (open circle) this value was calculated using antidromic cortical volleys evoked by stimulation of the corticospinal tract at two spinal levels.

171

The largest proportion of the adult corticospinal tract is made up of small, slowly conducting fibres, some of which may be unmyelinated (Ralston and Ralston 1985, Ralston *et al.* 1987). Compared to the minority of large fibres, the function of these slow fibres is still poorly understood. In neither adult nor neonate is there any information about the natural activity conveyed by such fibres. We do not even know whether this system is active at birth, and if not, when activity begins.

Relationship between behavioural maturation and the development of the corticospinal system

The different features of corticospinal development described above are really only markers of the developmental timetable. The key issue is whether such changes are either necessary or sufficient for the normal maturation of skilled finger movements. Kuypers (1962) and Lawrence and Hopkins (1976) proposed that maturation of CM connections is essential for such movements. Lawrence and Hopkins had hand-reared infant monkeys from birth, and investigated the maturation of different aspects of their motor behaviour. At 3–4 weeks of age, the first signs of reaching were evident, although this was inaccurate and grasping was very clumsy. It formed part of a rather gross whole arm and hand movement. Smoother reaching was achieved in the third month and it was at this stage that the earliest signs of relatively independent finger movements (RIFMs) were considered to be present. Mature RIFMs were judged to be present at 7–8 months of age. A similar conclusion was reached by Galea and Darian-Smith (1995). Hinde *et al.* (1964) observed that infant monkeys first begin to groom other monkeys at around 6 months of age, and RIFMs are essential for grooming (Porter and Lemon 1993). Since, in the macaque monkey, CM projections to the hand are very weak at birth but are already clearly present at 2.5 months, it is possible that the establishment of CM connections could precede the onset of RIFMs, as defined by Lawrence and Hopkins (1976). The earliest signs of EMG responses to TMS were also seen at 3 months of age.

Lawrence and Hopkins went on to demonstrate that if monkeys were subjected to a bilateral pyramidotomy at birth, they were unable to perform RIFMs at a later age. This emphasizes the relatively late stage of corticospinal development at birth: a pyramidal lesion at this stage cannot be compensated for (Carr *et al.* 1993; see also Chapter 9). In assessing the contribution of the maturing CM system to the acquisition of hand skill in the normal infant, however, we must reiterate our earlier point that this is only one of many influential factors. As we stated (Armand *et al.* 1996):

". . it was not only the presence of the CM connections, but the manner in which these connections were used by the motor system that ultimately determined the motor behavior observed in the developing animal. It can be argued that the influence of important factors contributing to the execution of RIFM, such as the use of tactile feedback, visuomotor coordination, and, at higher levels of organization, the impact of experience, mimicry, and culture, cannot be expressed unless the motor pathways linking the cortex to the final common path are developed."

Concluding remarks

Recent research into the development of the corticospinal system have highlighted the protracted nature of the structural and functional changes involved. Rather than there being a sudden change at a particular age, there are gradual changes which last for several years (Eyre *et al.* 1991, Müller and Hömberg 1992, Armand *et al.* 1994, Müller *et al.* 1994). It is evident that the capacity to perform a precision grip is present long before the conduction velocity of the fastest fibres reaches an adult value, and this means that the corticospinal system is functional long before full myelination of the axons is complete. These longer and slower changes are of course paralleled by gradual and protracted improvements in motor skill (Halverson 1943, Forssberg *et al.* 1991, Müller and Hömberg 1992). Such changes may be important in determining the fine temporal structure of the motor programmes, leading to smoother coordination as well as better anticipatory control of reafferent sensory inputs generated by finger movement.

ACKNOWLEDGEMENTS

We thank The Wellcome Trust, Action Research and the CNRS–Royal Society Exchange Scheme for financial support.

REFERENCES

Adams, C.E., Mihailoff, G.A., Woodward, D.J. (1983) 'A transient component of the developing corticospinal tract arises in visual cortex.' *Neuroscience Letters*, **36**, 243–248.

Alisky, J.M., Swink, T.D., Tolbert, D.L. (1992) 'The postnatal spatial and temporal development of corticospinal projections in cats.' *Experimental Brain Research*, **88**, 265–276.

Armand, J. (1982) 'The origin, course and terminations of corticospinal fibers in various mammals.' *Progress in Brain Research*, **57**, 329–360.

—— Edgley, S.A., Lemon, R.N., Olivier, E. (1994) 'Protracted postnatal development of corticospinal projections from the primary motor cortex to hand motoneurones in the macaque monkey.' *Experimental Brain Research*, **101**, 178–182.

—— Olivier, E., Edgley , S.A., Lemon, R.N. (1996) 'The structure and function of the developing corticospinal tract. Some key issues.' *In:* Wing A.M., Haggard P., Flanagan, J.R. (Eds.) *Hand and Brain. The Neurophysiology and Psychology of Hand Movements.* San Diego: Academic Press, pp. 125–145.

—— —— —— —— (1997) 'The postnatal development of corticospinal projections from motor cortex to the cervical enlargement in the macaque monkey.' *Journal of Neuroscience*, **17**, 251–266.

Baldissera, F., Cavallari, P. (1993) 'Short-latency subliminal effects of transcranial magnetic stimulation on forearm motoneurones.' *Experimental Brain Research*, **96**, 513–518.

Baker, S.N., Olivier, E., Lemon, R.N. (1994) 'Recording an identified pyramidal volley evoked by transcranial magnetic stimulation in a conscious macaque monkey.' *Experimental Brain Research*, **99**, 529–532.

Barkovich, J.A., Lyon, G., Evrard, P. (1992) 'Formation, maturation, and disorders of white matter.' *American Journal of Neuroradiology*, **13**, 447–461.

Biber, M.P., Kneisley, L.W., LaVail, J.H. (1978) 'Cortical neurons projecting to the cervical and lumbar enlargements of the spinal cord in young and adult rhesus monkeys.' *Experimental Neurology*, **59**, 492–508.

Bortoff, G.A., Strick, P.L. (1993) 'Corticospinal terminations in two new-world primates: further evidence that corticomotoneuronal connections provide part of the neural substrate for manual dexterity.' *Journal of Neuroscience*, **13**, 5105–5118.

Brody, B.A., Kinney, H.C., Kloman, A.S., Gilles, F.H. (1987) 'Sequence of central nervous system myelination in human infancy. I. An autopsy study of myelination.' *Journal of Neuropathology and Experimental Neurology*, **46**, 283–301.

Cabana, T., Martin, G.F. (1984) 'Developmental sequence in the origin of descending spinal pathways. Studies using retrograde transport techniques in the North American opossum (*Didelphis virginiana*).' *Brain Research*, **317**, 247–263.

—— —— (1985) 'Corticospinal development in the North-American opossum: evidence for a sequence in the growth of cortical axons in the spinal cord and for transient projections.' *Brain Research*, **355**, 69–80.

Carr, L.J., Harrison, L.M., Evans, A.L. Stephens, J.A. (1993) 'Patterns of central motor reorganization in hemiplegic cerebral palsy.' *Brain*, **116**, 1223–1247.

D'Amato, C.J., Hicks, S.P. (1978) 'Normal development and post-traumatic plasticity of corticospinal neurons in rats.' *Experimental Neurology*, **60**, 557–569.

Dekkers, J., Becker, D.L., Cook, J.E., Navarrete, R. (1994) 'Early postnatal changes in the somatodendritic morphology of ankle flexor motoneurons in the rat.' *European Journal of Neuroscience*, **6**, 87–97.

Dum, R.P., Strick, P.L. (1991) 'The origin of corticospinal projections from the premotor areas in the frontal lobe.' *Journal of Neuroscience*, **11**, 667–689.

Edgley, S.A., Eyre, J.A., Lemon, R.N., Miller, S. (1990) 'Excitation of the corticospinal tract by electromagnetic and electrical stimulation of the scalp in the macaque monkey.' *Journal of Physiology*, **425**, 301–320.

Evans, A.L., Harrison, L.M., Stephens, J.A. (1990) 'Maturation of the cutaneomuscular reflex recorded from the first dorsal interosseous muscle in man.' *Journal of Physiology*, **428**, 425–440.

Eyre, J.A., Miller, S., Ramesh, V. (1991) 'Constancy of central conduction delays during development in man: investigation of motor and somatosensory pathways.' *Journal of Physiology*, **434**, 441–452.

Felix, D., Wiesendanger, M. (1971) 'Pyramidal and non-pyramidal motor cortical effects on distal forelimb muscles of monkeys.' *Experimental Brain Research*, **12**, 81–91.

Flament, D., Hall, E.J., Lemon, R.N. (1992) 'The development of cortico-motoneuronal projections investigated using magnetic brain stimulation in the infant macaque.' *Journal of Physiology*, **447**, 755–768.

Forssberg, H., Eliasson, A.C., Kinoshita, H., Johansson, R.S., Westling, G. (1991) 'Development of human precision grip. 1: Basic coordination of force.' *Experimental Brain Research*, **85**, 451–457.

Galea, M.P., Darian-Smith, I. (1995) 'Postnatal maturation of the direct corticospinal projections in the macaque monkey.' *Cerebral Cortex*, **5**, 518–540.

Goldstein, L.A., Kurz, E.M., Kalkbrenner, A.E., Sengelaub, D.R. (1993) 'Changes in dendritic morphology of rat spinal motoneurons during development and after unilateral target deletion.' *Developmental Brain Research*, **73**, 151–163.

Gracies, J.M., Meunier, S., Pierrot-Deseilligny E. (1994) 'Evidence for corticospinal excitation of presumed propriospinal neurones in man.' *Journal of Physiology*, **475**, 509–518.

Gribnau, A.A.M., De Kort, E.J.M., Dederen, P.J.W.C., Nieuwenhuys, R. (1986) 'On the development of the pyramidal tract in the rat. II. An anterograde tracer study of the outgrowth of the corticospinal fibers.' *Anatomy and Embryology*, **175**, 101–110.

Halverson, H.M. (1943) 'The development of prehension in infants.' *In:* Barker, R.G., Kounin, J.S., Wright, H.F. (Eds.) *Child Behavior and Development.* New York: McGraw Hill, pp. 49–65.

Heffner, R.S., Masterton, R.B. (1975) 'Variation in form of the pyramidal tract and its relationship to digital dexterity.' *Brain, Behavior and Evolution*, **12**, 161–200.

———— (1983) 'The role of the corticospinal tract in the evolution of human digital dexterity' *Brain, Behavior and Evolution*, **23**, 165–183.

Hinde, R.A., Rowell, T.E., Spencer-Booth, Y. (1964) 'Behaviour of socially living rhesus monkeys in their first six months.' *Proceedings of the Zoological Society of London*, **143**, 609–649.

Holt, A.B., Cheek, D.B., Mellits, E.D., Hill, D.E. (1975) 'Brain size and the relation of the primate to the non-primate.' *In:* Cheek, D.B. (Ed.) *Fetal and Postnatal Cellular Growth.* New York: John Wiley, pp. 23–44.

Humphrey, T. (1960) The development of the pyramidal tracts in human fetuses, correlated with cortical differentiation. *In:* Tower, D.B., Schadé, J.P. (Eds.) *Structure and Function of the Cerebral Cortex.* Amsterdam: Elsevier, pp. 93–103.

Jenny, A.B., Inukai, J. (1983) 'Principles of motor organization of the monkey cervical spinal cord.' *Journal of Neuroscience*, **3**, 567–575.

Joosten, E.A.J., Gribnau, A.A.M., Dederen, P.J.W.C. (1987) 'An anterograde tracer study of the developing corticospinal tract in the rat: three components.' *Brain Research*, **433**, 121–130.

Kalil, K. (1985) 'Development and plasticity of the sensorimotor cortex and pyramidal tract.' *In: Development, Organization and Processing in Somatosensory Pathways.* New York: Alan R. Liss, pp. 87–96.

Khater-Boidin, J., Duron, B. (1991) 'Postnatal development of descending motor pathways studied in man by percutaneous stimulation of the motor cortex and the spinal cord.' *International Journal of Developmental Neuroscience*, **9**, 15–26.

Koh, T.H.H.G., Eyre, J.A. (1988) 'Maturation of corticospinal tracts assessed by electromagnetic stimulation of the motor cortex.' *Archives of Disease in Childhood*, **63**, 1347–1352.

Kudo, N., Furukawa, F., Okado, N. (1993) 'Development of descending fibers to the rat embryonic spinal cord.' *Neuroscience Research*, **16**, 131–141.

Kuypers, H.G.J.M. (1962) 'Corticospinal connections: postnatal development in the rhesus monkey.' *Science*, **138**, 678–680.

—— (1981) 'Anatomy of the descending pathways.' *In:* Brookhart, J.M., Mountcastle, V.B. (Eds.) *Handbook of Physiology – The Nervous System II.* Bethesda, MD: American Physiological Society, pp. 597–666.

Langworthy, O.R. (1933) 'Development of behavior patterns and myelinization of the nervous system in the human fetus and infant.' *Contributions to Embryology*, **24**, 1–58.

Lawrence, D.G., Hopkins, D.A. (1976) 'The development of motor control in the rhesus monkey: evidence concerning the role of corticomotoneuronal connections.' *Brain*, **99**, 235–254.

—— Kuypers, H.G.J.M. (1968) 'The functional organization of the motor system in the monkey. I. The effects of bilateral pyramidal lesions.' *Brain*, **91**, 1–14.

Lemon, R.N. (1993) 'The G.L. Brown Prize Lecture. Cortical control of the primate hand.' *Experimental Physiology*, **78**, 263–301.

Ludolph, A.C., Hugon, J., Spencer, P.S. (1987) 'Non-invasive assessment of the pyramidal tract and motor pathway of primates.' *Electroencephalography and Clinical Neurophysiology*, **67**, 63–67.

Matthews, M.A., Duncan, D. (1971) 'A quantitative study of morphological changes accompanying the initiation and progress of myelin production in the dorsal funiculus of the rat spinal cord.' *Journal of Comparative Neurology*, **142**, 1–22.

Mihailoff, G.A., Adams, C.E., Woodward, D.J. (1984) 'An autoradiographic study of the postnatal development of sensorimotor and visual components of the corticopontine system.' *Journal of Comparative Neurology*, **222**, 116–127.

Müller, K., Hömberg, V. (1992) 'Development of speed of repetitive movements in children is determined by structural changes in corticospinal efferents.' *Neuroscience Letters*, **144**, 57–60.

—— —— Lenard, H-G. (1991) 'Magnetic stimulation of motor cortex and nerve roots in children. Maturation of cortico-motoneuronal projections.' *Electroencephalography and Clinical Neurophysiology*, **81**, 63–70.

—— Ebner, B., Hömberg, V. (1994) 'Maturation of fastest afferent and efferent central and peripheral pathways: no evidence for a constancy of central conduction delays.' *Neuroscience Letters*, **166**, 9–12.

Nathan, P.W., Smith, M.C., Deacon, P. (1990) 'The corticospinal tracts in man. Course and location of fibres at different segmental levels.' *Brain*, **113**, 303–324.

Oka, H., Samejima, A., Yamamoto, T. (1985) 'Post-natal development of pyramidal tract neurones in kittens.' *Journal of Physiology*, **363**, 481–499.

Olivier, E., Lemon, R.N., Edgley, S.A., Armand, J. (1994) 'Development of the primate corticospinal tract: changes in the conduction velocity of corticospinal fibres in anaesthetized neonatal and infant macaque monkeys.' *Journal of Physiology*, **476**, 27P.

—— Edgley, S.A., Armand, J., Lemon, R.N. (1997) 'An electrophysiological study of the postnatal development of the corticospinal system in the macaque monkey.' *Journal of Neuroscience*, **17**, 267–276.

Palmer, E., Ashby, P. (1992) 'Corticospinal projections to upper limb motoneurones in humans.' *Journal of Physiology*, **448**, 397–412.

Passingham, R.E. (1985) 'Rates of brain development in mammals including man.' *Brain, Behavior and Evolution*, **26**, 167–175.

Phillips, C.G. (1971) 'Evolution of the corticospinal tract in primates with special reference to the hand.' *In: Proceedings of the 3rd International Congress of the Primatological Society, Zurich. Vol. 2.* Basel: Karger, pp. 2–23.

Porter, R., Lemon, R.N. (1993) *Corticospinal Function and Voluntary Movement.* Oxford: Oxford University Press.

Ralston, D.D., Ralston, H.J. (1985) 'The terminations of corticospinal tract axons in the macaque monkey.' *Journal of Comparative Neurology*, **242**, 325–337.

—— Milroy, A.M., Ralston, H.J. (1987) 'Non-myelinated axons are rare in the medullary pyramids of the macaque monkey.' *Neuroscience Letters*, **73**, 215–219.

Reh, T., Kalil, K. (1981) 'Development of the pyramidal tract in the hamster. I. A light microscopic study.' *Journal of Comparative Neurology*, **200**, 55–67.

—— —— (1982) 'Development of the pyramidal tract in the hamster. II. An electron microscopic study.' *Journal of Comparative Neurology*, **205**, 77–88.

Schreyer, D.J., Jones, E.G. (1982) 'Growth and target finding by axons of the corticospinal tract in prenatal and postnatal rats.' *Neuroscience*, **7**, 1837–1853.

—— —— (1988) 'Axon elimination in the developing corticospinal tract of the rat.' *Brain Research*, **466**, 103–119. (*Erratum* appears in *Brain Research*, **467**, 320.)

Stanfield, B.B., O'Leary, D.D.M. (1985) 'The transient corticospinal projection from the occipital cortex during the postnatal development of the rat.' *Journal of Comparative Neurology*, **238**, 236–248.

Tanji, J. (1994) 'The supplementary motor area in the cerebral cortex.' *Neuroscience Research*, **19**, 251–268.

Theriault, E., Tatton, W.G. (1989) 'Postnatal redistribution of pericruciate motor cortical projections within the kitten spinal cord.' *Developmental Brain Research*, **45**, 219–237.

Tower, S.S. (1940) 'Pyramidal lesion in the monkey.' *Brain*, **63**, 36–90.

Weidenheim, K.M., Kress, Y., Epshteyn, I., Rashbaum, W.K., Lyman, W.D. (1992) 'Early myelination in the human fetal lumbosacral spinal cord: characterization by light and electron microscopy.' *Journal of Neuropathology and Experimental Neurology*, **51**, 142–149.

Yakovlev, P.I., Lecours, A-R. (1967) 'The myelogenetic cycles of regional maturation of the brain.' *In:* Minkowski, A. (Ed.) *Regional Development of the Brain in Early Life.* Oxford: Blackwell Scientific, pp. 3–70.

9

THE DEVELOPMENT OF DESCENDING MOTOR PATHWAYS IN CHILDREN WITH HEMIPLEGIC CEREBRAL PALSY: THE EFFECTS OF EARLY BRAIN DAMAGE

L.J. Carr and J.A. Stephens

The acquisition of motor skills requires the integration of many factors, including both peripheral and central sensory and motor systems. Any of these may be disrupted by injury. In man, the age at which a central lesion occurs appears to influence the functional outcome: outcome is generally better if damage is sustained early in development (Gardner *et al.* 1955, Teuber 1974, Finger and Wolf 1988). This is said to be due to the greater plasticity of the developing central nervous system (CNS). In man this hypothesis is supported by clinical observation and recent neurophysiological findings. Similar observations have been made in animals and are backed by histological evidence for CNS reorganization.

Animal evidence for CNS reorganization
Motor systems
The concept of plasticity of the developing CNS was championed by Kennard (1942), who compared the effects of ablation of the sensorimotor cortex in adult and infant macaque monkeys. She concluded that: 'In mammals comparable lesions of the cerebral cortex affecting motor status have far less permanent and severe effect when the injury is sustained in infancy than when it occurs in maturity.' These observations were not without precedent; Soltmann (1876) made unilateral lesions in the motor cortex of dogs at different ages. In one puppy, who walked normally following such a lesion, he showed that stimulation of the undamaged motor cortex elicited bilateral limb movements. This was not seen in dogs lesioned as adults. He postulated that the undamaged motor cortex had taken over the function of the damaged cortex (see Finger and Wolf 1988).

Animal evidence has now emerged indicating that after early CNS damage, cortical reorganization and novel corticospinal projections may be seen. Rats subjected to hemispherectomies in infancy may develop an anomalous corticospinal projection arising from the intact ipsilateral cortex (Hicks and D'Amato 1970, Leong and Lund 1973, Ono *et al.* 1994). Tracing studies have shown that, in addition, normally decussated corticospinal axons may recross the spinal cord into denervated areas (Reinoso and Castro 1989, Barth and Stanfield 1990, Rouiller *et al.* 1991). After unilateral pyramidotomies in young hamsters, immunohistochemical studies suggest that corticospinal fibres from the undamaged tract may show compensatory sprouting into the denervated cord, at the same time as branching in the normal side, thus making bilateral connections (Kuang and Kalil 1990). These workers further showed that sprouting was most robust following the earliest lesions and was not seen following pyramidotomies in the mature hamster (Merline and Kalil 1990).

Studies suggest that the anomalous ipsilateral corticospinal projections may make functional connections. Following unilateral CNS lesions in the young rat or hamster, such ipsilateral projections are associated with sparing of many aspects of forelimb function (Hicks and D'Amato 1970, Reh and Kalil 1982, Barth and Stanfield 1990). In rats, intracortical microstimulation of the intact hemisphere may evoke movements of the ipsilateral forelimb at low threshold (Kartje-Tillotson et al. 1985). Such findings are not reported in normal rodents or in rodents who sustain lesions when mature.

The above studies support the hypothesis that reorganization of neural connections is more likely if brain damage occurs early in development. However, when comparing rodents with man, it should be noted that in rodents the CNS is relatively immature at the time of birth; the brain is only a small proportion of the final adult size and the corticospinal tract has not decussated (this occurs postnatally on day 1 in the rat and day 3 in the hamster). Thus at the time of birth the maturity of the rodent CNS is approximately equivalent to that of a 16 week human fetus. Cats and primates may therefore provide better models for comparison, since here the corticospinal tract decussates before birth. In cats following neonatal hemispherectomy, corticospinal projections from the intact hemisphere may also develop into the ipsilateral spinal cord (Gómez-Pinilla et al. 1986). When compared with cats lesioned as adults, performance was significantly better in these cats in a range of tasks which evaluate movement, posture and sensory functions (Villablanca et al. 1986).

To date, primate studies have failed to demonstrate motor reorganization histologically. No anomalous corticospinal projections were detected in ten rhesus monkeys following unilateral ablation of the sensorimotor cortex between 6 days and 3 months of age (Sloper et al. 1983). Although ablation performed in infancy initially had a less disruptive effect, the eventual outcome was similar in both infant and adult lesioned monkeys (Passingham et al. 1983). Passingham and colleagues argued that Kennard may have misinterpreted this delayed manifestation of clinical signs as a permanent absence of deficits.

Cognitive function

Preservation of cognitive function has been reported by Goldman and Galkin (1978) in the case of a rhesus monkey who underwent bilateral resection of the prefrontal cortices antenatally (day 106 post conception). Its subsequent performance on delayed response tasks matched that of normal monkeys. Goldman found that the thalami, the principle source of projections to the prefrontal cortex, did not show the degeneration typically seen following postnatal lesions. Ectopic sulci and gyri were noted in the frontal, temporal and occipital lobes. This would suggest that anatomical and behavioural reorganization may occur in primates, but critically depends on the maturity of the brain at the time of damage. If one measures cortical maturity by the relative size of the brain compared to its final adult size, maturity at day 106 in the monkey matches that of a newborn human (see Passingham et al. 1983).

Sensory systems

In developing mammals neurons in the somatosensory cortex form discrete vertical columns, connected by gap junctions. These domains do not appear to be simple subsections of cortical maps and their functional significance remains unclear (Yuste *et al.* 1992). Following peripheral deafferentation or CNS ablation, cortical maps may show extensive reorganization in the primate somatosensory cortex. For example, following section of the median nerve at the wrist the cortex loses sensory input from the glabrous surface of the medial digits. After a period of recovery the deprived cortex becomes responsive to stimuli from other parts of the hand, outside median nerve territory. Conversely, following ablation of the area of cortex sensitive to light touch to the glabrous surface of the third digit, adjacent cortical sites become responsive to stimulation of this digit (Kaas 1991). Some changes occur very rapidly after the lesion has been made, suggesting that some of this plasticity results from the unmasking of weaker inputs from the surrounding cortical networks, rather than true structural reorganization (Merzenich and Sameshima 1993). However, structural reorganization is reported, particularly after early lesions; for example, Schneider (1979) found histological and behavioural evidence of anomalous axonal growth in the visual pathways of Syrian hamsters following early lesions. These changes were not found in hamsters lesioned in adult life.

Evidence for CNS reorganization in man

There is much clinical evidence to suggest that in man early CNS damage may result in reorganization and sparing of function. Recent advances in neuroimaging and neurophysiological techniques have provided futher evidence for CNS reorganization. Studies have particularly looked at the development of speech and of sensory and motor functions and are briefly reviewed below.

Speech

In 1861 Broca localized the area of speech production to the third left frontal convolution. Soon afterwards he noted that following damage to this area subsequent recovery of language appeared to be age dependent; after left-sided stroke adults generally remained aphasic whereas those with congenital left-sided lesions developed speech. He speculated that in young children the third right convolution may substitute for the left (Berker *et al.* 1986). It is now recognized that the left hemisphere is the dominant side in around 95% of the population. More recent studies confirm that articulate language may remain largely intact following unilateral lesions of the dominant hemisphere and that this phenomenon appears to be crucially age dependent (Woods 1980, Vargha-Khadem *et al.* 1985).

Sensory function

Writing in 1885, Gowers observed: 'It is a curious fact that lesions of the brain occurring in infancy or early childhood seem never to cause permanent loss of sensibility, although they must sometimes involve the sensory paths or centres.' Gardner *et al.* (1955) compared the outcome of patients undergoing hemispherectomy for infantile hemiplegia and for tumour and found that sensory modalities were better retained in subjects with infantile hemiplegia. Uvebrant (1988) confirms that sensory function is significantly better in those with congenital lesions, particularly if born preterm. A recent case report suggests that retained sensory function may be associated with bilateral neural reorganization. Magnetoencephalography and magnetic resonance imaging were used to localize somatosensory function in the cortex of a young adult with a congenital middle cerebral artery infarction which had destroyed both primary and secondary somatosensory areas in the left hemisphere (Lewine *et al.* 1994). Clinical examination of the hemiplegic right hand revealed only mild impairment of pain, touch and temperature. Stereognosis and graphaesthesia were near normal. Electrical stimulaton of the right median nerve evoked activity in two areas: an intact region of the contralateral left inferior temporal gyrus, not normally responsive to somatosensory stimulation, and also ipsilaterally over the primary somatosensory cortex of the intact right hemisphere. Bilateral somatosensory evoked potentials have also been reported in four patients after hemispherectomy (Mauguière and Desmedt 1989).

Interestingly some children with early brain damage have hyperaesthesia, with enhanced light touch and two-point discrimination (Rudel *et al.* 1966). This could also result from reorganization of somatosensory pathways.

Motor function
It has long been recognized that congenital hemiplegia is never manifest by the severe hemiparesis seen in adults acquiring similar sized lesions. Important factors affecting motor outcome after focal CNS damage are likely to include the time, site and extent of the lesion. In addition, sensory abnormalities and visual deficits, as well as cognitive and behavioural problems will all influence motor function. Considering only the motor system, there is variation between subjects in the site and extent of lesions, and until recently, accurate timing of early insults was difficult. The detailed functional assessment of subjects undergoing hemispherectomy has provided valuable insight into the particular importance of the timing of the lesion (Gardner *et al.* 1955). Motor outcome was compared in two groups of adults after hemispherectomy: those with a history of epilepsy associated with infantile hemiplegia and those with glioma. Gardner *et al.* concluded from their own and earlier studies that in subjects with infantile hemiplegia, hemispherectomy rarely caused more than a transient increase in the existing hemiplegia, and noted that useful hand function was often preserved. This suggests that in these subjects the unaffected hemisphere was already driving motor function on the hemiplegic side. The results are in marked contrast to the poor motor outcome of adults with gliomas. Recent studies confirm that motor impairment is more severe in children with postnatal hemiplegia than in those with congenital hemiplegia, and least severe in those with a clear preterm insult (Uvebrant 1988).

Altered neuronal connections are futher suggested by anomalous motor outcome. In childhood hemiplegia, particularly if manifest within the first year, a high incidence of persistent mirror movements is noted (Woods and Teuber 1978). These are illustrated in Figure 9.1b, where surface EMG was recorded from the left and right hands of a child with congenital hemiplegia and mirror movements. When moving the fingers of his unaffected left hand, symmetrical involuntary EMG activity is also seen in the fingers of the right hand. The activity is of similar duration on both sides. This contrasts with a healthy child making

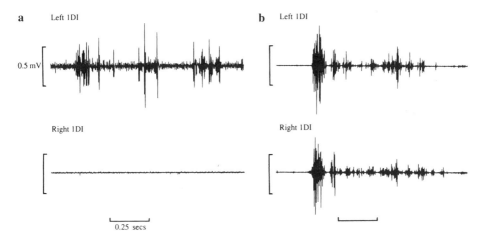

Fig. 9.1. EMG activity in left and right intrinsic hand muscles. Subjects opposed the thumb and index finger of the left hand with the right hand relaxed. Surface EMG was recorded from the left and right 1DI muscles. *(a)* Recording from a healthy 8-year-old child: EMG activity is restricted to the left hand. *(b)* Recording from a 5-year-old child with a congenital right-sided hemiplegia and strong mirror movements (Group A) shows simultaneous and symmetrical EMG activity in the left and right 1DI muscles.

similar voluntary movements of the left hand (Fig. 9.1a), where EMG activity is restricted to the left hand.

Mirror movements are described during normal development but are pathological if they are pronounced and persistent (Connolly and Stratton 1968, Schott and Wyke 1981). They are typically strongest in the hands and forearms. Observations from our group and those of other colleagues (personal communications) would suggest that around 15% of children with hemiplegic cerebral palsy show strong mirror movements, though the study of Woods and Teuber suggested a higher incidence approaching 50%.

Neuroradiological studies suggest that the unaffected hemisphere may play a role in the recovery of motor function of adults after stroke (Chollet *et al.* 1991). In subjects with good recovery from striatocapsular motor stroke, positron emission tomography has shown abnormal bilateral activation of motor pathways on performing tasks with the recovered hand, with the recruitment of additional motor areas. Patients also showed extension of the hand representation area of the unaffected somatosensory cortex (Weiller *et al.* 1992, 1993). Sabatini *et al.* (1994) used positron emission tomography to study hand function in a man with an early left-sided hemiplegia and good motor recovery. Activation of either the left or right hand led to increased cerebral blood flow in the left premotor and sensorimotor cortices only, with no detectable flow changes in the right hemisphere.

Recent advances in neurophysiological techniques now allow detailed *in vivo* assessment of many aspects of motor function. Three techniques will be described in detail since these formed the basis of our study of motor pathway organization in children with hemiplegia (Carr *et al.* 1993).

This technique has been developed as a safe and painless method of noninvasively exciting the motor cortex in man (Barker *et al.* 1985). Previously electrical stimulation had been used to study corticospinal projections and to map the sensory and motor homunculi (Penfield and Boldrey 1937, Merton and Morton 1980), but when used transcranially this technique is painful. The basic laws of electromagnetism describe how a time-varying magnetic field will induce an electric field in any medium through which it passes. If the medium is conductive, current will flow. Magnetic fields of the frequency required to cause neuromuscular stimulation pass through body structures without signficant attenuation, so that the high resistance of the skull does not affect the distribution of the magnetic field below the stimulating coil (Barker *et al.* 1990). The shape, position and orientation of the stimulating coil affect the characteristics of the electric field induced in the cortex and may be calculated from mathematical models (Roth *et al.* 1991). If applied over the motor cortex, transcranial magnetic stimulation evokes electromyographic (EMG) responses at short latency. It is assumed that these responses are mediated by the large diameter, fast conducting corticomotoneuronal fibres of the corticospinal tract. Evidence for this is provided by the short central conduction time of these responses (Edgley *et al.* 1990) and the gradient of the threshold and distribution of responses, which concurs with our knowledge of corticomotoneuronal projections (see Thompson *et al.* 1990).

The development of transcranial cortical stimulation has been particularly important in demonstrating functional corticospinal projections. In man, magnetic stimulation has been used to study maturation of these tracts (Koh and Eyre 1988, Eyre *et al.* 1991, Müller *et al.* 1991) and the disruptive effects of various pathological conditions, such as demyelinating disease (Boniface *et al.* 1991) and motoneuron disease (Berardelli *et al.* 1991). Transcranial stimulation has been used as a prognostic indicator in adults following stroke (Dominkus *et al.* 1990, Hömberg *et al.* 1991, Heald *et al.* 1993). Heald *et al.* found that measurement of the central motor conduction time within 72 hours of the stroke was predictive of functional outcome at 12 months. Patients with a normal central motor conduction time rapidly made a good functional recovery. Those with delayed central conduction time or raised threshold to stimulation made a slower recovery although final outcome was similar. Patients in whom central motor conduction was absent were at high risk of stroke-related death or made a slow, poor functional recovery. Recently magnetic stimulation has provided evidence for plasticity of motor maps in man in a number of pathological conditions including amputation, spinal cord injury, congenital mirror movements and after early hemispherectomy (Cohen *et al.* 1991). Brouwer and Ashby (1990) found evidence for altered corticospinal projections in children with spastic diplegia. Benecke *et al.* (1991) demonstrated abnormal ipsilateral EMG responses in upper limb muscles following early hemispherectomy, as did Farmer *et al.* (1991) in children with congenital hemiplegia.

CUTANEOMUSCULAR REFLEXES

Assessment of cutaneous and stretch reflexes have been part of clinical examination since the 19th century when it was recognized that they may be altered in certain neurological conditions. Examining the stretch reflex in human biceps, Hammond (1960) recognized

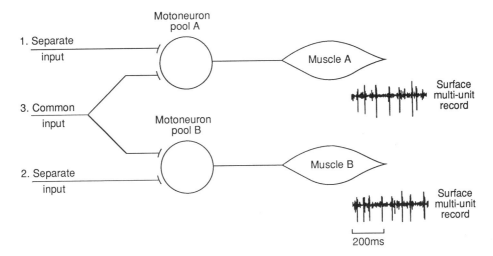

Fig. 9.2. Schematic representation of the last order inputs to two motoneuron pools A and B, which supply muscles A and B respectively. Cross-correlograms may be constructed by comparing the times of occurrence of motor unit spikes in the two multi-unit records. If motoneuron pools A and B share branches of a common stem presynaptic input (input 3) their discharges will show short-term synchronization, resulting in a short duration central peak in the cross-correlogram. This is not present if the inputs to the motoneurons are separate (inputs 1 and 2).

that it contained long-latency components that could not be readily explained by activity in fast conducting spinal pathways. Similar long-latency components were seen in the cutaneous reflex recorded from the contracting muscles of the hand (Caccia *et al.* 1973). The physiology of these late components has been the subject of intense debate as to whether they result from a slow afferent loop or a transcortical reflex (see Matthews 1991).

Stephens and his group have extensively examined the cutaneomuscular reflex (see Chapter 7). The reflex shows a maturational profile: initially it is monophasic with only an early excitatory (E1) component; this diminishes in size as the child matures, and the later components (I1 and E2) become more prominent (Issler and Stephens 1983, Evans *et al.* 1990). The late components of the reflex may be attenuated or abolished by CNS lesions of dorsal columns, sensorimotor cortex or corticospinal tract (Jenner and Stephens 1982). These observations have led to the hypothesis that the late E2 component has a transcortical pathway, while the E1 and I1 components are spinal reflexes.

CROSS-CORRELATION ANALYSIS OF EMG

Stimulation techniques are arguably an artificial way of examining the neural mechanisms that generate voluntary movements. Recording from different muscles during spontaneous movements, cross-correlation analysis of motor unit discharges allows exploration of the underlying muscle synergies, particularly the distribution of shared synaptic drive to the respective motoneuron pool. Moore *et al.* (1970) were the first to use this technique to investigate neural connections. The authors showed that when correlograms were constructed between the spike trains of two neurons, their different primary and secondary features could be used to infer the underlying synaptic connections generating the correlation. One such example is demonstrated in Figure 9.2, where two motoneurons (A and B) both receive an excitatory input from a branched last-order common-stem presynaptic fibre (input 3). Such an arrangement can be expected to produce a short duration peak in the cross-correlogram of discharges from the two cells, centred around time zero. Kirkwood and Sears (1978) developed a theoretical framework showing that the time course of such a correlogram peak was dependent on the size and shape of the common excitatory postsynaptic potentials and on the firing characteristics of the motoneurons. Thus short duration central peaks in cross-correlograms constructed between different motor units may be taken as likely evidence of activity in branched monosynaptic inputs to the motoneurons (Sears and Stagg 1976, Datta and Stephens 1990, Kirkwood and Sears 1991).

Study

Our recent study (Carr *et al.* 1993) examined 33 subjects with hemiplegia using the three techniques described above. It aimed to examine the effects of early brain damage on the development of the central motor pathways to the upper limbs, to determine whether re-organization might occur and if so, whether this had any functional effect.

Farmer *et al.* (1991) had previously used these techniques to assess four children all of whom had strong mirror movements and congenital hemiplegia. In these subjects they found evidence for anomalous motor pathways, suggesting that corticospinal projections from the undamaged cortex had branched abnormally to supply homologous motoneuron pools bilatcrally. Our study, summarized below, confirms and extends these observations.

Methods

The 33 hemiplegic subjects were aged from 2 to 26 years. Nine subjects had acquired a hemiplegia (between the ages of 4 months and 23 years). The remaining 24 subjects had congenital hemiplegia, where damage had occurred before the end of the neonatal period (28 days), usually pre- or perinatally. The timing of the CNS insult was gauged from clinical history and neuroimaging if available. The hemiplegia was right-sided in 22 subjects and lcft-sidcd in 11. For comparison 17 healthy subjects aged 2–21 years were also studied.

Subjects with mirror movements were actively recruited to the study. The intensity of any unintentional movements in the opposite hand were graded from 0 to 4 in all subjects, where 0 = no clearly imitative movement; 1 = barely discernible but repetitive movement; 2 = slight but unsustained movement or stronger, but briefer repetitive movement; 3 = strong sustained repetitive movement; and 4 = movement equal to that expected for the intended hand (Woods and Teuber 1978). The ability to perform discrete independent finger movements with the hemiplegic hand was also assessed.

Surface EMG was recorded using Neurolog modules from left and right forearm extensor muscles and left and right first dorsal interosseus (1DI) muscles in all subjects. Recording electrodes were made from neonatal ECG electrodes, cut down to reduce their recording area. The filtered, amplified EMG was saved on magnetic tape for future analyses (Racal Store 4).

Magnetic brain stimulation was performed using a Magstim 200 stimulator and a 'figure of eight' coil. The coil design allows focal cortical stimulation, since the peak magnetic field (2.2 tesla) lies beneath the intersection of the two loops. The coil was placed tangentially over the hand area of each motor cortex in the sagittal plane. Any EMG responses were recorded from left and right 1DI, usually with a low level of ongoing background EMG, since muscle preactivation is often necessary if responses are to be elicited in younger subjects (Koh and Eyre 1988). In each subject the mean latency and area of at least three responses was calculated using computer software (SIGAVG program, CED).

Cutaneomuscular reflexes were evoked by stimulating the digital nerves of the index finger using ring electrodes (Medelec E/DS-K16639). Stimulation was at around twice threshold for perception with a frequency of 3 per second and pulse width of 100 ms. The reflex was then recorded from the preactivated muscles of the hand or forearm (IDI or forearm extensors) on both the stimulated and non-stimulated sides. The rectified EMG was time-locked to the stimulus and the result of around 500 stimulations averaged using computer software (SIGAVG program, CED). This averaging is usually necessary to show the reflex clearly; it takes a few minutes and is well tolerated by children.

Cross-correlograms were constructed by comparing the time of occurrence of motor unit spikes. Medium and large amplitude spikes were selected from multi-unit EMGs recorded from left and right upper limbs using a level detector (Neurolog NL 200). The resulting trigger pulses were passed into a microcomputer via a CED 1401 laboratory interface. At least 2000 spikes were used to construct cross-correlograms of 1 ms bin width.

Results

The clinical and neurophysiological findings identified four separate groups of hemiplegic subjects (A, B, C and D). Table 9.1 summarizes the clinical features and results of these four groups. The distinguishing features of each group will be discussed in turn.

CONTROL SUBJECTS

Mirror movements were absent or weak in all subjects (grades 0–2, n = 17).

Focal magnetic stimulation of either motor cortex evoked EMG responses of short latency in the contralateral 1DI (range 13–26 ms, n = 11). Ipsilateral responses were not seen. A typical example is shown in Figure 9.3.

Following stimulation of the digital nerves, in all control subjects (n = 12) the cutaneomuscular reflex was seen on the stimulated side only. In the ten older subjects the late I1 and E2 components had developed. An example is shown in Figure 9.4.

Cross-correlograms were constructed from multi-unit EMG recordings taken from homologous muscle pairs. In all control subjects (n = 14) correlograms were flat, indicating that during voluntary activity there was no evidence for activity in common-stem presynaptic fibres supplying left and right homologous motoneuron pools of the hands and forearms. An example is shown in Figure 9.5.

GROUP A

The 11 hemiplegic subjects all had congenital hemiplegia with very strong mirror move-

185

TABLE 9.1
Summary of clinical features and results

Group	N	RIFM	Strong MM	Peak in L/R correlogram	I1,E2 non-stim	Response to magnetic stimulation of: Undamaged MC Ipsi	Undamaged MC Contra	Damaged MC Ipsi	Damaged MC Contra
A	11	5	11	11	7/7	10/10	10/10	0/10	0/10
B	10	3	0	0	0	10/10	10/10	0/10	4/10
C	3	0	0	0	0	0/3	3/3	0/3	0/3
D	9	9	0	0	0	0/9	9/9	0/9	9/9
						Left MC		*Right MC*	
Control	17	N/A	0	0	0	0/12	12/12	0/12	12/12

RIFM = the ability to make relatively independent finger movements with the hemiplegic hand.
Strong MM = mirror movements grade 3–4.
Peak in L/R correlogram = central peak seen in cross-correlograms constructed between motor unit spikes of left and right 1DI muscles.
I1,E2 non-stim = I1,E2 components of cutaneomuscular reflex recorded on non-stimulated side following stimulation of digital nerves of unaffected hand, expressed as a fraction of the number of subjects with an I1,E2 component on the stimulated side.
MC = motor cortex. Ipsi/Contra = ipsilateral/contralateral 1DI.

ments (grades 3–4), of which an example is shown in Figure 9.1b. Five subjects were able to make relatively independent finger movements of the affected hand.

Focal magnetic stimulation of the damaged motor cortex failed to evoke EMG responses in any subject (n = 10). In contrast, stimulation of the undamaged motor cortex always evoked bilateral responses in both contralateral and ipsilateral 1DI (n = 10). An example is shown in Figure 9.6. In each subject the EMG responses were of similar size on the two sides and of similar short latency (responses ranged from 14–24 ms, with the ipsilateral response occurring from 2 ms before to 2.6 ms after the contralateral response). Paired t tests failed to show significant differences between the area or latency of responses on the two sides ($p > 0.05$).

• *Cutaneomuscular reflexes.* These were recorded following stimulation of the digital nerves of the unaffected hand in nine subjects. In seven subjects a mature triphasic reflex was evoked on the stimulated side and in six of these the I1 and E2 components were recorded simultaneously on the non-stimulated side (see Figure 9.4). In the remaining subject only the I1 component was recorded bilaterally. The E1 component was never recorded bilaterally. In two young subjects only the early E1, I1 components were evoked on the stimulated side and there was no modulation of EMG on the nonstimulated side.

Stimulation of the hemiplegic hand evoked a cutaneomuscular reflex in eight subjects. This was always restricted to the stimulated side and only the early components of the reflex were evoked, namely an E1 component (n = 5) or an E1 and I1 component (n = 3).

• *Cross-correlation analysis.* In all subjects from Group A (n = 11) there were short-duration peaks centred at time zero when cross-correlograms were constructed between motor unit spikes of homologous left and right 1DI. An example is shown in Figure 9.6. Similar results were obtained when cross-correlograms were constructed for left and right forearm

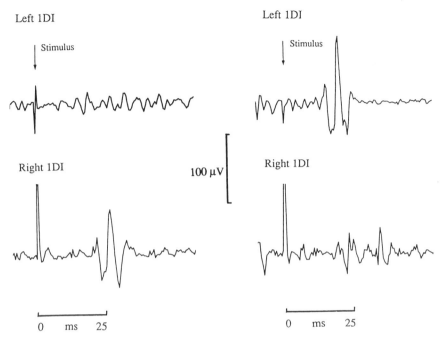

A Stimulate left motor cortex   **B** Stimulate right motor cortex

Left 1DI   Left 1DI

Stimulus   Stimulus

Right 1DI   100 µV   Right 1DI

0   ms   25   0   ms   25

Fig. 9.3. Focal magnetic transcranial stimulation in a healthy 10-year-old child. The coil was discharged over the hand area of the motor cortex at time zero and EMG recorded from left and right 1DI, while the subject gently abducted the index fingers. *(a)* Stimulation of the left motor cortex evokes a response in the contralateral right 1DI. *(b)* Stimulation of the right motor cortex evokes a response in the contralateral left 1DI.

extensors (10/11 subjects) and left and right abductor digiti minimi (3/3 subjects). The duration of these peaks ranged from 12–27.3 ms (mean 17.5 ms). Central peaks were never present in correlograms constructed between nonhomologous muscle pairs.

GROUP B
This group comprised ten subjects of whom eight had a congenital hemiplegia and two had acquired their hemiplegia later in life, at 9 months and 7 years respectively. Mirror movements were absent or weak in these subjects (grades 0–2). Three subjects were able to make relatively independent movements of the fingers of the hemiplegic hand.
• *Focal magnetic brain stimulation.* Stimulation of the damaged motor cortex failed to evoke any EMG response in six subjects. In four subjects responses were seen in the contralateral 1DI *(i.e.* in the hemiplegic hand) ranging from 17–22 ms. Interestingly, three of these subjects had good function of the hemiplegic hand.
    Stimulation of the undamaged motor cortex evoked bilateral responses in both contralateral and ipsilateral 1DI in all subjects (n = 10). However, in contrast to Group A, ipsilateral

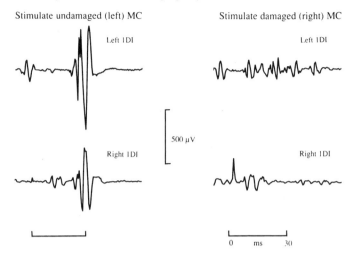

AB: 14 years. Left sided hemiplegia, pronounced mirror movements.

Stimulate undamaged (left) MC   Stimulate damaged (right) MC

Left 1DI   Left 1DI

500 μV

Right 1DI   Right 1DI

0   ms   30

Fig. 9.4. Cutaneomuscular reflexes recorded from left and right 1DI, following stimulation of the digital nerves of the right index finger at 3/second. The reflex is shown in a healthy control subject and in subject AB from Group A, who has a congenital left-sided hemiplegia and strong mirror movements. Rectified EMG was averaged from at least 500 stimulations, time-locked to the stimulus. In the control subject a triphasic response (E1, I1 and E2) is seen in right 1DI. There is no modulation of ongoing EMG in left 1DI. In subject AB stimulation of the unaffected right hand evokes a triphasic response in right 1DI. The I1 and E2 components are seen simultaneously in the unstimulated left 1DI.

responses were significantly later and smaller than contralateral responses (paired t test, $p<0.05$). On average the ipsilateral response occurred 4 ms later than the contralateral response (range 0.5–13.5 ms later, absolute latencies 14.5–31.5 ms) and was 50% smaller (the ipsilateral area ranged from 4% to 120% of the contralateral area). These differences were particularly marked in the two subjects with acquired hemiplegia. Figure 9.7 shows the results of magnetic stimulation in subject JA from Group B.

• *Cutaneomuscular reflexes.* Reflexes were recorded from nine subjects following stimulation of the digital nerves of the unaffected hand with a mature triphasic response in seven. In all subjects the reflex was only evoked on the stimulated side. Similarly when the hemiplegic hand was stimulated the reflex was restricted to the stimulated side (n = 10). In eight subjects only the early components were present. In two subjects a triphasic reflex was seen; both had good hand function.

• *Cross-correlation analysis.* In subjects from Group B all cross-correlograms constructed between EMGs of left and right muscle pairs were flat (n = 10), suggesting that the left and right motoneuron pools do not share common-stem last-order fibres. An example is shown in Figure 9.6.

GROUP C

As a group these three subjects were the most severely affected in the study. All had acquired

188

Cutaneomuscular reflex response to stimulation of right index finger

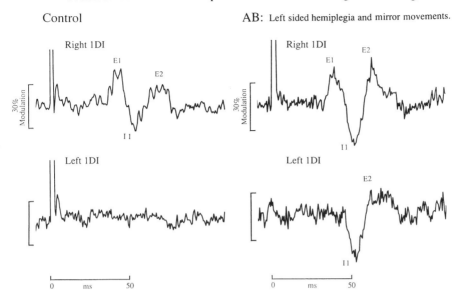

Fig. 9.5. Cross-correlograms constructed from motor unit spikes of multi-unit EMG recorded from left and right 1DI while both hands were active. Each cross-correlogram was constructed from at least 3500 spikes for each side. In a subject from Group A there is a central peak of around 15 ms duration. In contrast, no peaks are present in the correlograms of a healthy control subject or of a subject from Group B.

a dense hemiplegia after infancy, at 2 years, 10 years and 23 years. None could perform independent movements of the fingers of the hemiplegic hand. Mirror movements were absent or weak (grades 0–2).

• *Focal magnetic stimulation.* Responses were evoked only following magnetic stimulation of the undamaged motor cortex (n = 3). Responses were seen in the contralateral 1DI and were of short latency (range 18–22.5 ms). Ipsilateral responses were not seen. Stimulation of the damaged motor cortex failed to evoke any response.

• *Cutaneomuscular reflexes.* Following stimulation of the digital nerves of the unaffected hand a triphasic response was recorded on the stimulated side (n = 3). Stimulation of the hemiplegic hand evoked only the early E1, I1 components of the reflex (n = 3). The reflex was always entirely restricted to the stimulated side.

• *Cross-correlation analysis.* Cross-correlograms between EMGs of left and right muscle pairs were flat.

GROUP D

This group of nine subjects had the mildest hemiplegia overall. The hemiplegia was congenital in six subjects and acquired before 3 years of age in three subjects. All subjects could perform independent finger movements with the hemiplegic hand. Mirror movements were absent or weak (grades 0–2).

Control. LP: 10 years. Healthy child.

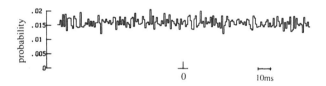

Group A. MP: 17 years. Hemiplegia, pronounced mirror movements.

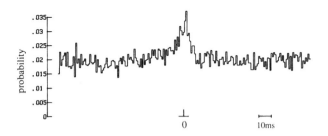

Group B. JA: 16 years. Hemiplegia, no mirror movements.

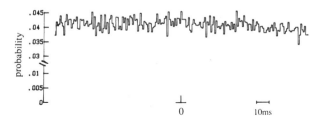

Fig. 9.6. Focal magnetic transcranial stimulation in a 14-year-old subject from Group A with a congenital left-sided hemiplegia and strong mirror movements. Stimulation of the undamaged motor cortex evokes an EMG response in both the contralateral right 1DI and the ipsilateral left 1DI. The two responses are of similar size and latency. No responses are evoked from the damaged motor cortex.

Magnetic stimulation of either motor cortex evoked short-latency responses in the contralateral 1DI (range 13.5–18 ms), as had been seen in control subjects. No ipsilateral responses were seen.

• *Cutaneomuscular reflexes.* In these subjects (n = 9) the cutaneomuscular reflex was always restricted to the stimulated side. The configuration of the reflex showed some asymmetry between the affected and unaffected sides; the E2 component was present on the unaffected side in eight subjects, but in only five subjects on the affected side.

190

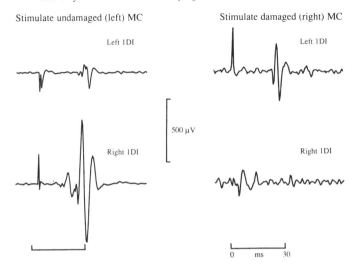

JA: 16 years. Left sided hemiplegia, no mirror movements.

Stimulate undamaged (left) MC   Stimulate damaged (right) MC

Left 1DI   Left 1DI

500 μV

Right 1DI   Right 1DI

0   ms   30

Fig. 9.7. Focal magnetic transcranial stimulation in a 16-year-old subject from Group B with a congenital left-sided hemiplegia but no mirror movements. Stimulation of the undamaged motor cortex evokes an EMG response in both the contralateral right 1DI and the ipsilateral left 1DI. The ipsilateral response is smaller and of longer latency than the contralateral response. Stimulation of the damaged motor cortex evokes a response in the contralateral 1DI at short latency.

• *Cross-correlation analysis.* In subjects from Group D cross-correlograms were flat between EMGs of left and right muscle pairs.

Discussion

The principle conclusion of the study is that considerable reorganization of descending motor pathways may follow early CNS damage. To summarize the results: evidence of novel corticospinal projections was found in 21 of the 33 hemiplegic subjects (those from Groups A and B). The two groups showed different clinical and neurophysiological features, suggesting that two distinct patterns of reorganization may occur.

Subjects from Group A all had strong mirror movements. Cortical stimulation of the undamaged motor cortex evoked symmetrical responses in both the contralateral and ipsilateral hands. Cross-correlation analysis of multi-unit EMG indicated the presence of common last-order inputs to homologous left and right motoneuron pools. Taken together the results suggest that corticospinal axons have branched bilaterally to supply both left and right motoneuron pools of distal upper-limb muscles. This conclusion corroborates the findings of the earlier study by Farmer *et al.* (1991).

Subjects from Group B did not have strong mirror movements. They showed ipsilateral responses following stimulation of the undamaged motor cortex, but these responses were smaller and later than the contralateral responses. Branched last-order presynaptic inputs were not detected using cross-correlation analysis. Thus it would appear that corticospinal

191

axons from the undamaged cortex are distributed bilaterally as separate, non-branched projections.

Subjects in Groups C and D did not show neurophysiological evidence of reorganization of central motor pathways. The former group were clinically the most severely affected in the study. Cortical stimulation failed to evoke EMG responses in the hemiplegic hand. In adults with unilateral stroke this finding is associated with severe clinical deficits (Berardelli *et al.* 1991, Hömberg *et al.* 1991, Heald *et al.* 1993). Subjects from Group D all had mild hemiplegia. The results of cortical stimulation were indistinguishable from those of the control subjects. In adults this result is associated with mild clinical deficits (Hömberg *et al.* 1991).

EVIDENCE FOR REORGANIZATION OF MOTOR PATHWAYS

• *Magnetic brain stimulation and cross-correlation analysis.* In hemiplegic subjects from Groups A and B, stimulation of the undamaged motor cortex evoked bilateral responses in both ipsilateral and contralateral 1DI muscles (n = 20). A number of mechanisms could account for the abnormal ipsilateral responses. Firstly they may simply result from stimulus spread to the contralateral cortex. A number of considerations make this unlikely, in particular the observation that ipsilateral EMG responses were evoked in none of the control subjects (n = 12) and in only 20 of the hemiplegic subjects given magnetic stimulation (n = 32). Only following stimulation of the undamaged motor cortex were ipsilateral responses seen, indeed no EMG responses were evoked in 19 of the hemiplegic subjects following maximal stimulation of the damaged motor cortex. (For a more detailed discussion, see Carr *et al.* 1993.)

It is therefore more likely that the ipsilateral EMG responses seen in subjects from Groups A and B reflect the presence of abnormal corticospinal projections that have developed from the undamaged motor cortex to supply ipsilateral motoneuron pools of the hemiplegic hand. To consider the underlying pathophysiology: one possibility is that corticospinal axons have branched abnormally to supply motoneuron pools on both sides of the spinal cord. As discussed above there is evidence that collateral sprouting of axons across the cord may follow unilateral damage in subprimate species (Gómez-Pinilla *et al.* 1986, Kuang and Kalil 1990). If this were the case in our subjects one would predict that unilateral cortical stimulation would result in symmetrical, bilateral motor evoked responses. Such branching would also result in short duration central peaks in cross-correlograms constructed between homologous left and right muscle pairs. This combination of observations was found in subjects from Group A. Cross-correlogram peaks in these subjects were of a mean duration of 17.5 ms. Multi-unit data, as used in the present study, lead to some dispersion of the central peaks, and values of around 17 ms would be consistent with the hypothesis that the peaks are generated largely by monosynaptic EPSPs arising from branched presynaptic inputs (Sears and Stagg 1976, Bremner *et al.* 1991, Farmer *et al.* 1991, Carr et al. 1993).

Central cross-correlogram peaks were seen only in subjects from Group A and only between homologous left and right muscle pairs. They were not present between nonhomologous muscle pairs. This suggests that the abnormal branched inputs are highly specific and supply only homologous motoneuron pools. This is supported clinically by the strong mirror movements seen in all these subjects, which show such precise symmetry.

In Group B the results suggest a different pattern of reorganization. In these subjects the ipsilateral and contralateral 1DI responses evoked by magnetic stimulation of the undamaged cortex showed significant differences in the latency and size of response on the two sides, implying that they are mediated by different fibres. This argument is strengthened by the results of cross-correlation analysis, which did not show evidence of activity in branched last-order inputs between homologous muscle pairs. Although the thresholds of response to magnetic stimulation were not examined in detail, no consistent differences were observed in the thresholds of the ipsilateral and contralateral EMG responses. This suggests that the fibres of the respective tracts have similar conduction velocities. In the absence of histological evidence, the precise anatomy of the ipsilateral pathways in Group B cannot be determined at this stage. However, there are a number of possibilities, outlined below.

(1) Enhancement of normal ipsilateral corticospinal projections. In primates ipsilateral corticospinal projections have their greatest influence over proximal muscles. They do not normally make direct corticomotoneuronal projections, but synapse with interneurons in the spinal cord and tend to be rather slowly conducting (Kuypers 1973). However, there is evidence that the ipsilateral corticospinal tract influences upper-limb function; Colebatch and Gandevia (1989) have shown that in adults with acquired hemiplegia the 'unaffected' arm is weak. Weakness is most marked proximally, but grip strength is also diminished. In healthy adults cortical stimulation does not normally evoke ipsilateral EMG responses. Futhermore, stimulation studies in adults recovering from stroke have failed to show abnormal ipsilateral EMG responses in biceps muscle (Palmer *et al.* 1992). It is possible that if damage occurs early these projections may be enhanced.

(2) Ipsilateral projections may have developed *de novo* from the undamaged motor cortex. This has been observed in lower mammals as discussed in the introduction but to date has not been observed in primates.

(3) Stabilization of ipsilateral projections which occur only transiently during normal development. During development in the opossum and the cat, transient ipsilateral corticospinal projections have been seen which are subsequently retracted (Cabana and Martin 1985, Alisky *et al.* 1992).

(4) Enhancement of cortical connections to brainstem pathways. The reticulospinal tract projects bilaterally and is rapidly conducting. If mediated by brainstem pathways the ipsilateral projection would be at least disynaptic, and hence the latency of ipsilateral cortically evoked responses would be greater than contralateral responses, as was indeed observed in subjects from group B.

• *Cutaneomuscular reflexes.* As discussed earlier, in patients with hemiplegia the cutaneomuscular reflex is often abnormal on the affected side, the I1 and E2 components being reduced or absent (Jenner and Stephens 1982, Evans *et al.* 1991). In the present study the E2 component was seen on the unaffected side in 25 subjects, but on the affected side in only eight. Such findings may be used to argue that the E2 component requires the integrity of the corticospinal tract to lower motoneurons. In the present study this hypothesis was tested directly using cortical stimulation. None of the subjects with absent EMG responses to stimulation of the damaged motor cortex showed an E2 component when the digital nerves of the affected hand were stimulated.

In six subjects from Group A, stimulation of the digital nerves of the unaffected hand evoked I1 and E2 components on both the stimulated and nonstimulated sides. In all these subjects cortical stimulation of the undamaged motor cortex evoked symmetrical bilateral EMG responses in 1DI, with no responses from the damaged motor cortex. One possible explanation is that there is an abnormality at the level of the motoneuron pool, with mingling of ipsilateral and contralateral projections. However, if this were the case one would predict bilateral EMG responses to stimulation of either motor cortex and to cutaneomuscular reflex testing of either hand, with all components bilaterally respresented. In the present study the E1 component was never recorded on the non-stimulated side. Taken with the evidence above, that the E2 component requires the integrity of the corticospinal–lower motoneuronal connection, the more likely explanation for the bilateral E2 components is that the cutaneous volley excites cells in the undamaged cortex which project bilaterally. Bilateral E2 components have also been reported in a patient with Klippel–Feil syndrome and strong mirror movements (Farmer *et al.* 1990).

The bilateral presence of the I1 component in seven subjects from Group A following stimulation of the unaffected hand raises the possibility that this component may also be transcortically mediated. A number of considerations make this unlikely, in particular if taken with the results of cortical stimulation. In six hemiplegic subjects an I1 component was recorded following stimulation of the affected hand, while cortical stimulation of the damaged motor cortex had failed to evoke any EMG response. This suggests that unlike the E2 component, the I1 component is not critically dependent on the integrity of the corticospinal–lower motoneuronal connection and would imply that the I1 response is not transcortically mediated. It seems more likely that spinal pathways, normally silent, have been facilitated (Carr *et al.* 1993; see also Chapter 7).

HAND FUNCTION AND CNS REORGANIZATION

Clinical observation of subjects from Groups A and B allows inferences to be drawn regarding the underlying corticoneuronal connections. Considering hand function in the two groups, five of 11 subjects in Group A and three of ten subjects in Group B were able to make relatively independent finger movements with the hemiplegic hand. This suggests that in these subjects there are monosynaptic corticomotoneuronal projections to the hemiplegic hand (see Chapter 8). In subjects from Group B good function of the hemiplegic hand was seen only if cortical stimulation had evoked responses from the contralateral damaged motor cortex, whereas in subjects from Group A responses were never evoked from the damaged motor cortex, yet half had good function of the hemiplegic hand. Futhermore, the strong symmetrical mirror movements present in all subjects from Group A were most marked in distal muscles to which corticomotoneuronal projections are most dense. This suggests that in subjects from Group A corticospinal axons have branched bilaterally and that some of these projections are corticomotoneuronal, whereas in subjects from Group B the novel ipsilateral projections are not monosynaptic.

TIMING OF CNS DAMAGE

Reorganization of central motor pathways was seen in subjects from Groups A and B.

Subjects from Groups C and D did not show neurophysiological evidence of reorganization. In the former group extensive CNS damage had been incurred after the age of 2 years and motor outcome was uniformly poor. Presumably the critical period for motor reorganization had been passed in these subjects. The increasing severity of hemiplegia across Groups A, B and C may reflect the functional benefits of the presence and type of reorganization. Animal studies suggest that any reorganization of motor pathways is critically age-dependent (see Gómez-Pinilla *et al.* 1986, Kuang and Kalil 1990). It is suggested that the ability of corticospinal axons to branch in response to CNS damage is lost once final synaptic connections are made, and that this is closely related to the time of completed axonal growth (Kalil 1988, Bregman *et al.* 1989). In man, caudal extension of corticospinal fibres into lumbosacral cord appears complete by 29 weeks gestation (Humphrey 1960), although the ability to perform fractionated finger movements (coincident with the development of direct corticomotoneuronal connections) develops at around 9 months postnatally. From clinical history and available neuroimaging we attempted to identify the critical periods for the presence and type of reorganization in the hemiplegic subjects.

In three subjects from Group A the CNS insult was known to have occurred around the time of preterm delivery at 26–27 weeks gestation. Thus at this stage in man the potential for collateral sprouting exists. In eight further subjects the timing of the insult was not clear, although none gave a history of any postnatal insult. Four scans were available for review; the distribution of damage and the general lack of gliosis indicated that in these subjects damage had occurred before the 34th week and generally before the 28th week of gestation. It is now generally accepted that in hemiplegic cerebral palsy the majority of cases are incurred prenatally (Nelson and Ellenberg 1986, Blair and Stanley 1988, Freeman and Nelson 1988). Taken with the arguments above it would seem that for collateral sprouting to occur in man, CNS damage must occur around the time of completed caudal extension, at or before 29 weeks gestation.

In subjects from Group B an abnormal ipsilateral projection was demonstrated from the undamaged cortex, but collateral sprouting was not shown. Eight of the subjects had a congenital hemiplegia; one had been born at 26 weeks gestation and four had presented in the neonatal period with convulsions or apnoea, suggestive of a perinatal event. Scans were available in five of these subjects; all were consistent with a vascular event occurring in a relatively mature brain, after 36 weeks gestation. In cats the ipsilateral corticospinal tract establishes final synaptic connections only after the contralateral tract has completed synaptogenesis (Alisky *et al.* 1992). This would support the hypothesis that in Group B CNS damage has occurred later than in Group A, where collateral sprouting of the contralateral corticospinal tract is no longer possible but enhanced synaptogenesis of the ipsilateral corticospinal tract may still occur.

One subject from Group B acquired a hemiplegia at 7 years of age, when the corticospinal tract is already relatively mature. Animal evidence suggests that axonal sprouting is limited in the adult CNS (Tsukahara and Murakami 1983), so that the mechanism for corticospinal reorganization may be different in this subject.

A number of studies have attempted to correlate scan findings with clinical outcome in congenital hemiplegia (Cohen and Duffner 1981, Kotlarek *et al.* 1981, Wiklund and

Uvebrant 1991, Fujimoto *et al.* 1992, Bouza *et al.* 1994). These studies have shown that the site and extent of the lesion are not consistently predictive of the nature or severity of motor outcome, nor of associated difficulties. Large cortical and subcortical lesions are generally associated with greater deficits, but such lesions also reflect a perinatal or late prenatal insult. In the present study, scan abnormalities were generally more extensive in subjects from Group B than in those from Group A. Cortical or subcortical cavitation and basal ganglia involvement was more common in the former group. Asymmetry of the cerebral peduncles was seen in both groups, indicating a loss of descending fibres. In adults with hemiplegia, if the size of the affected peduncle is less than 60% of the unaffected side, hand function is uniformly poor (Warabi *et al.* 1990), and Bouza *et al.* (1994) found that this was the most reliable indicator of motor outcome and upper limb involvement in childhood hemiplegia. In the present study the variations in scan technique and quality did not allow quantitive measurement of peduncle size, although there was no clear difference in the severity of cerebral peduncle shrinkage between subjects in Groups A and B. Interestingly the hemiplegia tended to be milder in subjects from Group A than in those from Group B, possibly reflecting the functional benefits of motor reorganization in this group.

Reorganization of motor pathways was not seen in subjects from Group D, in whom the hemiplegia was always mild. Asymmetry of the cerebral peduncles was not seen in any of the available scans (five subjects). Taken with the clinical observation of a mild hemiplegia, this would suggest that the corticospinal tracts remain relatively intact so that the stimulus for reorganization may be absent.

In conclusion this chapter has described some of the neurophysiological techniques used to assess motor pathways in man and shown how they may sometimes be predictive of outcome. It has reviewed the evidence for reorganization of motor pathways following CNS damage; both animal and human studies indicate that reorganization may occur, particularly if the damage is sustained early in development. These studies further suggest that such reorganization is often associated with preserved function. It is hoped that with the continuing refinement of neuroradiological and neurophysiological techniques, the mechanisms underlying such motor reorganization and their critical determinants may be elucidated.

ACKNOWLEDGEMENTS

We acknowledge the participation of Dr Linda M. Harrison, Dr A.L. Evans and Dr Simon F. Farmer in the study and their valuable support and criticism. We thank all the children and their families who participated in the study, and likewise the Bobath Centre for the Treatment of Children with Cerebral Palsy, the London Hemiplegia Register and Dr Lilly Dubowitz for their assistance. L.J. Carr was funded by an MRC Training fellowship.

REFERENCES

Alisky, J.M., Swink, T.D., Tolbert, D.L. (1992) 'The postnatal spatial and temporal development of corticospinal projections in cats.' *Experimental Brain Research*, **88**, 265–276.

Barker, A.T., Freeston, I.L., Jalinous, R., Merton, P.A., Morton, H.B. (1985) 'Magnetic stimulation of the human brain.' *Journal of Physiology*, **369**, 3P.

—— Freeston, I.L., Jarratt, J.A., Jalinous, R. (1990) 'Magnetic stimulation of the human nervous system: an introduction and basic principles.' *In:* Chokroverty, S. (Ed.) *Magnetic Stimulation in Clinical Neurophysiology.* London: Butterworths, pp. 55–72.

Barth, T.M., Stanfield, B.B. (1990) 'The recovery of forelimb-placing behavior in rats with neonatal unilateral cortical damage involves the remaining hemisphere.' *Journal of Neuroscience*, **10**, 3449–3459.

Benecke, R., Meyer, B-U., Freund, H-J. (1991) 'Reorganisation of descending motor pathways in patients after hemispherectomy and severe hemispheric lesions demonstrated by magnetic brain stimulation.' *Experimental Brain Research*, **83**, 419–426.

Berardelli, A., Inghilleri, M., Cruccu, G., Mercuri, B., Manfredi, M. (1991) 'Electrical and magnetic transcranial stimulation in patients with corticospinal damage due to stroke or motor neurone disease.' *Electroencephalography and Clinical Neurophysiology*, **81**, 389–396.

Berker, E.A., Berker, A.H., Smith, A. (1986) 'Translation of Broca's 1865 report. Localization of speech in the third left frontal convolution.' *Archives of Neurology*, **43**, 1065–1072.

Blair, E., Stanley, F.J. (1988) 'Intrapartum asphyxia: a rare cause of cerebral palsy.' *Journal of Pediatrics*, **112**, 515–519.

Boniface, S.J., Mills, K.R., Schubert, M. (1991) 'Responses of single spinal motoneurons to magnetic brain stimulation in healthy subjects and patients with multiple sclerosis.' *Brain*, **114**, 643–662.

Bouza, H., Dubowitz, L.M.S., Rutherford, M., Pennock, J.M. (1994) 'Prediction of outcome in children with congenital hemiplegia: a magnetic resonance imaging study.' *Neuropediatrics*, **25**, 60–66.

Bregman, B.S., Kunkel-Bagden, E., McAtee, M., O'Neill, A. (1989) 'Extension of the critical period for developmental plasticity of the corticospinal pathway.' *Journal of Comparative Neurology*, **282**, 355–370.

Bremner, F.D., Baker, J.R., Stephens, J.A. (1991) 'Correlation between the discharges of motor units recorded from the same and from different finger muscles in man.' *Journal of Physiology*, **432**, 355–380.

Broca, P. (1865) 'Sur le siège de la faculté de langage articulé.' *Bulletin of the Society of Anaesthetists*, **6**, 377–393.

Brouwer, B., Ashby, B. (1990) 'Do injuries to the developing human brain alter corticospinal projections?' *Neuroscience Letters*, **108**, 225–230.

Cabana, T., Martin, G.F. (1985) 'Corticospinal development in the North-American opossum: evidence for a sequence in the growth of cortical axons in the spinal cord and for transient projections.' *Brain Research*, **355**, 69–80.

Caccia, M.R., McComas, A.J., Upton, A.R.M., Blogg, T. (1973) 'Cutaneous reflexes in small muscles of the hand.' *Journal of Neurology, Neurosurgery and Psychiatry*, **36**, 960–977.

Carr, L.J., Harrison, L.M., Evans, A.L., Stephens, J.A. (1993) 'Patterns of central motor reorganization in hemiplegic cerebral palsy.' *Brain*, **116**, 1223–1247.

Chollet, F., DiPiero, V., Wise, R.J.S., Brooks, D.J., Dolan, R.J., Frackowiak, R.S.J. (1991) 'The functional anatomy of motor recovery after stroke in humans: a study with positron emission tomography.' *Annals of Neurology*, **29**, 63–71.

Cohen, L.G., Roth, B.J., Wasserman, E.M., Topka, H., Fuhr, P., Schultz, J., Hallett, M. (1991) 'Magnetic stimulation of the human cerebral cortex, an indicator of reorganization in motor pathways in certain pathological conditions.' *Journal of Clinical Neurophysiology*, **8**, 56–65.

Cohen, M.E., Duffner, P.K. (1981) 'Prognostic indicators in hemiparetic cerebral palsy.' *Annals of Neurology*, **9**, 353–357.

Colebatch, J.G., Gandevia, S.C. (1989) 'The distribution of muscular weakness in upper motor neuron lesions affecting the arm.' *Brain*, **112**, 749–763.

Connolly, K., Stratton, P. (1968) 'Developmental changes in associated movements.' *Developmental Medicine and Child Neurology*, **10**, 49–56.

Datta AK, Stephens JA (1990) 'Synchronization of motor unit activity during voluntary contraction in man.' *Journal of Physiology*, **422**, 397–419.

Dominkus, M., Grisold, W., Jelinek, V. (1990) 'Transcranial electrical motor evoked potentials as a prognostic indicator for motor recovery in stroke patients.' *Journal of Neurology, Neurosurgery, and Psychiatry*, **53**, 745–748.

Edgley, S.A., Eyre, J.A., Lemon, R.N., Miller, S. (1990) 'Excitation of the corticospinal tract by electromagnetic and electrical stimulation of the scalp in the macaque monkey.' *Journal of Physiology*, **425**, 301–320.

Evans, A.L., Harrison, L.M., Stephens, J.A. (1990) 'Maturation of the cutaneomuscular reflex recorded from the first dorsal interosseus muscle in man.' *Journal of Physiology*, **428**, 425–440.

—— —— —— (1991) 'Cutaneomuscular reflexes recorded from the first dorsal interosseus muscle of children with cerebral palsy.' *Developmental Medicine and Child Neurology*, **33**, 541–551.

Eyre, J.A., Miller, S., Ramesh, V. (1991) 'Constancy of central conduction delays during development in man: investigation of motor and somatosensory pathways.' *Journal of Physiology*, **434**, 441–452.

197

Farmer, S.F., Ingram, D.A., Stephens, J.A. (1990) 'Mirror movements studied in a patient with Klippel–Feil syndrome.' *Journal of Physiology*, **428**, 467–484.

—— Harrison, L.M., Ingram, D.A., Stephens, J.A. (1991) 'Plasticity of central motor pathways in children with hemiplegic cerebral palsy.' *Neurology*, **41**, 1505–1510.

Finger, S., Wolf, C. (1988) 'The 'Kennard effect' before Kennard. The early history of age and brain lesions.' *Archives of Neurology*, **45**, 1136–1142.

Freeman, J.M., Nelson, K.B. (1988) 'Intrapartum asphyxia and cerebral palsy.' *Pediatrics*, **82**, 240–249.

Fujimoto, S., Yokochi, K., Togari, H., Nishimura, Y., Inukai, K., Futamura, M., Sobajima, H., Suzuki, S., Wada, Y. (1992) 'Neonatal cerebral infarction: symptoms, CT findings and prognosis.' *Brain and Development*, **14**, 48–52.

Gardner, W.J., Karnosh, L.J., McClure, C.C., Gardner, A.K. (1955) 'Residual function following hemispherectomy for tumour and for infantile hemiplegia.' *Brain*, **78**, 487–502.

Goldman, P.S., Galkin, T.W. (1978) 'Prenatal removal of frontal association cortex in the fetal rhesus monkey: anatomical and functional consequences in postnatal life.' *Brain Research*, **152**, 451–485.

Gómez-Pinilla, F., Villablanca, J.R., Sonnier, B.J., Levine, M.S. (1986) 'Reorganization of pericruciate cortical projections to the spinal cord and dorsal column nuclei after neonatal or adult cerebral hemispherectomy in cats.' *Brain Research*, **385**, 343–355.

Gowers, W.R. (1885) *Lectures on the Diagnosis of Diseases of the Brain.* London: Churchill.

Hammond, P.H. (1960) 'An experimental study of servo action in human muscular control.' *In: Proceedings IIIrd International Conference in Medical Electronics.* London: Butterworths, pp. 190–199.

Heald, A., Bates, D., Cartlidge, N.E.F., French, J.M., Miller, S. (1993) 'Longitudinal study of central motor conduction time following stroke. 2. Central motor conduction measured within 72h after stroke as a predictor of functional outcome at 12 months.' Brain, 116, 1371–1385.

Hicks, S.P., D'Amato, C.J. (1970) 'Motor-sensory and visual behavior after hemispherectomy in newborn and mature rats.' *Experimental Neurology*, **29**, 416–438.

Hömberg, V., Stephan, K.M., Netz, J. (1991) 'Transcranial stimulation of motor cortex in upper motor neurone syndrome: its relation to the motor deficit.' *Electroencephalography and Clinical Neurophysiology*, **81**, 377–388.

Humphrey, T. (1960) 'The development of the pyramidal tracts in human fetuses, correlated with cortical differentiation.' *In:* Tower, D.B., Schade, J.P. (Eds.) *Structure and Function of the Cerebral Cortex.* Amsterdam: Elsevier, pp. 94–103.

Issler, H., Stephens, J.A. (1983) 'The maturation of cutaneous reflexes studied in the upper limb in man.' *Journal of Physiology*, **335**, 643–654.

Jenner, J.R., Stephens, J.A. (1982) 'Cutaneous reflex responses and their central nervous pathways studied in man.' *Journal of Physiology*, **333**, 405–419.

Kaas, J.H. (1991) 'Plasticity of sensory and motor maps in adult mammals.' *Annual Review of Neuroscience*, **14**, 137–167.

Kalil, K. (1988) 'Regeneration of pyramidal tract axons.' *Advances in Neurology*, **47**, 67–85.

Kartje-Tillotson, G., Neafsey, E.J., Castro, A.J. (1985) 'Electrophysiological analysis of motor cortical plasticity after cortical lesions in newborn rats.' *Brain Research*, **332**, 103–111.

Kennard, M.A. (1942) 'Cortical reorganization of motor function; studies on series of monkeys of various ages from infancy to maturity.' *Archives of Neurology and Psychiatry*, **48**, 227–240.

Kirkwood, P.A., Sears, T.A. (1978) 'The synaptic connexions to intercostal motoneurones as revealed by the average common excitation potential.' *Journal of Physiology*, **275**, 103–134.

—— —— (1991) 'Cross-correlation analyses of motoneuron inputs in a coordinated motor act.' *In:* Kruger, J. (Ed.) *Neuronal Cooperativity.* Berlin: Springer-Verlag, pp. 225–248.

Koh, T.H.H.G., Eyre, J.A. (1988) 'Maturation of corticospinal tracts assessed by electromagnetic stimulation of the motor cortex.' *Archives of Disease in Childhood*, **63**, 1347–1352.

Kotlarek, F., Rodewig, R., Brüll, D. (1981) 'Computed tomographic findings in congenital hemiparesis in childhood and their relation to etiology and prognosis.' *Neuropediatrics*, **12**, 101–109.

Kuang, R.Z., Kalil, K. (1990) 'Specificity of corticospinal axon arbors sprouting into denervated contralateral spinal cord.' *Journal of Comparative Neurology*, **302**, 461–472

Kuypers, H.G.J.M. (1973) 'The anatomical organization of the descending pathways and thier contributions to motor control especially in primates.' *In:* Desmedt, J.E. (Ed.) *New Developments in Electromyography and Clinical Neurophysiology, Vol 3.* Basel: Karger, pp. 36–68.

Leong, S.K., Lund, R.D. (1973) 'Anomalous bilateral corticofugal pathways in albino rats after neonatal lesions.' *Brain Research*, **62**, 218–221.

Lewine, J.D., Astur, R.S., Davis, L.E., Knight, J.E., Maclin, E.L., Orrison, W.W. (1994) 'Cortical organization in adulthood is modified by neonatal infarct: a case study.' *Radiology*, **190**, 93–96.

Matthews, P.B.C. (1991) 'The human stretch reflex and the motor cortex.' *Trends in Neurosciences*, **14**, 87–91.

Mauguière, F., Desmedt, J.E. (1989) 'Bilateral somatosensory evoked potentials in four patients with long-standing surgical hemispherectomy.' *Annals of Neurology*, **26**, 724–731.

Merline, M., Kalil, K. (1990) 'Cell death of corticospinal neurons is induced by axotomy before but not after innervation of spinal targets.' *Journal of Comparative Neurology*, **296**, 506–516

Merton, P.A., Morton, H.B. (1980) 'Stimulation of the cerebral cortex in the intact human subject.' *Nature*, **285**, 227.

Merzenich, M.M., Sameshima, K. (1993) 'Cortical plasticity and memory.' *Current Opinion in Neurobiology*, **3**, 187–196.

Moore, G.P., Segundo, J.P., Perkel, D.H., Levitan, H. (1970) 'Statistical signs of synaptic interaction in neurons.' *Biophysical Journal*, **10**, 876–900.

Müller, K., Hömberg, V., Lenard, H-G. (1991) 'Magnetic stimulation of motor cortex and nerve roots in children. Maturation of cortico-motoneuronal projections.' *Electroencephalography and Clinical Neurophysiology*, **81**, 63–70.

Nelson, K.B., Ellenberg, J.H. (1986) 'Antecedents of cerebral palsy. Multivariate analysis of risk.' *New England Journal of Medicine*, **315**, 81–86.

Ono, K., Watanabe, Y., Ishizuka, C., Uematsu, J., Aisaka, A., Yamano, T., Shimada, M. (1994) 'Axon ramification following unilateral cortical ablation in neonatal rats.' *Brain and Development*, **16**, 264–266.

Palmer, E., Ashby, P., Hajek, V.E. (1992) 'Ipsilateral fast corticospinal pathways do not account for recovery in stroke.' *Annals of Neurology*, 32, 519–525.

Passingham, R.E., Perry, V.H., Wilkinson, F. (1983) 'The long-term effects of removal of sensorimotor cortex in infant and adult rhesus monkeys.' *Brain*, **106**, 675–705.

Penfield, W., Boldrey, E. (1937) 'Somatic motor and sensory representation in the cerebral cortex of man as studied by electrical stimulation.' *Brain*, **60**, 389–443.

Reh, T.A., Kalil, K. (1982) 'Functional role of regrowing pyramidal tract fibers.' *Journal of Comparative Neurology*, **211**, 276–283.

Reinoso, B.S., Castro, A.J. (1989) 'A study of corticospinal remodelling using retrograde fluorescent tracers in rats.' *Experimental Brain Research*, **74**, 387–394.

Roth, B.J., Saypol, J.M., Hallett, M., Cohen, L.G. (1991) 'A theoretical calculation of the electric field induced in the cortex during magnetic stimulation.' *Electroencephalography and Clinical Neurophysiology*, **81**, 47–56.

Rouiller, E.M., Laing, F., Moret, V., Weisendanger, M. (1991) 'Trajectory of redirected corticospinal axons after unilateral lesion of the sensorimotor cortex in neonatal rat; a phaseolus vulgaris-leucoagglutinin (PHA-L) tracing study.' *Experimental Neurology*, **114**, 53–65.

Rudel, R.G., Teuber, H-L., Twitchell, T.E. (1966) 'A note on hyperesthesia in children with early brain damage.' *Neuropsychologia*, **4**, 351–356.

Sabatini, U., Toni, D., Pantano, P., Brughitta, G., Padovani, A., Bozzao, L., Lenzi, G.L. (1994) 'Motor recovery after early brain damage. A case of brain plasticity.' *Stroke*, **25**, 514–517.

Schneider, G.E. (1979) 'Is it really better to have your brain lesion early? A revision of the "Kennard principle".' *Neuropsychologia*, **17**, 557–583.

Schott, G.D., Wyke, M.A. (1981) 'Congenital mirror movements.' *Journal of Neurology, Neurosurgery and Psychiatry*, **44**, 586–599.

Sears, T.A., Stagg, D. (1976) 'Short-term synchronization of intercostal motoneurone activity.' *Journal of Physiology*, **263**, 357–381.

Sloper, J.J., Brodal, P., Powell, T.P.S. (1983) 'An anatomical study of the effects of unilateral removal of sensorimotor cortex in infant monkeys on the subcortical projections of the contralateral sensorimotor cortex.' *Brain*, **106**, 707–716.

Soltmann, O. (1876) 'Experimentalle Studien über der Functionem des Grosshirns der Neugeborenen.' *Jahrbuch Kinderheilkunde*, **9**, 106–148.

Teuber, H-L. (1974) 'Recovery of function after lesions of the central nervous system: history and prospects.' *Neurosciences Research Programme Bulletin*, **12**, 197–209.

Thompson, P.D., Rothwell, J.C., Day, B.L., Dressler, D., Maertens de Noordhout, A., Marsden, C.D. (1990) 'Mechanisms of electrical and magnetic stimulation of the human motor cortex.' *In:* Chokroverty, S. (Ed.) *Magnetic Stimulation in Clinical Neurophysiology*. London: Butterworths, pp. 121–143.

Tsukahara, N., Murakami, F. (1983) 'Axonal sprouting and recovery of function after brain damage.' *Advances in Neurology*, **39**, 1073–1084.

Uvebrant, P. (1988) 'Hemiplegic cerebral palsy. Aetiology and outcome.' *Acta Paediatrica Scandinavica*, Suppl. 345, 5–100.

Vargha-Khadem, F., O'Gorman, A.M., Watters, G.V. (1985) 'Aphasia and handedness in relation to hemispheric side, age at injury and severity of cerebral lesion during childhood.' *Brain*, **108**, 677–696.

Villablanca, J.R., Burgess, J.W., Olmstead, C.E. (1986) 'Recovery of function after neonatal or adult hemispherectomy in cats. 1. Time course, movement, posture and sensorimotor tests.' *Behavioural Brain Research*, **19**, 205–226.

Warabi, T., Inoue, K., Noda, H., Murakami, S. (1990) 'Recovery of voluntary movement in hemiplegic patients. Correlation with degenerative shrinkage of the cerebral peduncles in CT images.' *Brain*, **113**, 177–189.

Weiller, C., Chollet, F., Friston, K.J., Wise, R.J.S., Frackowiak, R.S.J. (1992) 'Functional reorganization of the brain in recovery from striatocapsular infarction in man.' *Annals of Neurology*, **31**, 463–472.

—— Ramsay, S.C., Wise, R.J.S., Friston, K.J., Frackowiak, R.S.J. (1993) 'Individual patterns of functional reorganization in the human cerebral cortex after capsular infarction.' *Annals of Neurology*, **33**, 181–189.

Wiklund, L-M., Uvebrant, P. (1991) 'Hemiplegic cerebral palsy: correlation between CT morphology and clinical findings.' *Developmental Medicine and Child Neurology*, **33**, 512–523.

Woods, B.T. (1980) 'The restricted effects of right-hemisphere lesions after age one; Wechsler test data.' *Neuropsychologia*, **18**, 65–70.

—— Teuber, H-L. (1978) 'Mirror movements after childhood hemiparesis.' *Neurology*, **28**, 1152–1158.

Yuste, R., Peinado, A., Katz, L.C. (1992) 'Neuronal domains in developing neocortex.' *Science*, **257**, 665–669.

10
POSTURAL ADJUSTMENTS ASSOCIATED WITH BALLISTIC MOVEMENTS IN ADULT HUMANS

P. Ashby, E. Cafarelli and E. Palmer

An apparently simple voluntary act, such as lifting up one arm quickly, is accompanied by a flurry of muscle activity on both sides of the body. The contraction of these distant muscles precisely counteracts any disturbance of equilibrium or displacement of body segments that might arise from the sudden arm movement. If the arm is weighted or if the position of the body changes, the pattern of distant muscle activation is automatically altered to deal with the new forces. How these 'associated postural adjustments', as they have been called (Cordo and Nashner 1982), are generated is still uncertain.

This chapter reviews some recent studies on the operation of this remarkable automatic motor system. For a detailed review the reader is referred to Massion (1992); see also Chapter 3. For the sake of readers unfamiliar with the terms used, definitions are given in Table 10.1.

Focal movements

If a person flexes the elbow as fast as possible there is a burst of EMG activity in the agonist biceps, a burst in the antagonist triceps and then a second burst in the biceps (Hallett *et al.* 1975a, Benecke *et al.* 1985, Forget and Lamarre 1987). This triphasic pattern appears to be typical of a ballistic movement into a target zone whether it be abduction of an entire arm (Palmer *et al.* 1994) or flexion of the distal phalanx of the thumb (Hallett and Marsden 1979). The first agonist burst, which accelerates the limb, is larger and longer for large amplitude movements (Benecke *et al.* 1985) and when the limb is weighted (Benecke *et al.* 1985, Manto *et al.* 1994). The antagonist burst, which decelerates the limb (Marsden *et al.* 1983) and is absent if the movement is made into a pillow (Forget and Lamarre 1987), is correlated with the size of the agonist burst and with the peak acceleration and peak velocity of the movement (Forget and Lamarre 1987). Curiously, the antagonist burst is smaller with larger amplitude movements, perhaps because the viscoelastic properties of the extended muscle contribute to the deceleration (Benecke *et al.* 1985).

If there was any background activity of the agonist before the movement began it is inhibited just before the first agonist burst occurs. This inhibition is most obvious with self-paced high velocity movements and may ensure that none of the agonist motoneurons are refractory at the time they are required for the agonist burst (Yabe 1976, Conrad *et al.* 1983, Mortimer *et al.* 1987). The antagonist is also inhibited from just before the agonist burst right up to the time that the antagonist burst occurs. This inhibition is larger for slow,

TABLE 10.1
Definitions of terms

Ballistic movement: a movement carried out as rapidly as possible

Focal movement: a directed movement of a body segment (Cordo and Nashner 1982)

Associated postural adjustment (APA): activation of postural muscles (usually) in advance of focal movements (Cordo and Nashner 1982)

Preparatory postural adjustment (PPA): activation of muscles to position the body prior to initiating a voluntary movement (Massion 1992). PPAs usually precede the focal movement by a longer interval (>100ms) than APAs

---

large amplitude movements and presumably makes a useful contribution to the force (Hufschmidt and Hufschmidt 1954, Hallett *et al.* 1975a, Agostino *et al.* 1992).

Generation of focal movements

The triphasic pattern, including the preceding inhibition of the antagonist, can be seen in deafferented subjects. Evidently the nervous system can generate the sequence of commands to accelerate and decelerate the limb in the absence of peripheral feedback. For this reason successive bursts are considered to be preprogrammed (Hallett *et al.* 1975a, Rothwell *et al.* 1982, Sanes and Jennings 1984, Forget and Lamarre 1987). This is not to say that afferent information cannot be incorporated into the programming of later bursts. In deafferented subjects the antagonist burst is smaller and not so well correlated with the agonist burst or with the acceleration of the movement, and its timing is more variable, suggesting that 'information from the moving limb is required to adjust the magnitude and time of onset of deceleration' (Forget and Lamarre 1987). This makes sense. If the nervous system overestimated the force required for a movement and generated too large an agonist burst the limb would be accelerated more than expected. Only if this error were detected could the braking forces be adjusted.

The motor cortex appears to be essential for the generation of ballistic movements. In the monkey, the firing rate of cortical neurons, including those with known projections to motoneurons, alters in the 100ms or so before a rapid movement in ways that can be related to the parameters of the movement (Cheney and Fetz 1980). This is still the case when the animal is deafferented and the cerebellum removed, while a lesion of the cortex abolishes previously learned ballistic movements of the contralateral limbs (Lamarre *et al.* 1978). In man, ballistic movements are slowed by conditions affecting corticospinal neurons (Hallett 1979, Horak *et al.* 1984) and can be delayed by stimulation over the motor cortex (Day *et al.* 1989). Whether the motor cortex is the site of origin of ballistic movements or simply one of the last stations in the output pathway remains to be elucidated.

The cerebellum seems to contribute to the timing and scaling of the bursts. When human subjects with cerebellar disorders make ballistic movements the agonist burst is late and too long, the premovement silence of the antagonist is lost, and the antagonist burst is late and does not increase appropriately with loading (Hallett *et al.* 1975b, Manto *et al.* 1994). Evidently the brain cannot make proper use of afferent information to calculate the braking action successfully. As a result ballistic movements are delayed and overshoot their target.

The role of the basal ganglia in the generation of ballistic movements is less clear. When subjects with parkinsonism attempt ballistic movements the latency and duration of the triphasic bursts are normal but the amplitudes of the bursts are small and movements are carried out by a succession of small triphasic pulses which apparently cannot be scaled up (Hallett *et al.* 1977).

In summary, the triphasic pattern of EMG activity associated with a ballistic movement of a body segment is carried out by a central programme which involves the motor cortex.

Associated postural adjustments (APAs)

Ballistic focal movements are preceded or accompanied by bursts of EMG in many distant muscles. These APAs serve to stabilize body segments against the reactive forces produced by the focal movement or to ensure that the body's centre of gravity remains within the base of support. A number of focal movements that are accompanied by APAs have been studied.

APAs associated with focal movements of the upper limbs
If a standing subject rapidly elevates one arm forward to the horizontal the burst of EMG in the anterior deltoid (representing the focal movement) is preceded by bursts in the ipsilateral leg muscles, biceps femoris and medial gastrocnemius and in the contralateral erector spinae and tensor fascia lata, and is followed by bursts in the contralateral biceps femoris and ipsilateral erector spinae (Belen'kii et al. 1967; Lee 1980; Bouisset and Zattara 1981, 1988; Horak *et al.* 1984; Lee *et al.* 1987). This pattern of APAs is modified by changes in the body's posture. When a subject standing on a movable platform elevates one arm the APAs occur in the ipsilateral biceps femoris if the platform is tilted forwards but in the ipsilateral tibialis anterior if the platform is tilted backwards (Gatev *et al.* 1991). When a seated subject elevates one arm, the pattern of APAs is different again (Moore *et al.* 1992, Palmer *et al.* 1994).

When a standing subject pulls on a handle with one arm the EMG burst in the biceps representing the focal movement is preceded by APAs in the ipsilateral hamstrings, gastrocnemius and erector spinae (Cordo and Nashner 1982, Friedli *et al.* 1984). If the trunk is supported these APAs disappear (Cordo and Nasher 1982). If the subject is walking on a treadmill the APAs associated with the arm pull vary continuously with the step cycle. In the early stance phase, when the leg is ahead of the centre of gravity, the potential forward movement of the trunk and pelvis is resisted by APAs in the hamstrings and gastrocnemius. In late stance when the leg is behind the centre of gravity the APAs occur in the tibialis anterior (Nashner and Forssberg 1986; Hirschfeld and Forssberg 1991, 1992).

Rapid movements at the wrist are accompanied by activity in proximal arm muscles. Interestingly, wrist flexion is associated with activity in the biceps when the forearm is supinated but with activity in the triceps when the forearm is pronated, while wrist extension is accompanied by activity in the triceps when the forearm is supinated but not when it is pronated (Aoki 1991).

Anticipatory activity of a somewhat different nature occurs when a muscle is unloaded by the subject's own volition as in the 'bimanual load lifting task'. If the subject is supporting a weight with the right arm and the weight is unexpectedly removed by another person, the EMG of the right elbow flexor muscles diminishes about 30 ms *after* the change in force. However, if the subject themself unloads the weight with their left arm the EMG of the right elbow flexors diminishes *before* the change of force. This occurs in deafferented subjects and is likely a central programme (Massion 1992). The unloading has to be an integral part of the voluntary movement: if the subject removes the load by deactivating an electromagnet, the anticipatory reduction in EMG does not occur (Dufossé *et al.* 1985). Similar anticipatory activity can be shown when a small hand muscle is unloaded (Kaluzny and Wiesendanger 1992).

APAs associated with movements of the trunk
With rapid forward flexion of the trunk the activity in the prime mover rectus abdominus is preceded by EMG activity in the tibialis anterior and vastus medialis as the hips and knees move backwards (Oddsson and Thorstensson 1986, Crenna *et al.* 1987, Oddsson 1990). With rapid backward extension of the trunk the activity of the prime mover erector spinae is associated with almost synchronous activity in the hamstrings and gluteus maximus (Crenna *et al.* 1987, Oddsson 1989), although trained gymnasts, who perform the movement with less change in the centre of gravity, show anticipatory activity in the gastrocnemius and in some cases the hamstrings (Pedotti *et al.* 1989).

Preparatory postural adjustments associated with movement of the lower limbs
For focal movements of the lower limbs it may be necessary to shift the centre of gravity *before* the movement can be safely commenced. Such movements, which really occur in two stages, may be organized in a different manner. The preliminary postural activity, which often occurs more than 100 ms before the activity giving rise to the focal movement, probably deserves a separate designation as a 'preparatory postural adjustment' (PPA) (Massion 1992).

If a subject, standing on both legs, is instructed to flex one leg as quickly as possible, the sartorius EMG burst associated with the movement is preceded by EMG bursts in the ipsilateral soleus and contralateral tibialis anterior. This preparatory activity shifts the centre of gravity over the supporting foot. (You cannot complete this manoeuvre with the side of the supporting foot flush against a wall). This preparatory activity is not seen if the subject is standing on one leg (Nouillot *et al.* 1992). Similarly, when standing subjects abduct one leg to 45° the transfer of weight to the supporting leg has to be almost complete before the abducting leg begins to move, as though the repositioning of the centre of gravity was a prerequisite for the leg movement to be performed (Mouchnino *et al.* 1992). It is interesting that naive subjects perform this movement by inclining the trunk over the supporting leg while trained dancers translate the hip to the side of the supporting leg and keep the trunk and head vertical. Naive subjects are unable to learn this in a short time indicating that the feed-forward programme generated by the dancers is a result of prolonged training (Mouchnino *et al.* 1992).

The act of rising up on the toes requires a forward shift of the centre of gravity. (You cannot carry out this movement if your toes are touching the wall). This movement also is carried out in two stages. First there is a silencing of any ongoing EMG activity in the soleus and bursts of EMG in the tibialis anterior, quadriceps and biceps femoris which move the centre of gravity forward and stabilize the knee. This activity is greater if the subject is leaning backwards. Only when the movement is complete is there EMG activity in the medial gastrocnemius, raising the body on the toes (Diener *et al.* 1993). This preparatory activity is abolished if the subject holds onto a frame (Nardone and Schieppati 1988). Similarly, rolling back on the heels involves a backward shift of the centre of gravity, in this instance effected by activity of the soleus prior to the execution of the movement by the activation of the tibialis anterior (Nardone and Schieppati 1988).

General characteristics of APAs

APAs show a number of notable features. The EMG bursts in the postural muscles usually precede the burst in the focal mover and occur before there is any disturbance of equilibrium (Cordo and Nashner 1982). APAs occur in deafferented subjects (Palmer *et al.* 1994), and APAs in groups of agonist and antagonist muscles may show the same triphasic pattern that is characteristic of focal movements (Friedli *et al.* 1984). For these reasons APAs are considered to be preprogrammed. This preprogramming is remarkably flexible. If the limb making the focal movement is loaded the APAs occur earlier (Friedli *et al.* 1984, Horak *et al.* 1984, Bouisset and Zattara 1988). The APAs also vary with the subject's perception of body support. If a standing subject is supported so that the trunk cannot move, a rapid flexion of the elbow is no longer associated with APAs in leg muscles (Cordo and Nashner 1982, Friedli *et al.* 1984); moreover, the biceps activity now occurs earlier, implying that, in the unsupported subject, it was delayed until potential disruptions of equilibrium had been dealt with (Cordo and Nashner 1982). APAs also vary with the moment to moment changes in the body's posture. APAs elicited in leg muscles while subjects walk on a treadmill are continuously modulated during the phases of stepping (Nashner and Forssberg 1986; Hirschfeld and Forssberg 1991, 1992). With novel tasks APAs adapt with practice over a few trials (Friedli *et al.* 1984, Oddsson and Thorstensson 1986, Pedotti *et al.* 1989), but new and more efficient patterns of APAs develop with years of practise in gymnasts (Pedotti *et al.* 1989) and dancers (Mouchnino *et al.* 1992). APAs are surprisingly well preserved in weightless spaceflight (Clément *et al.* 1984).

Generation of APAs

The site of origin of APAs is unknown. There are two main proposals: first, that they are generated at a lower hierarchical level of the nervous system and triggered as the focal movement is executed (Cordo and Nashner 1982, Friedli *et al.* 1984); and second, that they are generated as part of the overall ballistic movement (Bouisset and Zattara 1988). Recent studies in our laboratory (Palmer *et al.* 1994) support the second hypothesis. Seated subjects were asked to abduct the arm about 10° as rapidly as possible. This focal movement is associated with a typical triphasic pattern of activity in the agonist, deltoid, and antagonist, latissimus dorsi, muscles of the abducting arm (Fig. 10.1). But there are also bursts of EMG activity in the contralateral external oblique abdominal muscles and in the contralateral pectoralis major and latissimus dorsi. These bursts occur at about the same time as the first agonist

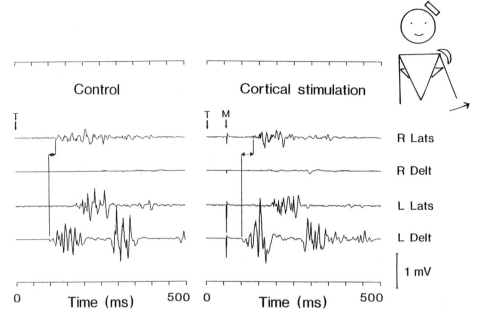

Fig. 10.1. *(Left)* Example of the EMG bursts in the deltoid and latissimus dorsi associated with a rapid abduction of the left arm in response to a tone at time zero. Note the 'triphasic' pattern of the left deltoid and left latissimus dorsi EMG bursts and the early EMG burst in the right latissimus dorsi. *(Right)* Effect of magnetic stimulation over the left motor cortex at time 60 ms on EMG bursts associated with abduction of the left arm in response to a tone at time zero. The triphasic pattern of the muscles of the left shoulder is unaltered but the EMG burst in the right latissimus dorsi is delayed. T = tone, M = magnetic stimulation. (Reproduced by permission from Palmer *et al.* 1994.)

burst of the focal movement. They probably serve to stabilize the trunk and shoulder girdle and can be considered to be examples of APAs. They can occur in a deafferented subject and are therefore likely preprogrammed. The fact that in this particular example the focal movement occurs on one side and the APAs on the other, provides an opportunity to explore the generation of these movements using the inhibitory effects of transcranial stimulation.

Currents induced in the brain by electrical or magnetic stimulation over the motor cortex cause an initial excitation of corticospinal neurons followed by a period in which voluntary muscle contractions are inhibited (Mills 1988, Cantello *et al.* 1992, Haug *et al.* 1992, Wilson *et al.* 1993) and a voluntary contraction in response to a 'go' signal is delayed (Day *et al.* 1989). The interruption of voluntary movement is not due to inhibition of spinal motoneurons, and it has been postulated that the activation of inhibitory neurons in the cortex somehow prevents the motor program from reaching cortical neurons (Day *et al.* 1989). In our experiments, when subjects abducted the left arm suddenly, magnetic stimulation over the left motor cortex delayed the EMG burst in the right latissimus dorsi, which was part of the associated postural response, relative to the burst in the left deltoid, which was responsible for the focal movement (Fig. 10.1). This delay was greatest when the stimulus

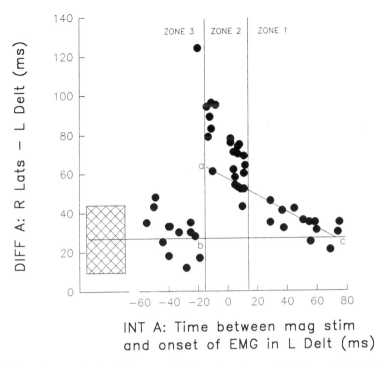

Fig. 10.2. Effect of magnetic stimulation over the left motor cortex on the timing of the EMG bursts in the left deltoid and right latissimus dorsi during abduction of the left arm in one subject. The difference in the onset latency of these EMG bursts (DIFF A) is plotted against the interval between the stimulus and the onset of EMG in the left deltoid (INT A). As this interval becomes shorter, *i.e.* as the stimulus is given nearer to the expected time of the left deltoid burst (zone 1), the delay of the right latissimus burst increases. The delay is greatest when the stimulus is given just before the expected time that the signal giving rise to the right latissimus burst would be traversing the cortex (zone 2). When both the EMG bursts occur before the stimulus (data points to the left side of the figure, zone 3), the difference in latency reverts to control values. (The shaded area represents the mean of the control values ±2 SD; N = 40.) (Reproduced by permission from Palmer *et al.* 1994.)

was given at the time when the neural activity giving rise to the latissimus burst would be expected to be traversing the cortex if the efferent pathway was the fast corticospinal tract. It diminished as the interval between the stimulus and this transit time became longer (Fig. 10.2). If subjects now made a ballistic abduction of the right arm, magnetic stimulation over the left motor cortex delayed the burst in the right deltoid, responsible for the focal movement, relative to the associated postural response in the left latissimus dorsi. This delay was also greatest when the stimulus was given just prior to the time that the neural activity giving rise to the burst in the right deltoid would be expected to be traversing the cortex, and declined as the interval between the stimulus and this transit time became larger (Fig. 10.3). It appears that the focal movement on one side and the APAs on the other are generated by the nervous system in exactly the same way in each case involving the contralateral motor cortex.

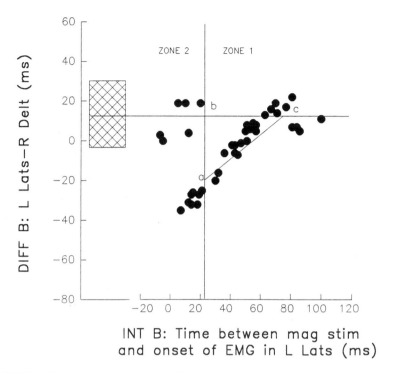

Fig. 10.3. Effect of magnetic stimulation over the left motor cortex on the timing of the EMG bursts in the right deltoid and left latissimus dorsi during abduction of the right arm in one subject. The difference in the onset latency of these EMG bursts (DIFF B) is plotted against the interval (INT B) between the stimulus and the onset of EMG in the left latissimus. As this interval becomes shorter, *i.e.* the stimulus is given nearer to the expected time of the left latissimus burst (zone 1), the right deltoid burst is progressively delayed until it occurs after the left latissimus burst (negative values of difference). When both the EMG bursts occur before the stimulus (data points to the left of the figure, zone 2) the difference in latency reverts to control values. (Shaded area represents the mean of the control values ±2 SD; N = 40.) (Reproduced by permission from Palmer *et al.* 1994.)

Are the focal movement and APAs preprogammed together on the basis of an internal representation of the body's current posture or is the focal movement dispatched along with some general signal (transmitted throught the cortex) that is directed to the appropriate postural muscles by channels automatically opened by the body's current position? Certainly descending activity reaching the cord must be influenced by the 'set' of spinal interneurons. However, APAs to abduction, adduction, flexion and extension of the arm in a standing subject are all different even though the standing posture is the same. Thus the important variable is the motor programme not the pattern of channels opened by the posture. Furthermore, APAs are altered when a subject anticipates that the limb will be loaded or that support is present whether or not this is true. Errors of focal movement are accompanied by parallel errors of APAs (Cordo and Nashner 1982). Thus, it seems likely that the focal movement and APAs are preprogrammed together.

Lesions of the cerebral hemispheres interfere with APAs. Pal'tsev and El'ner (1967) noted that when subjects with lesions of the frontal lobes lifted one arm, the APAs on the affected side were delayed or absent, and Horak *et al.* (1984) found that if subjects with left hemiplegia elevated the right arm, the APAs in the left paraspinal muscles and left biceps femoris opposite the affected hemisphere were delayed. When children with cerebral palsy flex the forearm against resistance the normal APAs are absent and EMG activity occurs in the biceps before the leg muscles (Nashner *et al.* 1983). When subjects with cortical lesions carry out the bimanual load lifting task, the anticipatory drop in EMG of the brachioradialis muscle supporting the weight is *less* with lesions of the supplementary motor area but *absent* contralateral to a lesion of the motor cortex (Viallet *et al.* 1992). Preparatory activity in the movement of rising on the toes is carried out more slowly in subjects with hemiplegia (Diener *et al.* 1993).

As with focal movements the cerebellum appears to be involved in the timing of APAs. When subjects with cerebellar atrophy elevate both arms forward to the horizontal, the general pattern of APAs (in tibialis anterior, erector spinae, hamstrings and quadriceps) is present but the time between the burst in the tibialis anterior and the bursts in the anterior deltoids is too long so the burst in the anterior deltoid is delayed (Diener *et al.* 1989). When subjects with cerebellar disease stand on their toes, the preparatory activity in the tibialis anterior and quadriceps is slow to build (or in some cases does not occur) and the activity in the triceps surae is delayed (Diener *et al.* 1992). The role of the basal ganglia in the generation of APAs is unclear. When subjects with parkinsonism elevate one arm (Dick *et al.* 1986, Rogers *et al.* 1987) or both arms (Diener *et al.* 1989) forwards, the APAs can be seen in the erector spinae and leg muscles just as in normal subjects. The APAs are slightly smaller and may occur less frequently, possibly because the focal movement itself is slower (Dick *et al.* 1986, Rogers *et al.* 1987). The APAs sometimes consist of repeated short bursts (Rogers *et al.* 1987). When parkinsonian patients performed the bimanual unloading task the anticipatory reduction in brachioradialis EMG occurred but was less pronounced and occurred less often (Viallet *et al.* 1987). Preparatory activity in the act of rising on the toes is present but slower to build up in parkinsonian subjects (Diener *et al.* 1990). Diener *et al.* concluded that APAs are not generated in either the basal ganglia or cerebellum but that the cerebellum coordinates the time between the components of the APAs and scales the force.

Development of focal movements and APAs
At what age do preprogrammed focal movements and APAs develop?

When asked to pick up an object between the finger and thumb, adults grip and lift in one smooth movement appropriate for the expected weight of the object—a focal movement that is presumably preprogrammed. Children below the age of 2 years grip first and then lift. The movement is slower, and there are stepwise force increases likely permitting peripheral feedback. Adults unsure of the physical properties of an object pursue a similar strategy (Forssberg *et al.* 1991). After the age of 2, the child can use information about the weight of the object obtained from the first trial to improve the motor programme for subsequent trials (Gordon *et al.* 1992), and after the age of 3 can, in addition, use visual information to predict the object's weight (Forssberg *et al.* 1992).

APAs in leg muscles prior to a focal movement of one arm occur at least as early as 6 years of age, although the latencies of the APAs and the focal movement are longer than in adults (Hirschfeld and Forssberg 1992). PPAs in the tibialis anterior prior to standing on tip-toes have been observed in the youngest children (4 years) able to follow the instruction consistently. The latency of the tibialis burst gradually shortens with age, but the delay between the PPAs in the tibialis anterior and the focal movement of the triceps surae increases in parallel with increasing body inertia (Haas *et al.* 1989).

Conclusion
On the basis of our experiments we postulate that:
1. Focal movements and their APAs (at least those APAs that stabilize body segments) are generated in the same way and are simply components of the overall ballistic movement.
2. When an instruction for a focal movement is given, the subject estimates the forces to be expected and their likely effects on the body's equilibrium, and prepares a programme for both the focal movement and the APAs.
3. On the 'go' signal this programme is released through *both* motor cortices to contralateral spinal neurons. The timing of each burst and the modification of the amplitude of subsequent bursts by afferent information may be carried out by the cerebellum.
4. The result of the first trial improves the estimates of the forces to be expected. In this way, short term adaptation can take place. Prolonged practice can result in even more efficient motor strategies.

ACKNOWLEDGEMENTS

The authors thank the Canadian Medical Research Council (Grant #6727) and the Parkinson's Foundation for financial support.

REFERENCES

Agostino, R., Hallett, M., Sanes, J.N. (1992) 'Antagonist muscle inhibition before rapid voluntary movements of the human wrist.' *Electroencephalography and Clinical Neurophysiology*, **85**, 190–196.

Aoki, F. (1991) 'Activity patterns of upper arm muscles in relation to direction of rapid wrist movement in man.' *Experimental Brain Research*, **83**, 679–682.

Belen'kii, V.Y., Gurfinkel, V.S., Pal'tsev, Y.I. (1967) 'Elements of control of voluntary movements.' *Biophysics*, **12**, 154–160.

Benecke, R., Meinck, H-M., Conrad, B. (1985) 'Rapid goal-directed elbow flexion movements: limitations of the speed control system due to neural constraints.' *Experimental Brain Research*, **59**, 470–477.

Bouisset, S., Zattara, M. (1981) 'A sequence of postural movements precedes voluntary movement.' *Neuroscience Letters*, **22**, 263–270.

—— —— (1988) 'Anticipatory postural adjustments and dynamic asymmetry of voluntary movements.' *In:* Gurfinkel, V.S., Ioffe, M.E., Massion, J., Roll, J.P. (Eds.) *Stance and Motion.* New York: Plenum Press, pp. 177–183.

Cantello, R., Gianelli, M., Civardi C., Mutani, R. (1992) 'Magnetic brain stimulation: the silent period after the motor evoked potential.' *Neurology*, **42**, 1951–1959.

Cheney, P.D., Fetz, E.E. (1980) 'Functional classes of primate corticomotoneuronal cells and their relation to active force.' *Journal of Neurophysiology*, **44**, 773–791.

Clément, G., Gurfinkel, V.S., Lestienne, F., Lipshits, M.I., Popov, K.E. (1984) 'Adaptation of postural control to weightlessness.' *Experimental Brain Research*, **57**, 61–72.

Conrad, B., Benecke, R., Goehmann, M. (1983) 'Premovement silent period in fast movement initiation.' *Experimental Brain Research*, **51**, 310–313.

Cordo, P.J., Nashner, L.M. (1982) 'Properties of postural adjustments associated with rapid arm movements.' *Journal of Neurophysiology*, **47**, 287–302.

Crenna, P., Frigo, C., Massion, J., Pedotti, A. (1987) 'Forward and backward axial synergies in man.' *Experimental Brain Reserch*, **65**, 538–548.

Day, B.L., Rothwell, J.C., Thompson, P.D., Maertens De Noordhout, A., Nakashima, K., Shannon, K., Marsden, C.D. (1989) 'Delay in the execution of voluntary movement by electrical or magnetic brain stimulation in intact man. Evidence for the storage of motor programs in the brain.' *Brain*, **112**, 649–663.

Dick, J.P.R., Rothwell, J.C., Berardelli, A., Thompson, P.D., Gioux, M., Benecke, R., Day, B.L., Marsden, C.D. (1986) 'Associated postural adjustments in Parkinson's disease.' *Journal of Neurology, Neurosurgery and Psychiatry*, **49**, 1378–1385.

Diener, H-C., Dichgans, J., Guschlbauer, B., Bacher, M., Langenbach, P. (1989) 'Disturbances of motor preparation in basal ganglia and cerebellar disorders.' *Progress in Brain Research*, **80**, 481–488.

—— —— —— —— Rapp, H., Langenbach, P. (1990) 'Associated postural adjustments with body movement in normal subjects and patients with parkinsonism and cerebellar disease.' *Revue Neurologique*, **146**, 555–563.

—— —— —— —— —— Klockgether, T. (1992) 'The coordination of posture and voluntary movement in patients with cerebellar dysfunction.' *Movement Disorders*, **7**, 14–22.

—— Bacher, M., Guschlbauer, B., Thomas, C., Dichgans, J. (1993) 'The coordination of posture and voluntary movement in patients with hemiparesis.' *Journal of Neurology*, **240**, 161–167.

Dufossé, M., Hugon, M., Massion, J. (1985) 'Postural forearm changes induced by predictable in time or voluntary triggered unloading in man.' *Experimental Brain Research*, **60**, 330–334.

Forget, R., Lamarre, Y. (1987) 'Rapid elbow flexion in the absence of proprioceptive and cutaneous feedback.' *Human Neurobiology*, **6**, 27–37.

Forssberg, H., Eliasson, A.C., Kinoshita, H., Johansson, R.S., Westling, G. (1991) 'Development of human precision grip. I: Basic coordination of force.' *Experimental Brain Research*, **85**, 451–457.

—— Kinoshita, H., Eliasson, A.C., Johansson, R.S., Westling, G., Gordon, A.M. (1992) 'Development of human precision grip. II. Anticipatory control of isometric forces targeted for object's weight.' *Experimental Brain Research*, **90**, 393–398.

Friedli, W.G., Hallett, M., Simon, S.R. (1984) 'Postural adjustments associated with rapid voluntary arm movements. 1. Electromyographic data.' *Journal of Neurology, Neurosurgery and Psychiatry*, **47**, 611–622.

Gatev, P., Tankov, N., Gantchev, G., Krizkova, M. (1991) 'Postural adjustments upon arm movement during sinusoidal induced body oscillations.' *Acta Physiologica et Pharmacologica Bulgarica*, **17**, 3–6.

Gordon, A.M., Forssberg, H., Johansson, R.S., Eliasson, A.C., Westling, G. (1992) 'Development of human precision grip. III. Integration of visual size cues during programming of isometric forces.' *Experimental Brain Research*, **90**, 399–403.

Haas, G., Diener, H.C., Rapp, H., Dichgans, J. (1989) 'Development of feedback and feedforward control of upright stance.' *Developmental Medicine and Child Neurology*, **31**, 481–488.

Hallett, M. (1979) 'Ballistic elbow flexion movements in patients with amyotrophic lateral sclerosis.' *Journal of Neurology, Neurosurgery and Psychiatry*, **42**, 232–237.

—— Marsden, C.D. (1979) 'Ballistic flexion movements of the human thumb.' *Journal of Physiology*, **294**, 33–50.

—— Shahani, B.T., Young, R.R. (1975a) 'EMG analysis of stereotyped voluntary movements in man.' *Journal of Neurology, Neurosurgery and Psychiatry*, **38**, 1154–1162.

—— —— —— (1975b) 'EMG analysis of patients with cerebellar deficits.' *Journal of Neurology, Neurosurgery and Psychiatry*, **38**, 1163–1169.

—— —— —— (1977) 'Analysis of stereotyped voluntary movements at the elbow in patients with Parkinson's disease.' *Journal of Neurology, Neurosurgery and Psychiatry*, **40**, 1129–1135.

Haug, B.A., Schönle, P.W., Knobloch, C., Köhne, M. (1992) 'Silent period measurement revives as a valuable diagnostic tool with transcranial magnetic stimulation.' *Electrencephalography and Clinical Neurophysiology*, **85**, 158–160.

Hirschfeld, H., Forssberg, H. (1991) 'Phase-dependent modulations of anticipatory postural activity during human locomotion.' *Journal of Neurophysiology*, **66**, 12–19.

—— —— (1992) 'Development of anticipatory postural adjustments during locomotion in children.' *Journal of Neurophysiology*, **68**, 542–550.

211

Horak, F.B., Esselman, P., Anderson, M.E., Lynch, M.K. (1984) 'The effects of movement velocity, mass displaced, and task certainty on associated postural adjustments made by normal and hemiplegic individuals.' *Journal of Neurology, Neurosurgery and Psychiatry*, **47**, 1020–1028.

Hufschmidt, H-J., Hufschmidt, T. (1954) 'Antagonist inhibition as the earliest sign of a sensory-motor reaction.' *Nature*, **174**, 607.

Kaluzny, P., Wiesendanger, M. (1992) 'Feedforward postural stabilization in a distal bimanual unloading task.' *Experimental Brain Research*, **92**, 173–182.

Lamarre, Y., Bioulac, B., Jacks, B. (1978) 'Activity of precentral neurones in conscious monkeys: effects of deafferentation and cerebellar ablation.' *Journal of Physiology*, **74**, 253–264.

Lee, W.A. (1980) 'Anticipatory control of postural and task muscles during rapid arm flexion.' *Journal of Motor Behaviour*, **12**, 185–196.

—— Buchanan, T.S., Rogers, M.W. (1987) 'Effects of arm acceleration and behavioral conditions on the organization of postural adjustments during arm flexion.' *Experimental Brain Research*, **66**, 257–270.

Manto, M., Godaux, E., Jacquy, J. (1994) 'Cerebellar hypermetria is larger when the inertial load is artificially increased.' *Annals of Neurology*, **35**, 45–52.

Marsden, C.D., Obeso, J.A., Rothwell, J.C. (1983) 'The function of the antagonist muscle during fast limb movements in man.' *Journal of Physiology*, **335**, 1–13.

Massion, J. (1992) 'Movement, posture and equilibrium: interaction and coordination.' *Progress in Neurobiology*, **38**, 35–56.

Mills, K.R. (1988) 'Excitatory and inhibitory effects on human spinal motoneurones from magnetic brain stimulation.' *Neuroscience Letters*, **94**, 297–302.

Moore, S., Brunt, D., Nesbitt, M.L., Juarez, T. (1992) 'Investigation of evidence for anticipatory postural adjustments in seated subjects who performed a reaching task.' *Physical Therapy*, **72**, 335–343.

Mortimer, J.A., Eisenberg, P., Palmer, S.S. (1987) 'Premovement silence in agonist muscles preceding maximum efforts.' *Experimental Neurology*, **98**, 542–554.

Mouchnino, L., Aurenty, R., Massion, J., Pedotti, A. (1992) 'Coordination between equilibrium and head–trunk orientation during leg movement: a new strategy built up by training.' *Journal of Neurophysiology*, **67**, 1587–1598.

Nardone, A., Schieppati, M. (1988) 'Postural adjustments associated with voluntary contraction of leg muscles in standing man.' *Experimental Brain Research*, **69**, 469–480.

Nashner, L.M., Forssberg, H. (1986) 'Phase-dependent organization of postural adjustments associated with arm movements while walking.' *Journal of Neurophysiology*, **55**, 1382–1394.

—— Shumway-Cook, A., Marin, O. (1983) 'Stance posture control in selct groups of children with cerebral palsy: deficits in sensory organization and muscular coordination.' *Experimental Brain Research*, **49**, 393–409.

Nouillot, P., Bouisset, S., Do, M.C. (1992) 'Do fast voluntary movements necessitate anticipatory postural adjustments even if equilibrium is unstable?' *Neuroscience Letters*, **147**, 1–4.

Oddsson, L. (1989) 'Motor patterns of a fast voluntary postural task in man: trunk extension in standing.' *Acta Physiologica Scandinavica*, **136**, 47–58.

—— (1990) 'Control of voluntary trunk movements in man. Mechanisms for postural equilibrium during standing.' *Acta Physiologica Scandanivica*, **595** (Suppl.), 1–60.

—— Thorstensson, A. (1986) 'Fast voluntary trunk flexion movements in standing: primary movements and associated postural adjustments.' *Acta Physiologica Scandinavica*, **128**, 341–349.

Palmer, E., Cafarelli, E., Ashby, P. (1994) 'The processing of human ballistic movements explored by stimulation over the cortex.' *Journal of Physiology*, **481**, 509–520.

Pal'tsev, Y.I., El'ner, A.M. (1967) 'Preparatory and compensatory period during voluntary movement in patients with involvement of the brain of different localization.' *Biophysics*, **12**, 161–168.

Pedotti, A., Crenna, P., Deat, A., Frigo, C., Massion, J. (1989) 'Postural synergies in axial movements: short and long-term adaptation.' *Experimental Brain Research*, **74**, 3–10.

Rogers, M.W., Kukulka, C.G., Soderberg, G.L. (1987) 'Postural adjustments preceding rapid arm movements in parkinsonian subjects.' *Neuroscience Letters*, **75**, 246–251.

Rothwell, J.C., Traub, M.M., Day, B.L., Obeso, J.A., Thomas, P.K., Marsden, C.D. (1982) 'Manual motor performance in a deafferented man.' *Brain*, **105**, 515–542.

Sanes, J.N., Jennings, V.A. (1984) 'Centrally programmed patterns of muscle activity in voluntary motor behavior of humans.' *Experimental Brain Research*, **54**, 23–32.

Viallet, F., Massion, J., Massarino, R., Khalil, R. (1987) 'Performance of a bimanual load-lifting task by Parkinsonian patients.' *Journal of Neurology, Neurosurgery and Psychiatry*, **50**, 1274–1283.

212

———— ———— ———— ———— (1992) 'Coordination between posture and movement in a bimanual load lifting task: putative role of a medial frontal region including the supplementary motor area.' *Experimental Brain Reserach*, **88**, 674–684.

Wilson, S.A., Lockwood, R.J., Thickbroom, G.W., Mastaglia, F.L. (1993) 'The muscle silent period following transcranial magnetic cortical stimulation.' *Journal of the Neurological Sciences*, **114**, 216–222.

Yabe, K. (1976) 'Premotion silent period in rpaid voluntary movement.' *Journal of Applied Physiology*, **41**, 470–473.

11
DEVELOPMENT OF NEURAL MECHANISMS UNDERLYING GRASPING IN CHILDREN

A.M. Gordon and H. Forssberg

The ability to grasp and manipulate objects and to use objects as tools sets humans apart from nearly all other animals. The lateral position of the forearm relative to the trunk and unusual rotational capabilities of each limb segment allow humans extensive mobility. Furthermore, the relatively long thumb and short fingers, as well as neural substrates allowing independent opposition of the thumb to each of the fingers, underlie the ability to shape the hand to objects of various sizes and shapes. These behaviors were present and necessary for the survival of our earliest primate ancestors, who required them to retrieve food from branches of trees and for grooming (for review of evolution, see Marzke 1994). Further evolution of prehensile capabilities, along with increasing intelligence, have defined the distinctions between humans and the remainder of the animal kingdom.

Reaching serves to propel the hand to a desired location in space. Thus grasping and object manipulation require goal-directed reaching to place the hand in the appropriate spatial location. Grasping involves coordinating the digits according to the intrinsic properties of an object and precisely controlling fingertip forces once contact with an object is established. While these motor behaviors appear simple, they depend on complex neural mechanisms requiring profound sensorimotor interaction. Dexterous reaching and grasping movements are not present at birth in humans or other higher primates. They emerge in a series of steps during ontogeny. This chapter will focus on the development of the neural mechanisms underlying the control of prehension.

Neuro-anatomical substrates for prehension

The precision grip, with true opposition of the pulp of the thumb and index finger, is considered to be the hallmark of manual dexterity. It allows skillful manipulation of objects between the fingers and thumb with precise control of prehensile force (Napier 1956). This grasp pattern evolved relatively late during evolution, and is seen exclusively in some higher primates. In spite of a hand configuration similar to that of humans, the squirrel monkey (*Saimiri sciureus*), for example, grasps objects by closing all of the fingers and the hand together, irrespective of the size, shape and orientation of the object (Phillips 1971). The difference in grasping patterns, in spite of similar morphology, emphasizes the importance of the neural control apparatus that has evolved. Clinical evidence from humans, as well as experimental studies with old world monkeys (macaques), indicate that the motor cortex and corticospinal projections are essential for discrete movements of the fingers. Relatively independent finger movements are impaired or lost after lesions of the motor cortex or cortico-spinal tracts (Lawrence and Kuypers 1968, Lawrence 1994). Following corticospinal lesions in macaque monkeys, the precision grip is replaced by a whole hand grasp, similar to that of the squirrel monkey. Additional lesions show that the recovered whole-hand grasp is dependent on rubrospinal projections, while reaching movements are more dependent on other subcortical pathways (Lawence and Kuypers 1968). Later studies, which utilized electrophysiological techniques and histochemical staining, reveal a specific corticomoto-neuronal system, which preferentially innervates motoneurons to distal finger muscles (Fetz and Cheney 1980). Comparative anatomical studies have shown that corticomoto-neuronal projections reach their greatest density in anthropoid apes and humans, whereas there are few such projections in the squirrel monkey (Harting and Noback 1970). Based upon these investigations, as well as other anatomical, physiological and behavioral studies, it is generally accepted that the motor cortex and the corticomotoneuronal pathways constitute an essential part of the neural systems controlling the precision grip and object manipulation with independent finger movements (Schieber 1990).

The ability to perform independent finger movements and grasp with the precision grip is not present when voluntary reaching and grasping emerge. In humans, the precision grip appears around 9–12 months after birth, and its development parallels the development and maturation of corticomotoneuronal connections. We do not contend that development of these structures occurs in the absence of socially and environmentally driven experiences. Indeed, sensory and motor maps are dynamically maintained and driven by function (for reviews, see Merzenich and Jenkins 1993, Donoghue 1995). Nevertheless, appropriate maturation of neuronal structures is necessary for development of independent finger move-ment. The development of these pathways and their significance for the development of manual dexterity are discussed in Chapter 8.

Coordination of reaching and grasping

During reaching, the configuration of the hand begins long before the object is contacted. First, there is a progressive opening of the grip with extension of the fingers, followed by flexion which serves to preshape the fingers according to the size of the object (Jeannerod 1981, 1984). Visuomotor channels are thought to process 'extrinsic' object properties (*e.g.* position and orientation in extrapersonal space) and 'intrinsic' object properties (*c.g.* size and shape), which are used to regulate transport and grasp respectively (Jeannerod 1981, 1984). Although it has been proposed that the channels are separate, they are likely to be interdependent since perturbation of the object or the arm influences both reach and finger aperture (Paulignan *et al.* 1990, Haggard and Wing 1991, Castiello *et al.* 1993). In monkeys, neurons in the inferior parietal lobe and the inferior premotor area are responsive to the size, shape and orientation of objects, as well as the specific types of grip that are to be used (Rizzolatti *et al.* 1988). In humans, neuropsychological studies of patients with lesions suggest that the identification of the intrinsic properties of objects involves the occipitotem-poral pathway, while object localization and grasping are processed in the posterior parietal cortex (see Jeannerod *et al.* 1995).

The random appearance of limb movements in newborn infants suggests that they are not goal-directed. While infants may not position the hand in a manner which is conducive to grasping, the limb, however, may be partially directed toward fixated objects moving in the environment (von Hofsten 1979). The hand opens before or during the reach, but the fingers do not close when the object is approached. While some infants may exhibit crude hand-shaping to an object during the first weeks after birth (see Bower 1970), these finger movements are very immature. The movements may represent a preformed proximodistal motor pattern, eventually evolving into prehension (Trevarthen 1984). The distance and direction of the reach improve around 4–5 months of age, but the hand orientation and finger closure are still rather restricted (von Hofsten 1982, von Hofsten and Rönnqvist 1988). By 9 months, the fingers begin to be shaped according to the size of the object, and this ability develops further during ontogeny (von Hofsten and Rönnqvist 1988).

Coordination of grasping and object manipulation

Grasping in infants is governed largely by tactile and proprioceptive reflexes (Peiper 1963, Twitchell 1970). Stimulation of the palm elicits closure of the fingers, while stimulation of the dorsal hand may inhibit a grasp reflex or elicit a reflexive opening of the hand. Stretching the flexor muscles by traction of the arm also induces hand closure as part of a flexor synergy, in which all flexor muscles about the shoulder, elbow and wrist are contracted along with the finger flexors. Gradually, these reflexive behaviors become less stereotyped, and normal prehension develops in several steps.

The grasp reflex may disappear before voluntary grasping emerges (Illingworth 1975), though some researchers postulate that the reflex remains and interacts purposefully with motor commands (*e.g.* Twitchell 1970). In contrast to monkeys deafferented surgically *in utero*, monkeys that have experienced reflexive grasping during infancy recover manipulative function following deafferentation (Taub 1976). In humans, the palmar grasp, in which all the fingers are voluntarily clasped around an object, emerges at around 4 months of age (Halverson 1931). At about the same time there is a progressive dissociation of the grasping reflex and the traction response (Twitchell 1970). Gradually, in the latter part of the first year, independent finger movements emerge and children begin to grasp between the tips of the thumb and index finger (precision grip). As development continues, the grip becomes more defined and children gradually become capable of using several grip patterns (Napier 1956, Connolly and Elliott 1972).

Sequential coordination of fingertip forces

Once an object is grasped, the fingertip forces must be coordinated appropriately, independent of whether the object is to be held stable, lifted or moved from one position to another. The coordination of these forces has been investigated extensively in human adults for more than a decade by Johansson and his colleagues (Johansson and Westling 1984, 1988; for reviews, see Johansson and Cole 1992, Johansson 1996) by asking subjects to grasp and lift a small instrumented object using the precision grip. Figure 11.1 shows the instrumented object and a recording of a grip–lift movement in an adult. The initiation of finger closure during reaching to match the intrinsic properties of the object (Jeannerod 1981, 1984) results in only a short delay between contact of the index finger and thumb (T0-1). Following

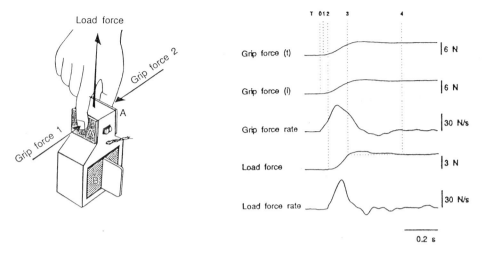

Fig. 11.1. *(Left)* Schematic drawing of the instrumented grip object: (A) exchangeable grip surfaces covering strain-gauge force transducers for measuring grip and lift force; (B) exchangeable mass. *(Right)* Grip force from the thumb (t) and index finger (i), grip force rate, load force and load force rate as a function of time for an adult. The object is contacted first by one finger (T0). Both grip forces begin to increase (T1), before the onset of positive load force (T2). The grip force and load force increase in parallel during the loading phase until lift-off (T3). (Modified from Gordon 1994.)

contact of the object by both fingers, there is a small increase in grip (pinch) force during the *preload phase* (T1-2), establishing a firm grasp before the onset of positive load (vertical lift) force increase (T2). During the following *loading phase* (T2-3), the grip and load force increase simultaneously until the load force overcomes the gravitational force on the object, and it is lifted from its support (T3). The object is transported to the desired position during the *transition phase* (T3-4), and held stationary in the air during the subsequent *static phase*, before being replaced on the support surface and released (not shown).

Each phase of the grip/lift movement is characterized by a specific pattern of muscular activity and force development, which is programmed to achieve a particular goal (*e.g.* to establish grip contact or lift the object from its support). The completion of the goal is reflected by transient mechanical events giving rise to phase-specific patterns of discrete sensory inputs. This sensory information is used to monitor the progress of the movement, and may trigger subsequent movement phases. Thus, the entire reaching–grasping–lifting behavior appears to consist of a series of prestructured motor commands, which are activated in a sequence upon signaling of specific sensory inputs reflecting the success of the previous command.

This sensorimotor interaction is exemplified by the response of tactile afferents at the fingertips (recorded using microneurography). The initial response of tactile afferents from the fingertips contacting the object (particularly, fast adapting type I afferents; FA I) signals that a stable contact from opposing fingers (Johansson 1991) as well as appropriate placement of the fingers (Gordon and Soechting 1995) have been achieved. The subsequent release

217

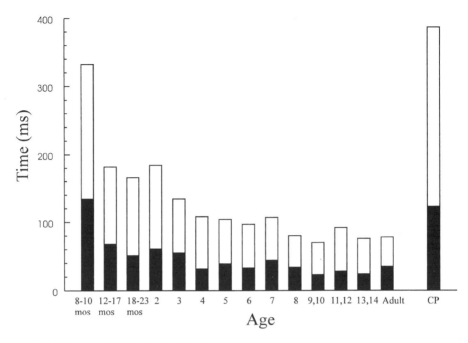

Fig. 11.2. Histogram showing the duration between contact of the thumb and index finger *(filled bars)* and the duration of the preload phase *(unfilled bars)* as a function of age. [Adapted from data in Eliasson *et al.* (1991) and Forssberg *et al.* (1991).]

of motor commands initiating the lifting drive is prolonged greatly when this information is suppressed by anesthetizing the fingertips (Johansson and Westling 1984). Fast adapting type II afferents (FA II) are particularly sensitive to mechanical transients, and signal when the object lifts off from its support (Westling and Johansson 1987, Johansson 1991). These afferent responses can indicate if an object has started to move earlier than anticipated when the object is lighter than expected, and trigger an abrupt termination of the muscle commands driving the loading phase within 60–90 ms after lift-off. Conversely, if the object is heavier than expected and the lift-off does not occur at the predicted load force, the absence of the movement is confirmed through the lack of transient FA II response. In this event, a new control mode is initiated in which the forces are increased slowly in small discontinuous steps until the object is lifted (Johansson and Westling 1988; Gordon *et al.* 1991b, 1993). The programmed motor command that drives the unloading phase when the object is replaced on the support surface similarly is triggered by somatosensory information signaling the touch down of the object (Johansson and Westling 1988).

In a recent series of studies, we have examined the development of the coordination of fingertip forces in healthy children (Forssberg *et al.* 1991, 1992, 1995; Gordon *et al.* 1992, 1994; Gordon 1994; Eliasson *et al.* 1995a) and in children with infantile cerebral paresis (Eliasson *et al.* 1991, 1992, 1995b). In children, the various movement phases of the lift described above are much longer than in adults, especially in those below 2 years of age.

This is due partly to prolonged delays from the mechanical events signaling the termination of one phase and the onset of the motor activity beginning the next phase (Forssberg *et al.* 1991). This can be seen in Figure 11.2, which shows the latencies between contact of each finger and the duration of the preload phase for each age group studied. For the youngest children (below 1 year), the latency between the contact of the two fingers was more than three times longer than in adults, and the preload phase duration was more than four times longer. Together, these phases are nearly twice as long in children below 3 years of age than they are in adults, but they quickly approach adult values thereafter. The youngest children often require several touches of the object before they can establish a stable grasp and initiate the loading phase. This probably reflects an inefficient shaping and closure of the hand during the reaching phase (von Hofsten and Rönnqvist 1988) as well as an inability to use quickly the tactile information obtained during finger contact to release the motor command for the loading drive. Similarly, the shift from the loading phase to the transition phase after lift-off in the youngest children is not smooth, as shown by a longer delay between lift-off and termination of the grip force increase.

Children with spastic hemiplegia and diplegia aged between 6 and 8 years have not yet developed the capacity to form smooth transitions between phases comprising the grip/lift movement (Eliasson *et al.* 1991). As is also evident in Figure 11.2, the delay from initial finger contact to the onset of the loading phase is much longer in the children with cerebral palsy (CP) than in healthy children of a similar age, and even longer than in infants less than 1 year old. The latency between lift-off of the object from its support and termination of the grip force increase is also prolonged (not shown). These children often have disturbed tactile sensation at the fingertips, which further emphasizes the importance of such sensory information for triggering prestructured motor commands comprising each phase of the grip/lift movement.

Parallel coordination of fingertip forces
During the loading phase, adults normally generate the grip force and load force in parallel until the object lifts off from its support (Johansson and Westling 1984). This can be seen in Figure 11.3, which shows the grip force plotted against load force during the preload and loading phases for three superimposed trials for adults and for children of various ages. There is a linear relationship between the two forces for the adults. The parallel development of grip force and load force reflects a functional synergy in which the grip and load forces are coupled, thus simplifying the movement. These two forces also are coupled during the movement of grasped objects (Flanagan *et al.* 1993, Flanagan and Tresilian 1994). In contrast, when the precision grip first emerges, young children do not generate the forces in parallel (Forssberg *et al.* 1991). Instead, they initiate the grip force in conjunction with a negative load force, pressing the object against its support. By the onset of positive load force, there is already a large grip force, and subsequent increases in the isometric grip and load force during the loading phase are not in parallel. This is reflected by curvilinear traces in the figure. During the latter part of the second year, the grip and load forces begin to increase more in parallel, and the coupling between them increases until adolescence.

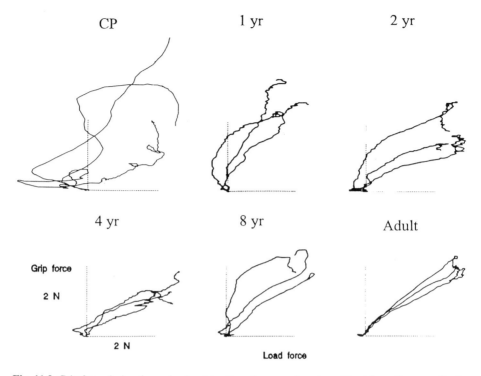

Fig. 11.3. Grip force during the preload and loading phase as a function of load force for normally developing children of various ages, an 8-year-old child with CP (diplegia), and an adult. [Modified from Eliasson *et al.* (1991) and Forssberg *et al.* (1991).]

In contrast, the grip force and load force often remain uncoupled in children with CP who have impaired manual dexterity (Fig. 11.3). These children exhibit a similar sequential onset of grip and load force, in conjunction with a large negative load force during the preload phase, which is even more exaggerated than in young infants. The sequential activation of the forces and excessive grip force at the onset of the lift drive in young children and children with CP probably allows additional information regarding the surface friction to be obtained and the grasp to be stabilized, as well as providing a strategy less dependent on anticipatory control.

Variability in force coordination
In adults, the generation of grip and load forces is highly automated and invariant between trials. This can be seen in Figure 11.4, which shows, for five superimposed lifts by subjects aged 1 year to adulthood, the grip force from the thumb and index finger, the load force, the first derivative of grip force (grip force rate) and the position of the object during the lift. The adult plots show very low variability between lifts. In contrast, those for the young children exhibit marked variability between trials, with excessive grip forces which oscillate during the static phase when the object is held in the air. In addition, there is a

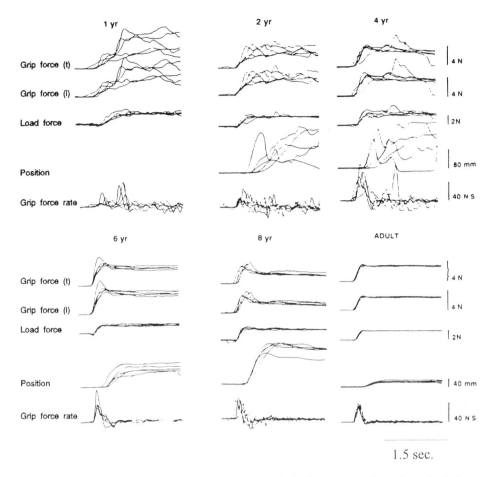

1.5 sec.

Fig. 11.4. Grip force from the thumb (t) and index finger (i), load force, vertical position and grip force rate as a function of time during several trials for one child of each age and an adult. Position signals are omitted for the 1-year-old since these children often grasped the object from the experimenter's palm. (Modified from Forssberg *et al.* 1991.)

large intrasubject variability in the force amplitudes and temporal parameters. A similar large variability of motor output in children is also seen in other motor tasks, including postural control and locomotion (Forssberg and Nashner 1982; Forssberg 1985; Hadders-Algra *et al.* 1996). Despite the negative consequences of being unable to reproduce reliably a force pattern over successive lifts of an object, the increased variability seen in children may serve as an adaptive strategy. It may allow the CNS to explore and evaluate different response patterns, and relate the intended movement to the motor consequences (Touwen 1978, Sporns and Edelman 1993). This would facilitate the establishment of relationships between movement parameters and interactions with the environment. The variability also may reflect constant adaptation to a rapidly changing system (*i.e.* changes in limb length and mass).

Gradually, the force output becomes more stable and stereotypical, with subtle improvements continuing until adolescence.

Anticipatory control of force output

During lifts of an object, its precise weight cannot be determined until after lift-off since information signaling the required force to displace the object is necessary. Similarly, frictional information is unavailable until after 0.1–0.2 seconds following initial contact with the object (Johansson and Westling 1984, Edin *et al.* 1992). Excessive force development may result in brisk lifting movements and potential damage to fragile objects, while too slow a force development may increase the risk of dropping the object. In order to avoid these possibilities, the development of isometric force during the loading phase must be scaled (planned) prior to the initiation of the movement to match the object's expected weight and friction based on previous manipulatory experience. Similar anticipatory force control is seen during mastication (Ottenhoff et al. 1992, Trulsson and Johansson 1996) and when catching a ball (Lacquaniti *et al.* 1992). The latter study suggests that such anticipatory control must take into account the geometry and dynamics of the limb in addition to the physical properties of the object. Anticipatory control of the force output is characterized by grip and load force-rate profiles which are mainly bell-shaped (similar to the continuous velocity profiles during arm movements; cf. Brooks 1984) with the amplitude scaled from the onset towards the target load force. This can be seen in Figure 11.5 (adult traces), which shows the grip and load forces and their derivatives during consecutive lifts of an object with slippery (satin: *dotted traces*) and rough (sandpaper: *solid traces*) contact surfaces. The peak force rate amplitudes are higher for the satin surfaces (cf. Johansson and Westling 1984, 1987). The force rates are appropriately decreased prior to lift-off to produce smooth, critically damped lifting movements (Johansson and Westling 1988, Gordon *et al.* 1993). Such anticipatory control of the force output is based on internal representations of the object's physical properties gained during previous experience with the object (Johansson and Westling 1988). Current visual information can also be used to retrieve appropriate internal representations for common objects (Gordon *et al.* 1993) or estimate the weight according to size–density cues (Gordon *et al.* 1991a,b,c). Knowledge about how useful such information will be during subsequent lifts with the object may influence the storage and retrieval of this information (Gordon *et al.* 1994).

In contrast, the force development for young children occurs in small increments, with multipeaked force-rate profiles (see Figs. 11.4, 11.5) (Forssberg *et al.* 1991). Similar force-rate profiles are observed when adults employ a 'probing strategy' in which coordinated grip and lifting force commands which yield low force rates are generated when lifting novel objects (Gordon *et al.* 1993), when they are uncertain about the object's physical properties (Gordon *et al.* 1991b) or when they encounter objects that are heavier than expected (Johansson and Westling 1988, Gordon *et al.* 1993). This reduces the dependence on anticipatory control at the expense of more slowly paced lifting, yet prevents large positional overshoots (or crushing the object) during the lifting movement. During the later part of the second year, the force-rate profiles become increasingly bell-shaped with small irregularities. Subsequent development is gradual and approximates adult-like coordination by the time

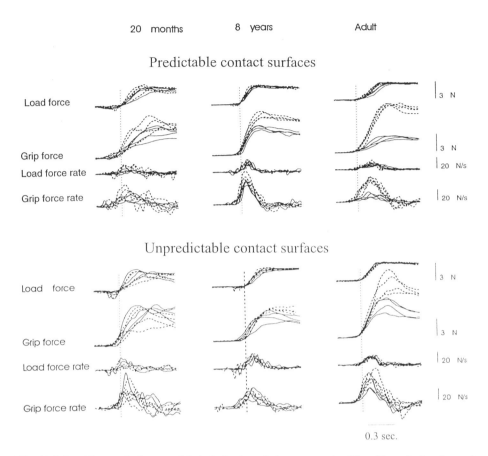

Fig. 11.5. Load force, grip force, and their derivatives during consecutive lifts with contact surfaces of either silk *(dashed lines)* or sandpaper *(solid lines)* during blocks of lifts in which the contact surfaces were predictable *(top)* and unpredictable *(bottom)* for a 20-month-old child, an 8-year-old child and an adult. (Modified from Forssberg *et al.* 1995.)

children reach 6–8 years of age, with subtle improvements until adolescence (Forssberg *et al.* 1991) (see Fig. 11.4).

During lifts in which the friction at the digit–object interface is completely predictable (numerous lifts with the same contact surfaces), the object's friction slightly influences the amplitude of the grip force rate in many children under 2 years of age (Fig. 11.5) (Forssberg *et al.* 1995). A similar scaling of both grip force and load force according to the object's weight is also seen at this age (Forssberg *et al.* 1992). Nevertheless, some children below the age of 18 months do not exhibit anticipatory control of the force output, and instead obtain higher forces mainly by prolonging the duration of isometric force increase. This suggests that anticipatory control of the force output used to manipulate objects likely emerges sometime during the second year of life, but at varying rates.

223

Predictable contact surfaces

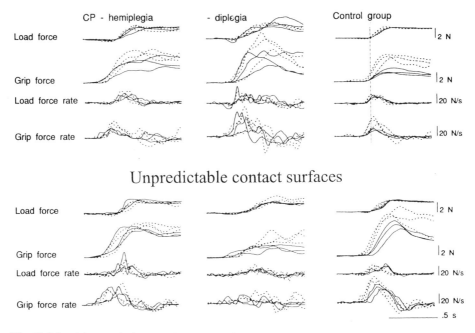

Fig. 11.6. Load force, grip force, and their derivatives during consecutive lifts with contact surfaces of either silk *(dashed lines)* or sandpaper *(solid lines)* during blocks of lifts in which the contact surfaces were predictable *(top)* and unpredictable *(bottom)* for a child with hemiplegia, another with diplegia, and a control subject. All children were between 6 and 8 years old. (Modified from Eliasson *et al.* 1995a.)

Despite the early evidence of anticipatory control of the force output in young children, the relative differences in force rates employed between objects of different frictions (or weights) is small in young children compared to adults. These differences generally become greater with increasing age concomitant with the emergence of more single-peaked force-rate profiles and the grip force/load force synergy described above. The small differences in force rates in these young children result in considerably slower accelerations of heavier objects (Forssberg *et al.* 1992), which are not temporally correlated with the occurrence of peak grip force (Paré and Dugas 1995) until the age of 6–8 years. Furthermore, anticipatory control is not seen in these children unless numerous trials with the same object characteristics are given, *i.e.* the weight and friction are predictable and remain stable from trial to trial (Forssberg *et al.* 1992, 1995). This can be seen in the lower portion of Figure 11.5, which shows the force traces during a series of lifts in which the contact surfaces were unpredictable from trial to trial. When the adults had two consecutive lifts with the same contact surfaces, they still scaled the grip force according to the contact surface in the preceding trial (*i.e.* higher grip force rates are seen for lifts with satin surfaces). No such force scaling was seen in younger children. This indicates that the mechanisms underlying the anticipatory control are not fully mature in these young children, and that they require several lifts with an object under conditions in which the object properties are kept constant (see Gordon *et al.* 1994) in order to store and retrieve appropriate representations of the object's physical characteristics. In contrast, only one or two lifts are required for adults to achieve appropriate representations of the object's physical characteristics (Johansson and Westling 1988, Gordon *et al.* 1993). Subtle improvements in the force coordination (Forssberg *et al.* 1991) and anticipatory control (Forssberg 1985, Forssberg *et al.* 1992) during precision grip in healthy children continue until adolescence.

Children with damage to cerebral structures and corticospinal pathways, such as in CP, often retain immature control strategies and some never develop proper anticipatory control of the finger-tip forces during precision grip (Eliasson *et al.* 1991, 1992, 1995b). This is illustrated in Figure 11.6, which shows the grip and load forces and their derivatives for one child with hemiplegia, one child with diplegia and one age-matched control subject (8 years old) during lifts with each contact surface. The influence of the object's friction on the force rates is small for the two CP children, and similar to that seen in the youngest children described above. Furthermore, these children also require several lifts of an object under predictable conditions, as seen by a lack of anticipatory control when the contact surfaces are unpredictable. This indicates a diminished capability to build appropriate internal representations of objects used for anticipatory control of the force output during subsequent manipulations. No influence of the object's weight on the force rates is seen in these children, even when the weights are presented in an entirely predictable order (not shown, see Eliasson *et al.* 1992).

Anticipatory control of the precision grip may develop later than anticipatory control underlying the hand closure relative to an object's size during reaching (von Hofsten and Rönnqvist 1988). However, visual information is continually available during reaching and this may guide the hand, as well as initiate and shape its closure. In contrast, anticipatory control of the force output during grasping is based on representations of the object's physical characteristics from previous lifts, or relationships between representations of weight and visual size/density cues.

While children begin to use anticipatory control to scale the force output in advance according to previously gained weight information during their second year, they are unable to use visual information regarding an object's current size until their third year (Gordon *et al.* 1992). This can be seen in Figure 11.7, which shows the relative difference in the peak load force rates employed for a small 300 g object and a proportionally larger 900 g object. Significant differences with this measure are not seen until the age of 2.5–3 years, whereas there are differences, based on the object's expected weight, by 1.5–2 years. This suggests that an additional year of development is necessary before children can make an associative transformation between the object's size and its weight. This probably involves additional demands on cortical processes, requiring further cognitive development. When the ability to use visual size cues emerges, children are much more influenced by this than adults are if the changes in size are not meaningful; that is if they do not covary with weight. This is in accordance with other studies showing children are less likely than adults to integrate sensory information from various modalities when they signal conflicting information (Forssberg and Nashner 1982).

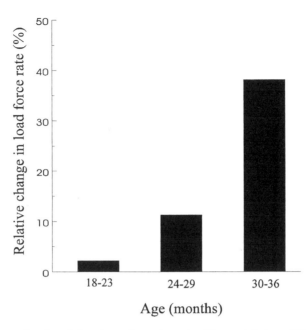

Fig. 11.7. Histogram showing relative change in maximum load force rate between lifts of a small (300 g) object and a large (900 g) object as a function of age. Zero per cent indicates no difference in load force rates. (Adapted from data in Gordon *et al.* 1992.)

Sensory adaptation of forces

In addition to triggering the release of prestructured motor commands during the early phases of a grip/lift movement, sensory information also is used intermittently to update the internal representation of the object's physical properties and regulate the force output during the current lift. Tactile afferent mechanoreceptors in the fingertips mediate the adaptation to the object's friction so that higher grip forces are employed for more slippery objects (Johansson and Westling 1984, Westling and Johansson 1984). This adaptation can be achieved independently at each object–digit interface (Edin *et al.* 1992) and results in only a small safety margin between the forces used and the force required to maintain grasp contact. Initial adjustments to new frictional conditions occur just 0.1 s after initial contact (Johansson and Westling 1984). Distinct bursts of slow (SA I) and fast (FA I) adapting afferents occur prior to the force adjustment, with the latter being especially sensitive to the slipperiness of the material (Westling and Johansson 1987). Thus tactile information is used to adjust the grip forces so that they are high enough to prevent accidental dropping of the object, and low enough to prevent unnecessary fatigue or to risk crushing fragile objects. Indeed, in healthy adult subjects only a small safety margin is employed, such that the grip force is only slightly higher than the force required to prevent dropping the object. Tactile afferent information signaling the extent to which the skin overlying the fingertip is indented may also be used to determine (perceive) the amount of force exerted at the fingertips (Henningsen *et al.* 1995).

Young children seemingly have a diminished capacity to adapt the grip forces according to frictional information at the fingertips (see Fig. 11.5). Children under 5 years of age employ considerably higher grip forces than adults (see Fig. 11.4) despite little difference in the slipperiness of the skin (Forssberg *et al.* 1995). This results in excessive safety margins, which are reduced in parallel with the maturation of force coordination (Forssberg *et al.* 1995, Paré and Dugas 1995). Despite the higher forces, most 1- to 2-year-old children employ slightly higher forces for more slippery objects when the contact surfaces are predictable (Fig. 11.5). However, only children over 2 years of age are able to adapt the grip forces by the end of the static phase following an unexpected frictional change. More rapid adjustments in grip force are seen only in adults.

The high safety margins of young children may partially reflect slow or inefficient responses to discrete sensory events such as slips at the object–digit interface. Discharges in tactile afferents normally trigger automatic force upgrades within 60–90 ms (Johansson and Westling 1984, 1987). These may partly involve supraspinal pathways involved in the long-latency component of cutaneous muscular reflexes (Jenner and Stephens 1982). These reflexes are weak or even absent in young children (Issler and Stephens 1983, Evans *et al.* 1990, Eliasson *et al.* 1995a). Alternatively, higher safety margins may be employed due to the large variations of within-trial grip forces exhibited in young children. This compensatory strategy, with excessive grip forces, would reduce the likelihood of dropping the object.

Large safety margins also are seen in subjects with a loss of tactile sensitivity at the fingertips. After digital anesthesia, adults lose their ability to regulate the grip force, and instead adopt an excessive grip force with a high safety margin (Johansson and Westling 1990). Similar behaviors are seen in elderly subjects (Cole 1991) as well as patients with damage to the median nerve (Johansson and Westling 1991). People with CP are thought to have impaired tactile sensory acuity in the fingertips (Tachdjian and Minear 1958, Lesný 1971, Uvebrant 1988). We found that children with CP have an impaired tactile regulation of the isometric fingertip forces during grasping (Eliasson *et al.* 1995b). Nearly all of the children with CP exhibited an excessive grip force during the static phase of the lift (up to 75% of their maximum grip force was employed to lift this 200 g object). Nevertheless, they did employ higher grip forces for more slippery objects, suggesting some maintained capability to use tactile afferent information.

Disturbed sensorimotor function in children with CP was also exhibited when the texture of the contact surfaces was unexpectedly altered between lifts (Eliasson *et al.* 1995b). Several children with CP do not adapt their grip forces to the actual friction even during the early static phase. It appears that they are unable to adapt quickly to a new texture, and require repeated trials or long lifting sequences before they can adjust the forces. A surprising finding was the poor relationship between two-point discrimination and the capability to adapt the grip force to the contact surfaces. This discrepancy suggests that the sensory pathways involved in the motor control of the hand and fingers are different than the neural pathways for tactile discrimination.

Conclusion
Coordinated grasping and manipulation of objects develops gradually over several years

of practice. It is dependent on the continuing development and maturation (*e.g.* myelination; cf. Müller *et al.* 1991) of the corticospinal tract and somatosensory systems that can effectively monitor sensory information from tactile afferents. The motor cortex and corticospinal tract directly control the precision grip (Lawrence and Kuypers 1968, Muir and Lemon 1983, Schieber 1990) and the force output of the distal muscles of the hand and wrist (Evarts 1968, Smith *et al.* 1975). Recent evidence suggests that the discharge of neurons in the motor cortex may also reflect the weight and friction of the object (Picard and Smith 1992). Indeed, early damage to these areas, such as in children with infantile CP, greatly impairs the ability to coordinate the force output in a functional synergy and to adapt the force during precision grip (Eliasson *et al.* 1991, 1992, 1995b). The regulation of forces during precision grip probably involves other cortical motor areas as well, such as the somatosensory cortex (Hepp-Reymond *et al.* 1989, Wannier *et al.* 1991). Cerebellar output may also reflect the physical properties of the object (Espinoza and Smith 1990, Dugas and Smith 1992). Thus maturation of these areas may be required before adult-like manual dexterity can be achieved. The maturation of peripheral mechanisms which reduce reflex latencies must also occur in order to skillfully manipulate objects. The prolonged reflex latencies in young children suggest a lack of sensorimotor integration (Issler and Stephens 1983, Evans *et al.* 1990, Eliasson *et al.* 1995a).

Despite the necessary maturation of neuronal structures needed for precise and dexterous finger movements and object manipulation, anticipatory control and sensory-driven control emerge early and gradually increase during ontogeny. Even before these behaviors approximate those of adults, young children may be able to compensate for their limited ability to use anticipatory and sensory-driven control by employing excessive forces, prolonging the movement phases, stabilizing the grasp by pushing the object against its support and exploring the relationship between the motor commands used and the movement outcome. Continued development of anticipatory control, the ability to integrate sensory information properly, and cognitive skills which allow predictive relationships between the object's physical characteristics may reflect the maturation of neural mechanisms controlling prehension.

REFERENCES

Bower, T.G.R., Broughton, J.M., Moore, M.K. (1970) 'Demonstration of intention in the reaching behaviour of neonate humans.' *Nature*, **228**, 679-681.

Brooks, V.B. (1984) 'How are "move" and "hold" programs matched?' *In:* Bloedel, J.R., Dichgans, J., Precht, W. (Eds.) *Cerebellar Functions.* Berlin: Springer, pp.1–23.

Castiello, U., Bennett, K.M.B., Stelmach, G.E. (1993) 'Reach to grasp: the natural response to perturbation of object size.' *Experimental Brain Research*, **94**, 163–178.

Cole, K.J. (1991) 'Grasp force control in older adults.' *Journal of Motor Behavior*, **23**, 251–258.

Connolly, K.J., Elliott, J. (1972) 'The evolution and ontogeny of hand function.' *In:* Blurton-Jones, C. (Ed.) *Ethological Studies of Child Behaviour.* Cambridge: Cambridge University Press, pp. 329–383.

Donoghue, J.P. (1995) 'Plasticity of adult sensorimotor representations.' *Current Opinion in Neurobiology*, **5**, 749–754.

Dugas, C., Smith, A.M. (1992) 'Responses of cerebellar Purkinje cells to slip of a hand-held object.' *Journal of Neurophysiology*, **67**, 483–495.

Edin, B.B., Westling, G., Johansson, R.S. (1992) 'Independent control of human finger-tip forces at individual digits during precision lifting.' *Journal of Physiology*, **450**, 547–564.

Eliasson, A-C., Gordon, A.M.Forssberg, H. (1991) 'Basic co-ordination of manipulative forces of children with cerebral palsy.' *Developmental Medicine and Child Neurology*, **33**, 661–670.

—— —— —— (1992) 'Impaired anticipatory control of isometric forces during grasping by children with cerebral palsy.' *Developmental Medicine and Child Neurology*, **34**, 216–225.

—— Forssberg, H., Ikuta, K., Apel, I., Westling, G., Johansson, R. (1995a) 'Development of human precision grip. V. Anticipatory and triggered grip actions during sudden loading.' *Experimental Brain Research*, **106**, 425–433.

—— Gordon, A.M., Forssberg, H. (1995b) 'Tactile control of isometric fingertip forces during grasping in children with cerebral palsy.' *Developmental Medicine and Child Neurology*, **37**, 72–84.

Espinoza, E., Smith, A.M. (1990) 'Purkinje cell simple spike activity during grasping and lifting objects of different textures and weights.' *Journal of Neurophysiology*, **64**, 698–714.

Evans, A.L., Harrison, L.M., Stephens, J.A. (1990) 'Maturation of the cutaneomuscular reflex recorded from the first dorsal interosseous muscle in man.' *Journal of Physiology*, **428**, 425–440.

Evarts, E.V. (1968) 'Relation of pyramidal tract activity to force exerted during voluntary movement.' *Journal of Neurophysiology*, **31**, 14–27.

Fetz, E.E., Cheney, P.D. (1980) 'Postspike facilitation of forelimb muscle activity by primate corticomotoneuronal cells.' *Journal of Neurophysiology*, **44**, 751–772.

Flanagan, J.R., Tresilian, J. (1994) 'Grip–load force coupling: a general control strategy for transporting objects.' *Journal of Experimental Psychology: Human Perception and Performance*, **20**, 944–957.

—— Wing, A.M (1993) 'Coupling of grip force and load force during arm movements with grasped objects.' *Neuroscience Letters*, **152**, 53–56.

Forssberg, H. (1985) 'Ontogeny of human locomotor control. I. Infant stepping, supported locomotion and transition to independent locomotion.' *Experimental Brain Research*, **57**, 480–493.

—— Nashner, L.M. (1982) 'Ontogenetic development of postural control in man: adaptation to altered support and visual conditions during stance.' *Journal of Neuroscience*, **2**, 545–552.

—— Eliasson, A.C., Kinoshita, H., Johansson, R.S., Westling, G. (1991) 'Development of human precision grip. I: Basic coordination of force.' *Experimental Brain Research*, **85**, 451–457.

—— Kinoshita, H., Eliasson, A.C., Johansson, R.S., Westling, G., Gordon, A.M. (1992) 'Development of human precision grip. II. Anticipatory control of isometric forces targeted for object's weight.' *Experimental Brain Research*, **90**, 393–398.

—— Eliasson, A.C., Kinoshita, H., Westling, G., Johansson, R.S. (1995) 'Development of human precision grip. IV: Tactlile adaptation of isometric finger forces to the frictional condition.' *Experimental Brain Research*, **104**, 323–330.

Gordon, A.M. (1994) 'Development of the reach to grasp movement.' *In:* Bennett, K.M.B., Castiello, U. (Eds.) *Insights into the Reach to Grasp Movement.* Amsterdam: Elsevier, pp. 37–56.

—— Soechting, J.F. (1995) 'Use of tactile afferent information in sequential finger movements.' *Experimental Brain Research*, **107**, 281–292.

—— Forssberg, H., Johansson, R.S., Westling, G. (1991a) 'Visual size cues in the programming of manipulative forces during precision grip.' *Experimental Brain Research*, **83**, 477–482.

—— —— —— —— (1991b) 'The integration of haptically acquired size information in the programming of precision grip.' *Experimental Brain Research*, **83**, 483–488,

—— —— —— —— (1991c) 'Integration of sensory information during the programming of precision grip: comments on the contributions of size cues.' *Experimental Brain Research*, **85**, 226–229.

—— —— Johansson, R.S., Eliasson, A.C.Westling, G. (1992) 'Development of human precision grip. III: Integration of visual size cues during the programming of isometric forces.' *Experimental Brain Research*, **90**, 399–403.

—— Westling, G., Cole, K.J., Johansson, R.S. (1993) 'Memory representations underlying motor commands used during manipulation of common and novel objects.' *Journal of Neurophysiology*, **69**, 1789–1796.

—— Forssberg, H., Iwasaki, N. (1994) 'Formation and lateralization of internal representations underlying motor commands during precision grip.' *Neuropsychologia*, **32**, 555–568

Hadders-Algra, M., Brogren, E., Forssberg, H. (1996) 'Ontogeny of postural adjustments during sitting in infancy: variation, selection and modulation.' *Journal of Physiology*, **493**, 273–288.

Haggard, P., Wing, A.M. (1991) 'Remote responses to perturbation in human prehension.' *Neuroscience Letters*, **122**, 103–108.

Halverson, H.M. (1931) 'Experimental study of prehension in infants by means of systematic cinema records.' *Genetic Psychology Monographs*, **10**, 107–286.

229

Harting, J.K., Noback, C.R. (1970) 'Corticospinal projections from pre- and postcentral gyri in the squirrel monkey (*Saimiri sciureus*).' *Brain Research*, **24**, 322–328.

Henningsen, H., Ende-Henningsen, B., Gordon, A.M. (1995) 'Contribution of tactile afferent information to the control of isometric finger forces.' *Experimental Brain Research*, **105**, 312–317.

Hepp-Reymond, M-C., Wannier, T.M.J., Maier, M.A., Rufener, E.A. (1989) 'Sensorimotor cortical control of isometric force in the monkey.' *In:* Allum, J.H.J., Hulliger, M. (Eds.) *Afferent Control of Posture and Locomotion. Progress in Brain Research Vol. 80.* Amsterdam: Elsevier, pp. 451–463.

Illingworth, R.S (1975) *The Development of the Infant and Young Child. Normal and Abnormal. 6th Edn.* Edinburgh: Churchill Livingstone.

Issler, H., Stephens, J.A. (1983) 'The maturation of cutaneous reflexes studied in the upper limb in man.' *Journal of Physiology*, **335**, 643–654.

Jeannerod, M. (1981) 'Intersegmental coordination during reaching at natural visual objects.' *In:* Baddeley, A. (Ed.) *Attention and Performance, Vol. 9.* Hillsdale: Erlbaum, pp. 153–168.

—— (1984) 'The timing of natural prehension movements.' *Journal of Motor Behavior*, **16**, 235–254.

—— Arbib, M.A., Rizzolatti, G.Sakata, H. (1995) 'Grasping objects: the cortical mechanisms of visuomotor transformation.' *Trends in NeuroSciences*, **18**, 314–320.

Jenner, J.R., Stephens, J.A. (1982) 'Cutaneous reflex responses and their central nervous pathways studied in man.' *Journal of Physiology*, **333**, 405–419.

Johansson, R.S. (1991) 'How is grasping modified by somatosensory input?' *In:* Humphrey, D.R., Freund, H-J. (Eds.) *Motor Control: Concepts and Issues.* Chichester: John Wiley, pp. 331–355.

—— (1996) 'Sensory control of dexterous manipulation in humans.' *In:* Wing, A.M., Haggard, P., Flanagan, J.R. (Eds.) *Hand in Brain: Neurophysiology and Psychology of Hand Movement.* San Diego: Academic Press, pp. 381–414.

—— Cole, K.J. (1992) 'Sensory-motor coordination during grasping and manipulative actions.' *Current Opinion in Neurobiology*, **2**, 815–823.

—— Westling, G. (1984) 'Roles of glabrous skin receptors and sensorimotor memory in automatic control of precision grip when lifting rougher or more slippery objects.' *Experimental Brain Research*, **56**, 550–564.

—— —— (1987) 'Signals in tactile afferents from the fingers eliciting adaptive motor responses during precision grip.' *Experimental Brain Research*, **66**, 141–154.

—— —— (1988) 'Coordinated isometric muscle commands adequately and erroneously programmed for the weight during lifting task with precision grip.' *Experimental Brain Research*, **71**, 59–71.

—— —— (1990) 'Tactile afferent signals in the control of precision grip.' *In:* Jeannerod, M. (Ed.) *Attention and Performance.* Hillsdale, NJ: Erlbaum, pp. 677–713.

—— —— (1991) 'Afferent signals during manipulative tasks in humans.' *In:* Franzen, O., Westman, J. (Eds.) *Information Processing in the Somatosensory System.* London: Macmillan, pp. 25–48.

Lacquaniti, F., Borghese, N.A., Carrozzo, C. (1992) 'Internal models of limb geometry in the control of hand compliance.' *Journal of Neuroscience*, **12**, 1750–1762.

Lawrence, D.G. (1994) 'Central neural mechanisms of prehension.' *Canadian Journal of Physiology and Pharmacology*, **72**, 580–582.

—— Kuypers, H.G.J.M. (1968) 'The functional organization of the motor system in the monkey. I.The effects of bilateral pyramidal lesions.' *Brain*, **91**, 1–14.

Lesný, I. (1971) 'Disturbance of two-point discrimination sensitivity in different forms of cerebral palsy.' *Developmental Medicine and Child Neurology*, **13**, 330–334.

Marzke, M.W. (1994) 'Evolution.' *In:* Bennett, K.M.B., Castiello, U. (Eds.) *Insights into the Reach to Grasp Movement.* Amsterdam: Elsevier, pp. 19–35.

Merzenich, M.M., Jenkins, W.M. (1993) 'Reorganization of cortical representations of the hand following alterations of skin inputs induced by nerve injury, skin island transfers, and experience.' *Journal of Hand Therapy*, **6**, 89–104.

Muir, R.B., Lemon, R.N. (1983) 'Corticospinal neurons with a special role in precision grip.' *Brain Research*, **261**, 312–316.

Müller, K., Hömberg, V., Lenard, H-G. (1991) 'Magnetic stimulation of motor cortex and nerve roots in children. Maturation of cortico-motoneural projections.' *Electroencephalography and Clinical Neurophysiology*, **81**, 63–70.

Napier, J.R. (1956) 'The prehensile movements of the human hand.' *Journal of Bone and Joint Surgery*, **38B**, 902–913.

Ottenhoff, F.A.M., Van Der Bilt, A., Van Der Glas, H.W., Bosman, F. (1992) 'Control of elevator muscle activity during simulated chewing with varying food resistance in humans.' *Journal of Neurophysiology*, **68**, 933–944.

Paré, M., Dugas, C. (1995) 'Developmental changes in prehension for children of 2–9 years old.' *Society for Neuroscience Abstracts*, **25**, 1920. *(Abstract)*

Paulignan, Y., MacKenzie, C., Marteniuk, R., Jeannerod, M. (1990) 'The coupling of arm and finger movements during prehension.' *Experimental Brain Research*, **79**, 431–435.

Peiper, A. (1963) *Cerebral Function in Infancy and Childhood.* New York: Consultants Bureau.

Phillips, C.G. (1971) 'Evolution of the corticospinal tract in primates with special reference to the hand.' *Proceedings of the International Congress of Primatology*, **2**, 2–23.

Picard, N., Smith, A.M. (1992) 'Primary motor cortical activity related to the weight and texture of grasped objects in the monkey.' *Journal of Neurophysiology*, **68**, 1867–1881.

Rizzolatti, G., Camarda, R.M., Fogassi, L., Gentilucci, M., Luppino, G., Matelli, M. (1988) 'Functional organization of inferior area 6 in the macaque monkey. II. Area F5 and the control of distal movements.' *Experimental Brain Research*, **71**, 491–507.

Schieber, M.H. (1990) 'How might the motor cortex individuate movements?' *Trends in NeuroSciences*, **13**, 440–445.

Smith, A.M., Hepp-Reymond, M-C., Wyss, U.R. (1975) 'Relation of activity in precentral cortical neurons to force and rate of force change during isometric contractions of finger muscles.' *Experimental Brain Research*, **23**, 315–332.

Sporns, O., Edelman, G.M. (1993) 'Solving Bernstein's problem: a proposal for the development of coordinated movement by selection.' *Child Development*, **64**, 960–981.

Tachdjian, M.O., Minear, W.L. (1958) 'Sensory disturbances in the hands of children with cerebral palsy.' *Journal of Bone and Joint Surgery*, **40A**, 85–90.

Taub, E. (1976) 'Movement in nonhuman primates deprived of somatosensory feedback.' *Exercise and Sport Sciences Reviews*, **4**, 335–374.

Touwen, B. (1978) 'Variability and stereotypy in normal and deviant development.' *In:* Apley. J. (Ed.) *Care of the Handicapped Child. Clinics in Developmental Medicine No. 67.* London: Spastics International Medical Publications, pp. 99–110.

Trevarthen, C. (1984) 'How control of movement develops.' *In:* Whiting, H.T.A. (Ed.) *Human Motor Actions: Bernstein Reassesed.* North-Holland: Elsevier Science, pp. 223–261.

Trulsson, M., Johansson, R.S. (1996) 'Forces applied by the incisors and roles of periodontal afferents during food-holding and -biting tasks.' *Experimental Brain Research*, **107**, 486–496.

Twitchell, T.E. (1970) 'Reflex mechanisms and the development of prehension.' *In:* Connolly, K. (Ed.) *Mechanisms of Motor Skill Development.* New York: Academic Press, pp. 25–45.

Uvebrant, P. (1988) 'Hemiplegic cerebral palsy. Aetiology and outcome.' *Acta Paediatrica Scandinavica*, Suppl. 345, pp. 5–100.

von Hofsten, C. (1979) 'Development of visually guided reaching: the approach phase.' *Human Movement Studies*, **5**, 160–178.

—— (1982) 'Eye–hand coordination in the newborn.' *Developmental Psychobiology*, **18**, 450–461.

—— Rönnqvist, L. (1988) 'Preparation for grasping an object: a developmental study.' *Journal of Experimental Psychology: Human Perception and Performance*, **4**, 610–621.

Wannier, T.M.J., Maier, M.A., Hepp-Reymond, M-C. (1991) 'Contrasting properties of monkey somatosensory and motor cortex neurons activated during the control of force in precision grip.' *Journal of Neurophysiology*, **65**, 572–589.

Westling, G., Johansson, R.S. (1984) 'Factors influencing the force control during precision grip.' *Experimental Brain Research*, **53**, 277–284.

—— —— (1987) 'Responses in glabrous skin mechanoreceptors during precision grip in humans.' *Experimental Brain Research*, **66**, 128–140.

12
THE DEVELOPMENT OF GRIP PATTERNS IN INFANCY

Karl M. Newell and P. Vernon McDonald

Prehension is the act of grasping and includes processes before and after the grip, such as the reach and withdrawal phases. Typically, humans utilize the hand for prehensile activity, although other organs such as the foot and the mouth may also be used for grasping. The many degrees of freedom of the arm(s) and hand(s) in both joint and muscle space contribute to the adaptability of the prehensile act in humans, and it is this functional flexibility that is a distinctive feature of human prehension when contrasted with the more limited prehensile actions of other primates. Grasping can be defined as the temporary union of hand and object (Bishop 1962, Malek 1981, MacKenzie and Iberall 1994). The grip pattern, therefore, describes the anatomical disposition of the fingers and thumb at the moment when they come into contact with the object, but it is only one aspect of the act of grasping. All grip patterns are dynamic action events and not merely static anatomical architectures.

The grasping actions of humans and other primates have been studied in detail by a number of investigators (*e.g.* Napier 1956, 1962, 1970; Landsmeer 1962; Elliott and Connolly 1984). Of the 58 possible movements of the hand, Napier (1970) claimed that prehensile grips fall into two basic functional categories—'precision' and 'power'. Napier distinguished these grips by the relative amount of finger versus palm prehension. In a precision grip the object is held between the tips of the fingers and the opposed thumb, whereas in the power grip the object is held between the ventral surface of the fingers and the palm. Napier held that the power grip was the first to appear during primate evolution, with the precision grip emerging later. He also proposed that this phylogenetic succession is observed in the ontogenetic development of human infants "whose precision grip only becomes effective long after the power grip is established". Some earlier investigators of prehension in human infants had distinguished these precision and power grips as 'pincer' and 'palmar', respectively; several other grip classification schemes have been proposed, including those by Landsmeer (1962), Kapandji (1970), Elliott and Connolly (1984), van Gemert (1984) and Cutkosky (1989). All of these classification approaches are based on anatomical or functional categorization schemes that vary in their characterization of the finger, thumb and palm contact patterns between object and hand.

In the prehensile progression traditionally described by developmentalists, a primitive grasp reflex is gradually transformed into voluntary prehension and a crude, clawing type of hand closure becomes a precise index finger–thumb opposition (Gesell 1928; Halverson 1931, 1937; Shirley 1931; Hooker 1938). According to Gesell (1928), maturation was the regulatory mechanism that stabilized the process of development and the emergence of the fundamental movement patterns, including prehension. Development itself was considered synonymous with growth and, therefore, was postulated to be a continuous process which, "beginning with conception proceeds stage by stage in orderly sequence, each stage representing a degree or level of maturity" (Gesell and Amatruda 1947). It was assumed that maturation was an unfolding process whereby the observed behavioral changes in development were presumably directly linked to concomitant neurological changes. Indeed, additional support for the assumptions of a maturational hypothesis was provided by those experimenters undertaking comparative studies of the development of the central nervous system (*e.g.* Coghill 1929, Bousfield 1953). The link between the maturation of the central nervous system and the emergence of behavior became the principal focus of much of the early motor development research (Gesell 1928; Halverson 1931, 1932; Shirley 1931; McGraw 1946). The maturational perspective, therefore, predicted a relatively orderly (invariant) sequence to the development of the fundamental motor patterns such as prehension, that was also regular (normative) in relation to developmental age.

More recent cognitive accounts of the ontogeny of hand function have also assumed a relatively invariant sequential order of progression to prehensile development and have chronicled the variations of power and precision grips, and their adaptations, over the early years of childhood (Bruner 1969, Connolly and Elliott 1972, Connolly 1973). These later studies attribute the prehensile progression to the development of perceptual-motor integration and increased cognitive capacity and mental representations in the older child. In this view, therefore, the order and regularity of the development of prehension is due to the acquisition of prescriptions for action that have been called, among other metaphors, plans, motor programs and subroutines (Newell and Barclay 1982).

Maturational and cognitive viewpoints have usually been seen as alternative explanations for the development of coordination, though they are not mutually exclusive. Current arguments regarding the nature of development are, in general, a matter of emphasis and, to some degree, a search from a variety of perspectives for the interactive effects between nature and nurture. The maturational perspective has retained its preeminence as the most widely used theoretical construct to account for infant motor development patterns despite the associated genetic determinism. This interpretation has lingered in motor development in spite of the subsequent theoretical contribution of Waddington's (1957) probabilistic epigenetic landscape and the empirical demonstrations of variations in the timing of the onset of patterns of coordination (Super 1981), and the more significant examples of omissions (Robson 1970, Touwen 1971) and reversals (Zingg 1940, Touwen 1971) in the developmental sequence.

In this chapter we will reexamine the assumption that there is a prescribed order in the development of grasping skills linking major shifts in grip patterns with the advance of chronological age. Also we will challenge the prescriptive, maturational and cognitive views as satisfactory accounts of the order and regularity observed in the development of prehension. Rather we will argue that prehensile skills are best viewed as an emergent property arising from the interaction of constraints imposed on the child rather than a direct consequence of prescriptions arising from a genetic algorithm or mental process. This interpretation for the observed order and regularity in the development of prehensile skills draws on the original propositions of the coordinative structure theory advanced by Kugler *et al.* (1980,

1982) and the more recent dynamical perspectives of coordination (Haken *et al.* 1985, Kugler and Turvey 1987, Beek and Beek 1988, Turvey 1990) and its development (Thelen *et al.* 1987, Thelen and Smith 1994) that have emerged since the beginnings of the paradigm shift to the self-organization metaphor.

The dynamical perspective suggests that organisms naturally adopt preferred patterns of coordination that are both stable and adaptive given the constraints imposed on action. In this view, the development of patterns of coordination are emergent properties of the principles of self-organizing biological systems, rather than reflections of prescriptions through symbolic knowledge structures (see also Kugler 1986). Understanding the constraints on action is central to discovering the way in which organismic, environmental and task constraints channel the dynamics of the patterns of coordination that emerge from the child–environment synergy (Newell 1984, 1986; Thelen 1986). Consequently, what follows is a review of traditional and contemporary studies of the development of grip patterns in order to reveal the impact that different constraints have on the sequence of grip patterns in infancy and early childhood.

A particular emphasis of this dynamical orientation to the development of prehension is an understanding of the role of body scale in determining the nature of the emergent grip patterns. Indeed, the interaction of task constraints (*e.g.* goal of the action), object properties (*e.g.* object size) and organismic constraints (*e.g.* hand size) appears to specify a preferred stable grip pattern of coordination. It is proposed that there are dimensionless body/object-scaled ratios that correspond to shifts in grip patterns for a given set of task constraints, which are to a large degree independent of developmental age.

The development of prehensile patterns
The literature on the development of prehension may be divided into three principal categories (after Castner 1932): naturalistic records of individual infants, psychometric investigations for the purpose of establishing norms of motor development, and cross-sectional experimental studies. These three operational approaches have typically examined prehension under different task constraints and have been guided by different theoretical persuasions. The findings from these studies are usually interpreted as supporting the prescriptive expectation of a sequential order to the appearance of grip patterns and the development of prehensile skills. However, there are a number of methodological limitations in these studies that are consistent with the suggestion that the order and regularity of children's grip patterns may be due to the narrow set of constraints imposed on the child, rather than the unfolding of the prescriptions of the genetic code as implied by the maturational theories or the development of new representations for action as proposed by cognitive theories.

Naturalistic studies
The earliest investigations of prehension preceded any theoretical views and consisted primarily of informal biographical records kept by parents. Accounts by Preyer (1890), Shinn (1893), Dearborn (1910) and others provide descriptions of the order in which certain prehensile behaviors appear. Castner (1932) suggested that such accounts be taken as atypical rather than typical instances of prehension due to the close relationship between the observers

and their infant subjects. In spite of this criticism, when the early naturalistic accounts are sufficiently complete and accurate, similar orders or sequences of behaviors are reported, although there are differences in the mean chronological ages noted for the onset of particular grasp patterns.

In general, the developmental order to grip patterns was seen to begin with reflex clasping, progressing through mechanical grasping of objects placed in the hand, to voluntary grasping of visually located objects (Preyer 1890, Shinn 1893). A number of discrepancies occur in the appearance of these various behaviors in terms of chronological age. For example, Moore (1896) placed the appearance of grasping to casual contact at 6 weeks, whereas other investigators did not observe this behavior until the 10th to 13th weeks (Preyer 1890, Shinn 1893). There is also a ten week discrepancy in the chronological ages recorded for the onset of visually directed grasping. Ament (1923) noted this behavior in infants at 10 weeks, whereas Simoneit (1928) did not observe it until 20 weeks. Other early observational studies suggested that the onset of visually directed reaching occurred between these two extreme chronological ages.

In these early studies, the type of grasp used by the child in action was not always reported with adequate detail. However, observations by Preyer (1890) and Dix (1911) noted the appearance of thumb opposition at 11 weeks and 16 weeks, respectively. Furthermore, Shinn (1893) described "good coordination between the fingers" and indicated that, at 34 weeks of age, the infant was unable to pick up tiny scraps, but at 36 weeks was able to pick up a small tack and pin. This observation places the emergence of the precision grip as late as 9 months.

In summary, these late 19th century naturalistic investigations provide descriptive records of the order of appearance and subsequent integration of many aspects of prehensile behavior, particularly during the period of infancy. However, even when grasping appears to have been carefully observed and recorded, details of the size and form of the object grasped are rarely provided, and no accounts reported anthropometric measurements of the infant's hand or arm. Finally, given that these early investigations of grasping spanned a period of 30 years in different environments and on individual cases, it is not surprising that divergent chronological ages were reported for the emergence of specific prehensile activities. Indeed, this variance in behavior in itself suggests that the development of prehension is not necessarily uniform and invariant and may be influenced by task, organismic and environmental constraints.

Psychometric investigations

In the 1920s and '30s there was a widespread concern among child psychologists for the establishment of norms of infant behavior, and prehension items were often included in the scales and tests. However, the issue at stake in these early tests was often not motor development as such but rather the maturation of the central nervous system as reflected in motor behavior. Consequently, prehensile activities were included under the general category of manipulative skills, which referred to both reaching and grasping. In addition, detailed examination was made of the other fundamental motor activity categories— namely, posture and locomotion.

Kuhlmann (1922) provided the earliest devised tests that included items requiring the prehension of objects during the first postnatal year. However, the tests in the lowest age groups, particularly at 3–6 months, were only roughly standardized. Furthermore, the tests were originally drawn up through a study of the informal records of Preyer (1890), Shinn (1893) and others and pilot-tested on a small unrepresentative group of infants. Little new knowledge was gained from Kuhlmann's tests about the development of prehension.

Gesell (1925, 1928) created a series of preschool tests for a number of developmental sequences, including prehension, which culminated in the construction of a tentative developmental scale of monthly increments from birth through 10 months of age. Gesell summarized the monthly increments in prehensile behavior under three broad categories: (1) the development of selective regard for objects from larger to smaller; (2) the development of reaching for objects from bilateral to unilateral; and (3) the development of grasping with hand and fingers from reflex, to grasp to tactile stimulation, to grasp to a visual cue. The grip itself was seen to develop from a crude primary grasp, to opposed thumb and then to precise pincer prehension.

A number of other psychometric investigations used procedures similar to those of Gesell. Linfert and Hierholzer (1928) based their tests in part on Gesell's scale so that equivalent age levels were reported. Although few prehension items were in their test battery, the study appears to be the only other psychometric investigation of this period that used an object as small as a pellet. Bühler (1930) based her infant tests in part on a more complete inventory of behavior during the first year. However, the prehension items were examined over a range only from 2 to 7 months (moving toward an object by changing position), and few new observations were furnished.

Although Gesell's investigations of grips patterns were the most controlled and extensive, some problems become apparent in attempting to summarize his results. Sometimes no grasp *pattern* is reported (*e.g.* Gesell 1928), it is merely stated that the infant grasped the object. On other occasions (*e.g.* Gesell and Thompson 1934), explicit reference is made to the relative amount of palmar *vs.* finger–thumb opposition. Given the variation in test objects used, the inconsistency of experimental conditions, and the resulting divergent findings regarding what prehensile activities are present at particular ages, it seems premature for Gesell to have proposed on the basis of these psychometric investigations that there is order and regularity in the development of prehension.

Experimental approach
EARLY EXPERIMENTS
Jones (1926) was one of the first investigators to manipulate experimentally the conditions under which human infant behavior was observed. Moreover, many more subjects were used than in any of the previous normative investigations. Almost 500 children were assessed, ranging in age from 11 to 41 weeks. A detailed study was made of thumb opposition in grasping a 2.5 cm cube, a 2.5 cm rubber ball, and a pencil. The focal question asked in the study was: does the thumb remain folded against the palm or fingers? Jones found that thumb opposition first appeared at 15 weeks, though it was not present in all cases until the 38th week. Unfortunately, which object elicited the early grasping was not reported.

236

Halverson's (1931, 1932, 1937) studies of prehension represent the first experimental investigations of the development of prehension as such. Twelve or more infants were tested at each of eight age levels: 16, 20, 24, 28, 32, 36, 40 and 52 weeks. Halverson was interested in three forms of behavior, the nature of visual attention (regard), the manner in which infants reach (approach), and the coordination pattern by which infants grasp (grip) a 2.5 cm cube. Unlike Jones (1926), Halverson did not find thumb opposition prior to 28 weeks. Instead, the young infants clamped the object into the palm by flexing the fingers, and although the thumb also flexed, it did not work in opposition. Halverson suggested that when opposition first appears at 28 weeks it is used only in association with a palmar grasp. By 36 weeks, fingertip grasping begins to emerge. An additional observation made by Halverson (1931) was that objects were moved distally and radially with respect to the palm. The relatively invariant developmental progression for prehension described by Halverson, and depicted schematically in Figure 12.1, is the description of grip patterns cited in developmental psychology textbooks.

Castner (1932) set out to map the course of fine prehension in children up to 1 year of age. Approximately ten subjects were tested at each of the following ages: 20, 28, 32, 36, 44 and 52 weeks. Castner examined the same three aspects of prehension as those recorded by Halverson (1931); namely, regard, approach, and grasp. Castner maintained that grasping the pellet was marked by increasing dominance and differentiation of the radial digits. Four types of grasp were observed: whole hand closure (20 weeks), palmar prehension (32–36 weeks), scissors closure (36–44 weeks), and pincer prehension (52 weeks). Castner's age estimates for the onset of specific prehensile skills lag behind those reported by Gesell (1928), who placed the emergence of the pincer grip of the pellet at 8 months (32 weeks), although deftness in this activity did not occur until 10 months (40 weeks).

A number of other investigators examined prehension as part of their more general developmental analysis of behavior. McGraw (1945) placed great emphasis on the collaboration of visual and motor mechanisms in the development of prehension. She outlined six phases of voluntary prehension: (1) newborn or passive, (2) object-vision, (3) visual-motor phase, (4) manipulation and deliberate, (5) visual release, and (6) mature. Although McGraw's outline may be useful for diagnostic purposes, little information was provided regarding either the objects used or the experimental situation. Similarly, Shirley (1931) stressed the role of vision in the development of prehension and also noted that a three-week difference occurred between the onset of grasping in a lying posture (15 weeks) and the onset of grasping in a sitting posture (18 weeks). Shirley, like McGraw, provided little information about experimental procedures, and it is therefore unclear as to what objects the infants were responding to. The types of grip were not alluded to apart from the observation that "thumb opposition is the first reaction in which the digits act separately", and this was placed at a median age of 18 weeks.

These early cross-sectional experiments represent the first systematic examinations of the development of grip patterns. They provide some useful information regarding the normative aspects of young infants' grasping behavior. However, the testing protocols were based on the earlier psychometric findings that resulted in only a small range of experimental manipulations being used. This narrow range of task conditions naturally affords a concom-

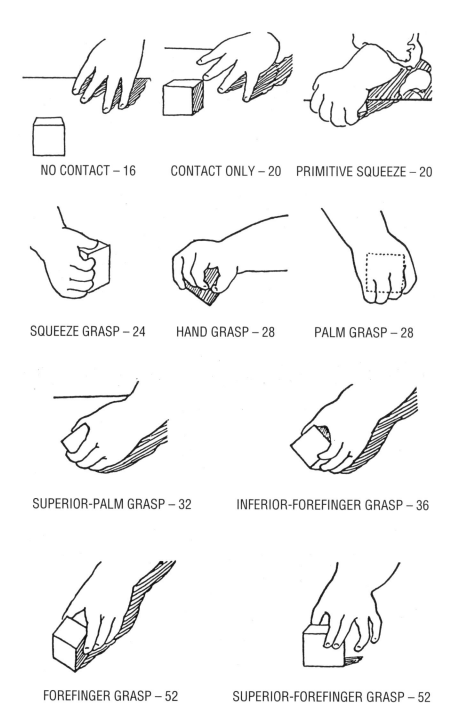

NO CONTACT – 16   CONTACT ONLY – 20   PRIMITIVE SQUEEZE – 20

SQUEEZE GRASP – 24   HAND GRASP – 28   PALM GRASP – 28

SUPERIOR-PALM GRASP – 32   INFERIOR-FOREFINGER GRASP – 36

FOREFINGER GRASP – 52   SUPERIOR-FOREFINGER GRASP – 52

Fig. 12.1. Schematic of the development of prehension. The number by each grip refers to the age in weeks at which the grip pattern appears. (Reproduced from Halverson 1931.)

itant narrow range of prehensile acts. As a consequence, the data that result from these tests tend to emphasize the priority of endogenous factors in the development of prehension and to many observers provide face if not construct validity for the maturational interpretation of the development of coordination (Gesell 1929, 1946).

Connolly (1970) has suggested that, as a consequence of the apparent success of the early developmental researchers (*e.g.* Gesell 1929, Halverson 1931) in answering the questions they posed, relatively little work was undertaken on motor skill development for almost 30 years. However, dissatisfaction with the assumption of genetic predeterminism stimulated a number of investigators in the 1960s to challenge the prevailing maturational interpretations of the development of behavior. In the area of prehension, the work of Bruner (1969), White (1970), Bower (1972) and Connolly (1973) offers the most systematic evidence re-evaluating the traditional sequence of prehensile skills proposed by Jones (1926), Halverson (1931) and Castner (1932), although the findings of some of these studies do not bear directly on the development of grip patterns.

White devoted much of his research effort toward establishing the role of experience in the development of human abilities (White *et al.* 1964, White 1970). White's work on human infancy "began with a study of the development of visual-motor capacities and in particular with the acquisition of visually directed reaching" (White 1970). White *et al.* (1964) developed a ten-step analysis of infants' prehension that culminated in the appearance of visually directed reaching just before 5 months. Subsequently, White and Held (1966) showed that prehension to visual stimuli can be significantly accelerated by modifying and enriching the environmental conditions in which the child is reared.

A number of investigators have more recently examined visually adapted reaching and pre-reaching in very young infants (Bower 1972; Field 1976, 1977; von Hofsten 1979, 1982, 1983, 1986; von Hofsten and Lindhagen 1979). This line of research suggests that even neonates (1–2 weeks) exhibit pre-reaching behavior and will make contact with an object. Furthermore, it has been found that infants vary their reaching behavior in accordance with the size and distance of the object (Bower 1972, Bruner and Koslowski 1972, Field 1976) and object direction (von Hofsten 1982). However, these studies were more concerned with the role of vision in the development of reaching than in documenting the influence of these different task constraints on the grip pattern *per se*.

There is evidence to suggest that manipulating the dynamic aspects of task constraints may also result in the earlier emergence of prehension. For example, von Hofsten (1982) used a moving rather than the traditional stationary object as the stimulus for a series of experiments in which the infant was required to intercept with the hand a brightly colored object moving in the horizontal plane. In these studies it was found that infants as young as 5 days would reach out and make contact with the moving object (von Hofsten 1982), a finding that has subsequently been replicated (von Hofsten 1986). In spite of the fact that the specific role for visual information in infants' pre-reaching and grasping activities has not been established (Lockman and Ashmead 1983), the emergence of prehensile skill earlier than proposed by the experimental studies (*e.g.* Halverson 1931) is consistent with the proposition that task constraints affect the observed onset of developmental motor patterns.

The objects used in the Bower and von Hofsten studies were quite large in relation to the size of the infants' hands. Therefore, when grasped, it is highly probable that a palmar or power grip was used, although neither von Hofsten nor Bower detail this. Nevertheless a chronological age of 1 week is considerably in advance of the age noted by Gesell, Halverson and others for initial reaching and grasping. Consequently, it seems reasonable to suggest that the emergence of thumb opposition and the precision grip may be advanced in certain circumstances.

In summary, these more recent investigations of prehension have indicated how reach and grasp behaviors may be influenced by environmental, organismic and task constraints, together with their interaction, but there has been little progress in understanding the development of the grip pattern itself.

The potential impact of anatomic and task constraints in prehensile skills has been studied by Connolly (1970, 1973; Connolly and Elliott 1972; Elliott and Connolly 1974). However, while recognizing that anatomy may impose limitations on movement (*e.g.* Elliot and Connolly 1974) and that size of objects may influence grips (*e.g.* Connolly 1973), Connolly never fully explored the significance of the hand-to-object size relationship. This omission may be due in part to his interest regarding the primacy of the cognitive control of the development of prehension. Thus, Connolly's research, along with that of Bruner (1969, 1972), seems to have been directed primarily toward examining the development of cognitive capacity as reflected in the development of prehension.

Connolly (1973) proposed that there was a sequence or dictionary of grips that developed during early childhood. This proposal was based on the observation of systematic changes over time in the grip configurations used by young children in the tasks of drawing and painting. These studies by Connolly and colleagues, however, are characterized by some of the same experimental design limitations as much of the earlier prehension research. For example, the experiments only compared infants' performance to that of adults under the *same* task constraints. Enumerating the grips utilized by young children in drawing led Connolly and Elliot (1972) to classify the grips according to their absolute difference to the adult grip, without reference to the body-scale of the objects to be grasped. Furthermore, the size of objects manipulated within an object category was quite limited.

The methods used in these more recent studies of prehension show significant improvement on those of earlier naturalistic and psychometric studies, although limitations still existed with respect to the range of task constraints manipulated and the failure to consider the role of body scale in the development of coordination. It is suggested that only a stronger manipulation of task, environmental and organismic constraints will reveal their full impact on the development of prehension (Newell 1986), regardless of chronological or maturational age. It is clear that a more considered empirical orientation to isolating the contribution of various constraints to the development of coordination in prehension is necessary. Otherwise it seems premature to conclude that the age-related invariant progressions in prehension during infancy and early childhood are reflections of the progressive development of prescriptions for prehension.

240

Limitations of research on the development of prehension

The early research on motor development, and on the development of prehension in particular, can be criticized on a number of grounds. The biographical investigations of the late 19th and early 20th centuries offer some insightful observations on the development of prehension, but their contribution is limited to descriptive records of the order of appearance of grasping patterns and other behaviors. Subsequent studies attempted to establish age norms for the emerging behavior and in so doing, frequently referred to these earlier works for purposes of comparison (Gesell 1929, Halverson 1931).

Such comparisons often reveal discrepant findings in assessments of the order and regularity of prehension development and these inconsistencies are not always due to the lack of formal investigative techniques. In particular, the divergent findings regarding the onset of prehensile behaviors may be attributable to differences in the way in which the experimental investigations were conducted, in spite of attempts at tighter control. Four major concerns regarding procedures are: the age of subjects, object characteristics, the mode of presentation of objects, and the postural position of subjects. The potential contribution of each of these experimental constraints will be examined in some detail to provide the background arguments for an alternative theoretical analysis of the development of prehension.

These methodological problems do not directly in and of themselves provide evidence against either the maturation hypothesis (Gesell 1929) or the cognitive orientation (Connolly and Elliott 1972) to the development of prehension. However, the fact that different prehensile grips appear when different constraints are imposed on the child suggests that there may be a systematic relation between the grip pattern and the confluence of constraints evident in the organism–environment synergy. The establishment of such a view would lend support to the dynamical perspective in which the patterns of coordination (*e.g.* grips) are emergent properties of the constraints imposed on action rather than products of prescriptions for action.

Age

Gesell's interest in collecting normative data necessitated the study of children from the earliest age possible (Gesell 1929, Gesell and Thompson 1934). Thus, Gesell and others who followed his lead in diagnostic enquiry (*e.g.* Shirley 1931, McGraw 1946) began their observations on newborn infants. Subsequent researchers, accepting the norms established for prehensile skills, began their studies on 4-month-old (Halverson 1931) and 5-month-old (Castner 1932) infants. The implicit assumption on which these investigators based their research was that the age norms reported by Gesell were indeed 'normative', thereby assuming chronological age to be an accurate indicator of both maturational level and prehensile capability. By ignoring inter-individual variability in assuming all 4-month-olds to be at the *same* developmental stage, these experimenters robbed the study of development of its very essence—intra-individual change over time (see Wohlwill 1973). This limitation has been perpetuated in many subsequent prehension studies. In addition to cross-sectional designs, there needs to be a return to the earlier type of longitudinal investigations that detailed the order of appearance of behaviors within individuals as a function of different task constraints. Connolly and Dalgleish (1989, 1993) reported the use of such a protocol with

241

respect to the development of spoon use and uncovered a set of very interesting findings on the development of prehension. However, the relation of subject age to the development of prehension is intricately interwoven with that of object characteristics because there is often a correlation between the age of a child and the size and shape of an object used in prehension.

Object characteristics

Gesell (1928) used a number of different objects, varying in both size and shape, in the examination of children's grasping activity. These initially included a bright red wooden embroidery ring of 11 cm diameter (this was attached to a string and dangled in front of the infant), a 2.5 cm bright red wooden cube, and an 8 mm white sugar pellet. Subsequently, other familiar objects were included such as a spoon, a rattle, a bell and a piece of paper. Gesell reported very different chronological ages for the emergence of voluntary grasping for the various objects used. At 4 months, both hands closed on the dangling ring when the infant was in the supine position. At 6 months, the cube was picked up from the table; and thumb opposition appeared first at about 9 months. At 7 months, infants could scoop or rake the pellet from the table; a partial pincer grip emerged at 8 months; and a precise pincer grip was evident by 10 months.

Subsequently, Halverson (1931) and Castner (1932) set out explicitly to examine cube and pellet prehension, respectively. The age norms established by Gesell were used as standards in their experiments. It is clear that different size objects afforded the onset of prehensile skills at different chronological ages and thus the wisdom in accepting Gesell's norms for motor development so literally should be questioned. The divergent responses as a function of age may be due entirely to the different task constraints. For example, grasping a 2.5 cm cube is a formidable task for a 4-month-old infant, but by scaling the size of the cube down in comparison to the size of the infant's hand, specific prehension grip patterns may be observed much earlier than expected from projections of the motor development sequence.

Halverson (1932) suggested that both hand size and object size may influence the type of grasp elicited, but in spite of this realization, he did not systematically manipulate the objects used in relation to the hand size of infants. Indeed, with reference to an apparent pincer grip used by infants of 12 weeks in grasping a small pellet, Halverson (1931) claims that this was not a reflection of a true precision grip. In a subsequent study on reaching (Halverson 1937), when no response was elicited within 9 seconds of presentation of a 7 mm pellet, the object was substituted by a 2.5 cm cube. A more gradual increment in object size may have revealed the influence of task constraints on the development of prehension.

A plausible reason for the delay in onset of thumb opposition in Halverson's study as opposed to the Jones (1926) report, may be due to the difference between placing the object in the hand (Jones 1926) and presenting the object on a table to await voluntary grasping (Halverson 1931). Alternatively, or additionally, the type of object may have affected the resultant observation. This is difficult to determine as Halverson primarily used a 2.5 cm cube and Jones failed to report the object size that first afforded thumb–index finger opposition. Also, the shift in position of the grasped cube relative to the palm may be influenced by the size of the object, in addition to progressive differentiation of thumb and finger movements.

Thus, although object characteristics such as size, shape, mass, coefficient of friction, etc., have been identified as key factors in determining the grasping pattern exhibited by young children (*e.g.* Gesell and Thompson 1934, McGraw 1946), there has been no systematic study of the effect of object characteristics and task constraints, in general, on the development of prehension. In particular, there has been no attempt to examine the role of body-scaled task constraints (*e.g.* object size to hand size) in the development of grip patterns exhibited by children of differing chronological ages, except for our preliminary work (Newell *et al.* 1989a,b) discussed later in this chapter.

Object presentation
The significance of task constraints is also evident in considering the mode of object presentation. Halverson (1931) addressed this issue when he alluded to the difference between a pencil placed in a child's hand (after Preyer 1890) and an object such as a cube placed on the table to await voluntary prehension. Unfortunately, rather than recognizing these different situations as potentially affording different actions, Halverson suggested that the thumb opposition elicited through the former situation was accidental in nature.

Another important aspect of object presentation is whether the object is static or dynamic. The customary mode of presentation in developmental prehension studies may be considered limited and slightly unnatural in that objects are typically placed in a stationary position on a table and infants given a fixed duration to exhibit a response. A more natural situation for infants may be to present objects in a dynamic, playful context. In addition, the dynamic display of stimuli may help overcome to some degree the performance limitations that may arise as a consequence of the poor visual acuity of the neonate and young infant (Dobson and Teller 1978, Boothe *et al.* 1985). The significance of dynamic stimulus contexts for prehension is an issue that has been addressed in some prehension studies (*e.g.* Bower 1972; von Hofsten 1979, 1986).

Postural position
One additional task constraint which has varied over investigations of prehension is the postural position of the children studied. For example, Gesell changed the postural position of the child according to his perception of the child's capabilities (Gesell 1929, Gesell and Thompson 1934). It appears that different postural positions were used for the various age groups. Gesell and Thompson (1934) reported that prior to 3 months infants lay supine, whereas after 3 months infants either sat strapped into a chair or sat erect alone, at a table. Although postural position may present more problems for the interpretation of reaching trajectories than grasping patterns, it has been suggested that posture also constrains the grasping action (Shirley 1931). The infant lying dorsally may be supported in a more stable manner than one in an upright position, and the influence of the force of gravity on the development of prehension interacts with postural position (Savelsbergh and van der Kamp 1994). A systematic way to examine the constraints imposed by postural position would be to use both supine and upright supported positions for prehension under a variety of task constraints.

243

Summary

The role in prehension of features external to the organism has largely been neglected in experimental tests of the maturational interpretation of the development of grip patterns, in spite of the explicit recognition of their potential in determining the pattern used. Even in the more recent experimental studies of prehension stimulated by a cognitive view of motor development, the range of task constraints manipulated has been very narrow. Undoubtedly, the collective evidence of the development of prehension in infancy suggests there is a ubiquity of order and regularity in the emergence of many fundamental motor skills in infancy regardless of methodological concerns. However, because order and regularity are observed at the behavioral level of analysis, this does not in itself provide sufficient evidence to infer that these patterns are reflections of some common prescription for action. Indeed, the normative developmental motor sequence observed in prehension and other phylogenetic activities may only exist by virtue of the common set of constraints typically imposed on infants and young children. The ensuing section briefly outlines the essence of the dynamical perspective in development as a basis for reinterpreting the progressions observed in the development of grip patterns.

Prehensile development: a dynamical perspective

In studies of the development of prehension, children typically exhibit movement sequences that are subsequently classified in terms of regard, approach and grasp. As we have seen in the previous synthesis, little experimental attention has been directed toward the systematic adaptations in children's prehensile actions to constraints such as object size and task goal, in spite of the apparent recognition of the potential influence of these factors (Halverson 1932, McGraw 1946). In assuming the unfolding neurological basis to the emergence of infant prehensile grip patterns, investigators have, in general, created experimental situations based on Gesell's (1928) age norms and task testing protocol.

In this section, we pursue the notion that the discrepancies in the onset times of particular grip patterns and the apparent order of the developmental progressions observed in the infant and early childhood studies of prehension reviewed above may well be driven to a large degree by the physical principles operating in the organism–environment interaction. Such an orientation (Kugler *et al.* 1980, 1982; Kugler and Turvey 1987) suggests that organisms exhibit behaviors that are stable and adaptive within the extant organismic, task and environmental constraints. In prehension, the interaction of task constraints, object properties and the organismic constraints of body growth and form appear candidate variables to consider the changing profile of grip patterns in infancy (Newell 1986).

The dynamical perspective to action

In the dynamical perspective of action, the patterns of coordination which develop are viewed as emergent properties of self-organization in biological systems, rather than as reflections of prescriptions of symbolic knowledge structures (Kugler *et al.* 1982, Kugler 1986, Thelen *et al.* 1987). In this viewpoint, the organizational principles of coordination and their resultant movement forms are specified in the dynamical stabilities and instabilities of the system—a system that is defined over the interaction of the organism and environment.

The evolving details of this theoretical framework have been developed in many papers over the past 15 years and they will not be repeated here (for recent reviews, see Turvey 1990, Thelen and Smith 1994). Rather, some key issues from this dynamical framework that pertain to the development of grip configurations in infancy are now briefly outlined.

It should be noted that the emphasis that the dynamical perspective gives to constraints in the development of coordination is different to that of the earlier maturational and the more contemporary cognitive frameworks. First, the dynamical perspective recognizes that it is the *confluence* of constraints that channels coordination dynamics—no emphasis is given to endogenous or exogenous factors as was the case in, respectively, the maturation and cognitive positions. Second, constraints provide boundary conditions to organizational principles in coordination through channeling the dynamics of the organism-environment system. As Kugler *et al.* (1980) proposed, it is not that actions are caused by constraints, rather that some actions are excluded by them. Third, the pattern of coordination is an emergent *a posteriori* property of system organization rather than an *a priori* prescription. These principles are particularly attractive in considering how new patterns of coordination, such as grip configurations, appear in the developmental sequence (see Kugler 1986, Newell 1986).

In this context Newell (1986) has proposed that it is useful to consider constraints to the development of coordination under three categories—organismic, environmental and task. Organismic constraints exist at all levels of analysis of the body and these were, to a large degree, the focus of the maturational approach to development in that Gesell (1928, 1929) recognized that children's biological equipment sets the primary limits, directions and modalities in which they react to their personal environments. Environmental constraints are generally recognized as those which are external to the organism and can, for example in grasping, be categorized into the ambient conditions for action and the more focal object constraints. Finally, task constraints are: (1) the goal of the task, and (2) the rules specifying or constraining movement dynamics in action. Stable and adaptive patterns of coordination and control for a given individual are realized from the *interaction* of these sources of constraint on action. In concert with the significance of initial conditions in nonlinear dynamic systems, it is the case that small quantitative changes in any of these sources of constraints could, in principle, lead to a qualitative transition in the movement form produced to realize the goal of the action.

The constraints on action should not be viewed as rigid, although some constraints are relatively less time-dependent than others. In development, the former group of constraints is often called structural while the latter group is viewed as functional. Thus, as Kugler (1986) has articulated, constraints tend to softly 'orient' the current state of the system towards preferred states through gradients that radiate out from the preferred (attractive) dynamic state. The flow patterns or morphologies that emerge define a self-organizing informational substrate that can be used to guide, or softly constrain, movement organizations. The above general principles of the dynamical perspective to action lead to a number of specific predictions for the development of coordination in infancy.

First, there is no rigidly determined or invariant order in the development of a movement sequence as is usually proposed for fundamental movement activities such as posture, locomotion and prehension. Rather, the order and regularity that is often observed in infancy is a consequence of a similar set of constraints on children developing in a variety of cultures (Newell 1986). The prediction is that stronger manipulations of the physical parameters that channel the dynamics of infant motor development would lead to the demonstration of a more flexible and adaptive motor system. Such a demonstration would prove difficult to explain using the principles of the prescriptive formulations of maturational or cognitive theories. For example, it would seem likely that the raising of an infant in a gravity-free environment would lead to the appearance of a 'new' motor development sequence (Newell 1986). Similarly, providing a different set of task constraints in prehension would lead to a different account of the development of prehension than that proposed by either Halverson (1931) or Connolly (1973). The dynamical perspective offers the prospects of a principled basis to account for the emergence of new action patterns in development, particularly the sudden appearance of new movement forms.

Second, the emergent forms of children's motor development are determined in large part by the dynamics of the organism–environment interaction. This implies that the informational and kinetic flow fields that arise in this interaction coalesce in a cooperative and competitive fashion to structure the patterns of coordination at the behavioral level exhibited by children under different task constraints. Both the maturational and cognitive theories are neutral with respect to the notion that biological constraints dictate that preferred action patterns will arise as a consequence of a certain confluence of constraints. For example, in the cognitive approach to motor development, there are no 'preferred' channels for the response dynamics other than those which are specified by prescriptive rules that are often arbitrary with respect to the laws of physical biology. Thus, the dynamical perspective offers predictions about the changes in the development of phylogenetic and ontogenetic coordination patterns that are driven and can be measured by physical principles (Kugler and Turvey 1987). The use of dimensional analysis (e.g. Bridgman 1922) to specify the boundaries to the grip patterns is one example of this orientation that is outlined subsequently in some detail.

Finally, the dynamical perspective to the development of coordination proposes that the child is sensitive to the invariant perceptual properties that specify the dynamics of the organism–environment interaction. This is consistent with Gibson's (1979) notion of affordances whereby the organism learns to detect the invariant informational properties that specify what activities an environment affords the individual. Candidate invariant informational properties may be found in geometrical, kinematic and kinetic features of organism–environment interaction. For example, Runeson and Frykholm (1983) have proposed that subjects can perceive the dynamics of an act through the kinematics. Furthermore, Bertenthal *et al.* (1985, 1987) have revealed that infants are sensitive to kinematic and kinetic invariants in various types of visual display. The link between information and movement dynamics is an important problem that is being approached through converging operations from perception and action (see Beek and Wieringen 1994).

Constraints and the development of grip patterns
The traditions of learning theory led to the manipulation of some environmental and task

constraints in examinations of the development of coordination (Peterson 1933). Indeed, one of the classic tests of the early maturation versus learning theory accounts of motor development was to manipulate the environment, either directly via training studies (*e.g.* McGraw 1935) or indirectly through the observation of differences in development between different cultures (Super 1981). However, from a physical principle perspective, the general impact of many of these interventions and cultural manipulations on motor development has been relatively weak. The apparently broad stability of the phylogenetic movement patterns in posture, locomotion and prehension has allowed the developmental sequence for coordination to appear orderly and regular across a wide range of cultural conditions. For example, the influence of training (*e.g.* Zelazo *et al.* 1972) and cultural background (Super 1981) on the motor development sequence appears to be primarily confined to the onset times of coordination patterns with developmental age, rather than to changes in the order or actual movement pattern in the developmental sequence.

The significance of task constraints in relation to the body scale of the child has been largely ignored in considerations of the developmental sequence of coordination (Newell 1984, 1986). Indeed, with respect to prehension, one might intuitively expect some body size to object size ratio to specify the grip pattern employed for a given set of functional task constraints. This is not to say that a child or adult cannot or will not employ different grip patterns in the same task situation, rather that there is a preferred stable and adaptive grip configuration for a given set of task constraints that an individual will typically gravitate toward using.

The significance of body size and shape in biological systems has been recognized for centuries by anatomists, artists, architects and philosophers. Indeed, the everyday units of scale are based to a large degree on anatomical properties of the body such as the foot, hand, arm span, etc. (Berriman 1953, Drillis 1963). This leads naturally to the idea of body scaled metrics such as those used in methods of similarity and dimensional analysis (*e.g.* Buckingham 1915, Thompson 1917, Bridgman 1922, Stahl 1962). Dimensionless body scaled ratios that correspond to shifts in gait patterns (*e.g.* Alexander 1984), the perception of effort in stair climbing (Warren 1984) and the perception by adults of the optimal size of objects for grasping (Hallford 1984) have previously been reported. Furthermore, a number of the traditional observations of the development of locomotion can be accounted for by the organismic constraints of growth and form. For example, the onset of voluntary locomotion appears to be related to weight/height and leg/trunk ratios (Shirley 1931, Norval 1947). Thus, the dynamics of coordination are strongly influenced by body scaling properties, and we should anticipate that these principles hold for the development of prehension. Indeed, a dimensionless body scaled ratio may emerge that corresponds to shifts in grasping patterns relatively independent of psychological or maturational age.

A preliminary examination of the influence of body scale on the development of prehension has been conducted by Newell *et al.* (1989b). The grip patterns of a group of children aged 2–4 years (N = 26) were contrasted with those of college students (N = 22) in picking up a cube from a table and placing it into another cube that had one side open and uppermost. Both cubes were situated at the body midline with the cube to be grasped nearest the subject. The size of the object was varied systematically (ten objects over a range of 0.8–24.2 cm),

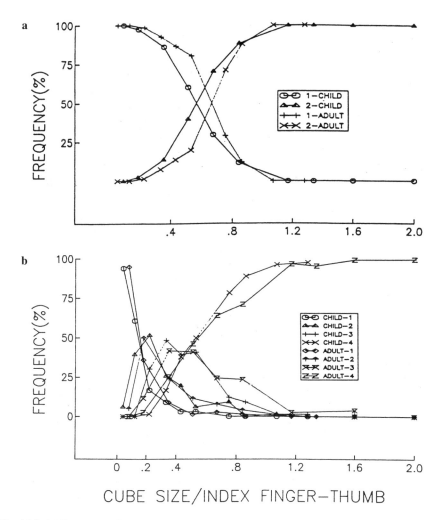

Fig. 12.2. *(a)* Frequency of hand use (1 = one hand, 2 = two hands) for 2- to 4-year-olds and adults as a function of the task/body ratio of object width/index finger–thumb range of motion. *(b)* Frequency of number of fingers used by 2- to 4-year-olds and adults as a function of the task/body ratio of object width/index finger–thumb range of motion. (Adapted by permission from Newell *et al.* 1989a.)

and subjects were required to displace the cube into an open-sided cube that was 2 cm larger than the cube to be grasped. No instructions or demonstrations were provided as to the grip pattern to be used. Subjects were videotaped and each grip was coded on a number of categories including: hand(s) used, number and type of digits in contact with object, depth of finger contact, contact of object with palm and angle of hand approach to object.

Figure 12.2 shows the frequency data for hand(s) used and number of fingers employed with the thumb, as a function of the ratio of the object width/thumb–middle finger range of motion. Figure 12.2a reveals that the frequency curves for hand use by children and adults are very similar both in pattern and absolute frequency when considered on an object/body scale. This suggests that object to hand size ratio strongly determines the use of one or two hands in grasping an object for a given set of task constraints, independent of developmental age. A similar trend is observed in Figure 12.2b which shows the number of fingers along with the thumb that grasp the object as a function of the same object to hand size ratio. These data, together with the similar trends observed on the other grip properties of hand orientation, depth of finger contact and palm contact, support the proposal that body scale is a strong determinant of the grip patterns utilized from the age of 2 years and into adulthood within a given set of functional constraints, such as the displacement task used here.

This experimental approach to the impact of body-scaled constraints on the development of prehension needs to be broadened to contrast the dimensionless ratios that specify grip pattern shifts across action categories, such as displacement, immobilization, manipulation, projection and catching. This would allow a contrast of the relative contribution of task goal and object properties to the grip pattern. Furthermore, it should be noted that the object to body ratio used to derive the abscissa in Figure 12.2 was determined on a single spatial dimension rather than a three-dimensional dynamic solution. Thus the approach here to body scaling was limited to the geometry of the object and hand without concern for the forces or the dynamics required to grip the object. However, this preliminary examination of the role of body scale and the development of prehension suggests that within the age boundaries studied, the grip pattern used may be independent of age when the object properties are body-scaled.

Another important feature to emerge from the data of the Newell *et al.* (1989b) experiment was that subjects tended to employ only a few grip patterns, in spite of the 28 biomechanical degrees of freedom that are available in joint space for each arm–hand biokinematic linkage. In fact, five grip patterns accounted on average for about 85% and 65% of the grip pattern variance in adults and children, respectively. This finding is consistent with the suggestion that there are only a few optimal boundary points that reflect preferred regions of stability and energy expenditure (Kugler 1986, Kugler and Turvey 1987). In summary, the findings from this experiment have provided strong evidence regarding the influence of body scale on the development of prehensile grip configurations.

The findings from the Newell *et al.* (1989b) experiment confirm that it is insufficient to study the development of prehension, as Halverson (1931) did, merely by comparison of an infant's grip of a 2.5 cm cube or a pellet and an adult's grip of the same objects. Objects also need to be scaled to body size to reveal the nature and importance of the organism/environment fit to coordination patterns. In many instances, this means that for studies on the development of prehension, objects need to be made smaller for infants and young children. A complementary comparison might be to scale the size of the object up in relation to the size of the hand. Indeed, if objects were 'scaled up' for adults to reflect the same body—object size ratios that infants face in grasping many everyday objects, it is most likely that adults would produce what are currently labeled 'child-like' grasping patterns. For example, it is probable that objects of a certain relative size for a given task goal afford a power type grip, *i.e.* the object would be so large as to be grasped in the palm and fingers.

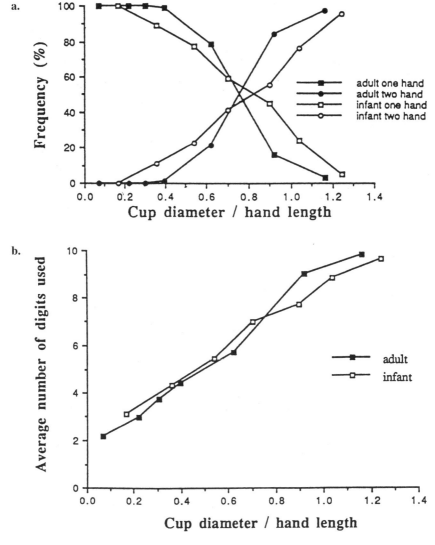

Fig. 12.3. *(a)* Frequency of hand use (one *vs* two hands) as a function of age group and object size. *(b)* Frequency of average number of digits used as a function of age group and object size. (Adapted by permission from Newell *et al.* 1993.)

The influence of object shape and size in determining grip configurations in infants (4–8 months) was examined by Newell *et al.* (1989a). Infants systematically changed the number of digits used in single hand grasping and the introduction of two hand grasping as a function of object size and shape. Indeed, apart from the increased variability of grip configurations in the 4-month-old group, the grip configurations for a given set of task constraints were remarkably similar across the 4–8 month age range. Furthermore, only the same five grip configurations (as reported above) were predominantly used by the infants over the seven object size/shape combinations used in the study. The major age difference occurred in the way the infants picked up information to determine the grip configurations. The younger infants predominantly used the haptic system in addition to the visual system, whereas by 8 months infants were predominately using vision to provide prospective control of the grip configuration. In summary, this experiment showed that infants as young as 4 months differentiate grip configurations as a function of task constraints, but it did not provide a sufficient test of the role of body scale in infant prehension.

A direct test of the influence of body scaling on infant grip configurations in prehension was reported by Newell *et al.* (1993). A group of 5- to 8-month-old infants and a group of adults engaged in a displacement grasping task with seven inverted cups that varied in size. The essential findings, shown in Figure 12.3, were that infant and adult grip configurations varied systematically with increasing object size. Furthermore, when object size was scaled to hand size, a common dimensionless ratio defined the transition from a one- to a two-hand grip (Fig. 12.3a), and the patterns of finger additions to the grip architecture (Fig. 12.3b) were remarkably similar for infants and adults over increments of object size. The data from this experiment clearly confirm the important role of body scale in determining the grip configuration used by young infants.

In more recent work we have extended the body scaling approach in prehension to consider the interaction of the task constraint (goal of the action) with the environmental constraint of object properties in determining the grip pattern in infants (Whyte *et al.* 1994). Data from the two infant studies reported above were reanalyzed to separate the data that were collected in regard to grasping in the service of mouthing from those data that relate to the act of displacing the object. Grasping is rarely carried out as an action in and of itself. It is nearly always conducted in the service of another activity such as throwing, catching, displacing, exploring or mouthing an object. Given the importance of the constraints relative to the channeling of the grip dynamics, the issue at stake was whether infants varied the grip to the same object as a function of the action goal that they intended to realize. The results showed that in the middle range of object sizes, infants tended to use different grips for mouthing and displacing actions even though the object size was identical. Future work needs to further examine this interaction of task and object influences on prehension in terms of the common language of the dynamics of the work space.

The findings from this series of grasping experiments on the role of body scale in the development of prehension are consistent with the notion that in considering the movement dynamics of biological systems one needs to examine the somatotypical features that are subject to the physical laws of growth and form (Thompson 1917, Pennycuick 1992). It should be noted that the length and width of the infant's hand increase on average by a factor of 200–300% during the first year of life and that these hand parameters increase by an additional factor of 200–300% by the age of 18 years (Hajnis 1969, Snyder *et al.* 1977, Flatt and Burmeister 1979). There are, unfortunately, no available estimates of the gains in finger size and strength during the first year of life.

Considering task constraints in isolation, it would be reasonable to speculate that a precision grip could be elicited prior to a power grip in infants. However, the general organismic constraint of anatomical and physiological development may be the limiting factor for such a reversal of prehensile coordination to occur (Lawrence and Kuypers 1968a,b; Lawrence and Hopkins 1972, 1976). Undoubtedly, in the young infant there are certain anatomical and neural features that underpin growth and development (see Lowry 1978); for example, reflex mechanisms provide an important contribution to the grasping skills of the neonate and young infant (Twitchell 1970). Thus, the organismic constraints imposed by a hand that has not yet fully developed structurally, clearly also contribute to possible differences in function between the infant's and adult's prehension.

In summary, the dynamical perspective predicts that the onset and order of prehensile development will reflect the constraints imposed on the child-environment synergy (Kugler 1986, Newell 1986). In this view, order and regularity occur in the development of the prehensile sequence because typically young children are acting under a similar relative set of organismic, environmental and task constraints. However, these patterns of coordination are flexibly assembled and not rigidly determined by maturational or cognitive prescriptions. There is a need to identify better and explore more fully the most significant constraints on motor development (Newell 1986, Thelen 1986) and to manipulate variables that can lead to predictable changes in the topological and scaling properties of the movement dynamics exhibited in infancy and early childhood. This approach also holds the promise of providing a principled examination of the role of individual differences in development (Kugler and Turvey 1987).

Conclusion

In this chapter we have argued that environmental, task and organismic constraints on the development of prehension may account for much of what has previously been attributed to the maturation of genetic neurological prescriptions for action (Gesell 1928, McGraw 1946) and the development of cognitive action plans (Bruner 1969, Connolly 1973). An important implication arising from this analysis of constraints on the development of prehension is that the order and regularity observed in prehensile patterns of coordination (and, in principle, other movement activities) may not be reflections of pre-established prescriptions for action. Rather, the development of grasping action patterns is consistent with the notion of properties of self-organizing principles in biological systems (Kugler *et al.* 1980, 1982; Kugler 1986; Thelen *et al.* 1987). According to this view, action patterns are emergent features of the constraints imposed on the organism–environment synergy, rather than prescriptions for action as is typically postulated by the maturation hypothesis and the extant cognitive formulations of motor development. Our recent findings on the influence of task constraints on the grip patterns of infants and young children (Newell *et al.* 1989a,b; 1993) provide encouragement for a general reconsideration from a dynamical perspective of the long-standing idea in development that there is a fundamental movement sequence in infancy and early childhood.

REFERENCES

Alexander, R.McN. (1984) 'Walking and running.' *American Scientist*, **72**, 348–354.
Ament, W. (1923) *The Mind of the Child: a Comparative History of Life*. London: Simpkin Marshall.

Beek, P.J., Beek, W.J. (1988) 'Tools for constructing dynamical models of rhythmic movement.' *Human Movement Science*, **7**, 301–342.

—— Wieringen, P.C.W. (1994) 'Perception–movement, information and dynamics. Special Issue.' *Human Movement Science*, **13**, 296–533.

Berriman, A.E. (1953) *Historical Metrology.* New York: Dutton.

Bertenthal, B.I., Proffitt, D.R., Spetner, N.B., Thomas, M.A. (1985) 'The development of infant sensitivity to biomechanical motions.' *Child Development*, **56**, 531–543.

—— —— Kramer, S.J., Spetner, N.B. (1987) 'Infants' encoding of kinetic displays varying in relative coherence.' *Developmental Psychology*, **23**, 171–178.

Bishop, A. (1962) 'Control of the hand in lower primates.' *Annals of the New York Academy of Sciences*, **102**, 316–337.

Boothe, R.G., Dobson, V., Teller, D.Y. (1985) 'Postnatal development of vision in humans and nonhuman primates.' *Annual Review of Neuroscience*, **8**, 495– 545.

Bousfield, W.A. (1953) 'The assumption of motor primacy and its significance for behavioral development.' *Journal of Genetic Psychology*, **83**, 79–88.

Bower, T.G.R. (1972) 'Object perception in infants.' *Perception*, **1**, 15–30.

Bridgman, P.W. (1922) *Dimensional Analysis.* New Haven, CN: Yale University Press.

Bruner, J.S. (1969) 'Processes of growth in infancy.' *In:* Ambrose, A. (Ed.) *Stimulation in Early Infancy.* New York: Academic Press, pp. 205–224.

—— (1972) 'Origins of problem solving in skill acquisition.' *In:* Rudner, R., Scheffler, I. (Eds.) *Logic and Art: Essays in Honor of Nelson Goodman.* Indianapolis: Bobbs–Merrill, pp. 100–126.

—— Koslowski, B. (1972) 'Visually preadapted constituents of manipulatory action.' *Perception*, **1**, 2–14.

Buckingham, E. (1915) 'On physically similar systems.' *Physiological Review*, **4**, 345–370.

Bühler, C. (1930) *The First Year of Life.* New York: Day.

Castner, B.M. (1932) 'The development of fine prehension in infancy.' *Genetic Psychology Monographs*, **12**, 105–193.

Coghill, G.E. (1929) *Anatomy and the Problem of Behaviour.* Cambridge: Cambridge University Press.

Connolly, K.J. (1970) 'Skill development: problems and plans.' *In:* Connolly, K.J. (Ed.) *Mechanisms of Motor Skill Development.* London: Academic Press, pp. 3–21.

—— (1973) 'Factors influencing the learning of manual skills by young children.' *In:* Hinde, R.A., Hinde, J.S. (Eds.) *Constraints on Learning.* London: Academic Press, pp. 337–365.

—— (1981) 'Maturation and the ontogeny of motor skills.' *In:* Connolly, K.J., Prechtl, H.F.R. (Eds.) *Maturation and Development: Biological and Psychological Perspectives. Clinics in Developmental Medicine No. 77/78.* London: Spastics International Medical Publications, pp. 216–230.

—— Dalgleish, M. (1989) 'The emergence of a tool using skill in infancy.' *Developmental Psychology*, **25**, 894–912.

—— —— (1993) 'Individual patterns of tool use by infants.' *In:* Kalverboer, A., Hopkins, B., Gueze, R. (Eds.) *Longitudinal Studies of Motor Development.* Cambridge: Cambridge University Press, pp. 174–204.

—— Elliott, J.M. (1972) 'Evolution and ontogeny of hand function.' *In:* Blurton-Jones, N. (Ed.) *Ethological Studies of Child Behaviour.* Cambridge: Cambridge University Press, pp. 329–383.

Cutkosky, M.R. (1989) 'On grasp choice, grasp models and the design of hands for manufacturing tasks.' *IEEE Transactions on Robotics and Automation*, **5**, 269– 279.

Dearborn, G.V.N. (1910) *Motor-sensory Development: Observations on the First Three Years of a Child.* Baltimore, MD: Warwick & York.

Dix, K.W. (1911) *Korperliche und peistige Entwicklung eines Kindes.* Leipzeig: Wunderlich.

Dobson, V., Teller, D.Y. (1978) 'Visual acuity in human infants: a review and comparison of behavioral and electrophysiological studies.' *Vision Research*, **18**, 1469–1483.

Drillis, R.J. (1963) 'Folk norms and biomechanics.' *Human Factors*, **5**, 427–441.

Elliott, J.M., Connolly, K.J. (1974) 'Hierarchical structure in skill development.' *In:* Connolly, K.J., Bruner, J. (Eds.) *The Development of Competence in Childhood.* London: Academic Press, pp. 135–168.

—— —— (1984) 'A classification of manipulative hand movements.' *Developmental Medicine and Child Neurology*, **26**, 283–296.

Field, J. (1976) 'The adjustment of reaching behavior to object distance in early infancy.' *Child Development*, **47**, 304–308.

—— (1977) 'Coordination of vision and prehension in young infants.' *Child Development*, **48**, 97–103.

253

Flatt, A.E., Burmeister, L. (1979) 'A comparison of hand growth in elementary schoolchildren in Czechoslovakia and the United States.' *Developmental Medicine and Child Neurology*, **21**, 515–524.

Gesell, A. (1925) *The Mental Growth of the Pre-school Child.* New York: Macmillan.

—— (1928) *Infancy and Human Growth.* New York: Macmillan.

—— (1929) 'Maturation and infant behavior pattern.' *Psychological Review*, **36**, 307–319.

—— (1946) 'The ontogenesis of infant behavior.' *In:* Carmichael, L. (Ed.) *Manual of Child Psychology.* New York: Wiley, pp. 295–331.

—— Amatruda, C. (1947) *Developmental Diagnosis. Normal and Abnormal Child Development.* New York: Harper & Row.

—— Thompson, H. (1934) *Infant Behavior. Its Genesis and Growth.* New York: McGraw-Hill.

Gibson, J.J. (1979) *The Perception of the Visual World.* Boston: Houghton Mifflin.

Hajnis, K. (1969) 'The dynamics of hand growth since the birth till 18 years of age.' *Panminerva Medica*, **11**, 123–132.

Haken, H., Kelso, J.A.S., Bunz, H. (1985) 'A theoretical model of phase transitions in human hand movements.' *Biological Cybernetics*, **51**, 347–356.

Hallford, E.W. (1984) 'Sizing up the world: the body as a referent in a size-judgment task.' Doctoral dissertation, Ohio State University.

Halverson, H.M. (1931) 'An experimental study of prehension in infants by means of systematic cinema records.' *Genetic Psychology Monographs*, **10**, 107–286.

—— (1932) 'A further study of grasping.' *Journal of General Psychology*, **7**, 34–63.

—— (1937) 'Studies of grasping responses of early infancy: I, II, III.' *Journal of Genetic Psychology*, **51**, 371–449.

Hooker, D. (1938) 'The origin of the grasping movement in man.' *Proceedings of the American Philosophical Society*, **79**, 597–606.

Jones, M.C. (1926) 'The development of early patterns in young children.' *Pedagogical Seminary*, **33**, 537–585.

Kapandji, I.A. (1970) *The Physiology of the Joints. Vol. 1.* Edinburgh: Churchill Livingstone.

Kugler, P.N. (1986) 'A morphological perspective on the origin and evolution of movement patterns.' *In:* Wade, M.G., Whiting, H.T.A. (Eds.) *Motor Development in Children: Aspects of Coordination and Control.* Boston: Martinus Nijhoff, pp. 459–525.

—— Turvey, M.T. (1987) *Information, Natural Law, and the Self-assembly of Rhythmic Movement.* Hillsdale, NJ: Erlbaum.

—— Kelso, J.A.S., Turvey, P.N. (1980) 'On the concept of coordinative structures as dissipative structures: I. Theoretical lines of convergence.' *In:* Stelmach, G.E., Requin, J. (Eds.) *Tutorials in Motor Behavior.* Amsterdam: North Holland, pp. 3–47.

—— —— —— (1982) 'On the control and coordination of naturally developing systems.' *In:* Kelso, J.A.S., Clark, J.E. (Eds.) The Development of Movement Control and Coordination. New York: Wiley, pp. 5–78.

Kuhlman, F. (1922) *A Handbook of Mental Tests: a Further Revision and Extension of the Binet–Simon Scale.* Baltimore: Warwick & York.

Landsmeer, J.M.F. (1962) 'Power grip and precision handling.' *Annals of Rheumatic Diseases*, **21**, 164–170.

Lawrence, D.G., Hopkins, D.A. (1972) 'Developmental aspects of pyramidal motor control in the rhesus monkey.' *Brain Research*, **40**, 117–118.

—— —— (1976) 'The development of motor control in the rhesus monkey: evidence concerning the role of corticomotoneuronal connections.' *Brain*, **99**, 235–254.

—— Kuypers, H.G.J.M. (1968a) 'The functional organization of the motor system in the monkey. I. The effects of bilateral pyramidal lesions.' *Brain*, **91**, 1–14.

—— —— (1968b) 'The functional organization of the motor system in the monkey. II. The effects of lesions of the descending brain-stem pathways.' *Brain*, **91**, 15–36.

Linfert, H.H., Hierholzer, H.M. (1928) 'A scale for measurement of the mental development of infants during the first year of life.' *Student Psychology and Psychiatry, Catholic University of America*, **1**, 1–179.

Lockman, J.J., Ashmead, D.H. (1983) 'Asynchronies in the development of manual behavior.' *In:* Lipsitt, L.P. (Ed.) *Advances in Infancy Research. Vol. 11.* Norwood, NJ: Ablex, pp. 113–136.

Lowry, G.H. (1978) *Growth and Development of Children.* Chicago: Year Book Medical.

MacKenzie, C.L., Iberall, T. (1994) *The Grasping Hand.* Amsterdam: North-Holland.

Malek, R. (1981) 'The grip and its modalities.' *In:* Tubiana, R. (Ed.) *The Hand.* Philadelphia: Saunders, pp. 469–476.

McGraw, M.B. (1935) *Growth: a Study of Johnny and Jimmy.* New York: Appleton-Century.

—— (1945) *The Neuromuscular Maturation of the Human Infant.* New York: Columbia University Press.

—— (1946) 'Maturation of behavior.' *In:* Carmichael, L. (Ed.) *Manual of Child Psychology.* New York: Wiley, pp. 332–369.

Moore, K.C. (1896) 'The mental development of a child.' *Psychological Reviews, Monographs Supplement,* **1**, No. 3.

Napier, J.R. (1956) 'The prehensile movements of the human hand.' *Journal of Bone and Joint Surgery,* **38B**, 902–913.

—— (1962) 'The evolution of the hand.' *Scientific American,* **207**, 156–162.

—— (1970) *The Roots of Mankind.* London: Allen & Unwin.

Newell, K.M. (1984) 'Physical constraints to development of motor skills.' *In:* Thomas, J.R. (Ed.) *Motor Development During Childhood and Adolescence.* Minneapolis: Burgess, pp. 105–120.

—— (1986) 'Constraints on the development of coordination.' *In:* Wade, M.G., Whiting, H.T.A. (Eds.) *Motor Development in Children: Aspects of Coordination and Control.* Boston: Martinus Nijhoff, pp. 341–360.

—— Barclay, C.R. (1982) 'Developing knowledge about action.' *In:* Kelso, J.A.S., Clark, J.E. (Eds.) *The Development of Movement Control and Coordination.* New York: Wiley, pp. 175–212.

—— Scully, D.M., McDonald, P.V., Baillargeon, R. (1989a) 'Task constraints and infant grip configurations.' *Developmental Psychobiology,* **22**, 817–831.

—— —— Tenenbaum, F., Hardiman, S. (1989b) 'Body scale and the development of prehension.' *Developmental Psychobiology,* **22**, 1–13.

—— McDonald, P.V., Baillargeon, R. (1993) 'Body scale and infant grip configurations.' *Developmental Psychobiology,* **26**, 195–206.

Norval, M.A. (1947) 'Relationship of weight and length of infants at birth to the age at which they begin to walk alone.' *Journal of Pediatrics,* **30**, 676–678.

Pennycuick, C.J. (1992) *Newton Rules Biology.* Oxford: Oxford University Press.

Peterson, J. (1933) 'Learning in children.' *In:* Murchinson, C. (Ed.) *A Handbook of Child Psychology.* New York: Russell & Russell, pp. 417–479.

Preyer, W. (1890) *The Mind of the Child.* (Translated by H.W. Brown.) New York: Appleton.

Robson, P. (1970) 'Shuffling, hitching, scooting or sliding: some observations in 30 otherwise normal children.' *Developmental Medicine and Child Neurology,* **12**, 608–617.

Runeson, S., Frykholm, G. (1983) 'Kinematic specification of dynamics as an informational basis for person and action perception: expectation, gender recognition, and deceptive intention.' *Journal of Experimental Psychology: General,* **112**, 710–720.

Savelsbergh, G.J.P., van der Kamp, J. (1994) 'The effect of body orientation to gravity on early infant reaching.' *Journal of Experimental Child Psychology,* **58**, 510–528.

Shinn, M.W. (1893) 'Notes on the development of a child.' *University of California Public Education,* **1**, 178–236.

Shirley, M.M. (1931) *The First Two Years: a Study of Twenty-five Babies. Vol. I. Locomotor Development.* Minneapolis: University of Minnesota Press.

Simoneit, M. (1928) *Die seelische Entwicklung des Menschen.* Berlin: Oehmigke.

Snyder, R.G., Schneider, L.W., Owings, C.L., Reynolds, H.M., Golomb, D.H., Schork, M.A. (1977) *Anthropometry of Infants, Children, and Youths to Age 18 for Product Safety Design SP-450.* Warrendale, PA: Society of Automotive Engineers.

Stahl, W.R. (1962) 'Similarity and dimensional methods in biology.' *Science,* **137**, 205–212.

Super, C.M. (1981) 'Cross-cultural research on infancy.' *In:* Triandis, H.C., Heron, A. (Eds.) *Handbook of Cross-cultural Psychology: Developmental Psychology. Vol. 4.* Boston: Allyn & Bacon, pp. 17–53.

Thelen, E. (1986) 'Development of coordinated movement: implications for early development.' *In:* Wade, M.G., Whiting, H.T.A. (Eds.) *Motor Development in Children: Aspects of Coordination and Control.* Boston: Martinus Nifhoff, pp. 107–124.

—— Smith, L.B. (1994) *A Dynamic Systems Approach to the Development of Cognition and Action.* Cambridge, MA: MIT Press.

—— Kelso, J.A.S., Fogel, A. (1987) 'Self-organizing systems and infant motor development.' *Developmental Review,* **7**, 39–65.

Thompson, D.W. (1917) *On Growth and Form.* London: Cambridge University Press.

Touwen, B.C.L. (1971) 'A study on the development of some motor phenomena in infancy.' *Developmental Medicine and Child Neurology,* **13**, 435–446.

Turvey, M.T. (1990) 'Coordination.' *American Psychologist,* **45**, 938–953.

255

Twitchell, T.E. (1970) 'Reflex mechanisms and the development of prehension.' *In:* Connolly, K.J. (Ed.) *Mechanisms of Motor Skill Development.* New York: Academic Press, pp. 25–37.

van Gemert, J.G.W.A. (1984) 'Arthrodesis of the wrist. A clinical, radiographic and ergonomic study of 66 cases.' *Acta Orthopaedica Scandinavica*, **55**, Suppl. 210.

von Hofsten, C. (1979) 'Development of visually directed reaching: the approach phase.' *Journal of Human Movement Studies*, **5**, 160–178.

—— (1982) 'Eye–hand coordination in the newborn.' *Developmental Psychology*, **18**, 450–461.

—— (1983) 'Catching skills in infancy.' *Journal of Experimental Psychology: Human Perception and Performance*, **9**, 75–85.

—— (1986) 'The emergence of manual skills.' *In:* Wade, M.G., Whiting, H.T.A. (Eds.) *Motor Development in Children: Aspects of Coordination and Control.* Boston: Martinus Nijhoff, pp. 167–185.

—— Lindhagen, K. (1979) 'Observations on the development of reaching for moving objects.' *Journal of Experimental Child Psychology*, **28**, 158–173.

Waddington, C.H. (1957) *The Strategy of the Genes.* London: George, Allen & Unwin.

Warren, W.H. (1984) 'Perceiving affordances: visual guidance of stair climbing.' *Journal of Experimental Psychology: Human Perception and Performance*, **10**, 683–703.

White, B.L. (1970) 'Experience and the development of motor mechanisms in infancy.' *In:* Connolly, K.J. (Ed.) *Mechanisms of Motor Skill Development.* London: Academic Press, pp. 95–136.

—— Held, R. (1966) 'Plasticity and sensorimotor development in the human infant.' *In:* Rosenblith, J.R., Allinsmith, W. (Eds.) *The Causes of Behavior: Readings in Child Development and Education Psychology.* London: McGraw-Hill, pp. 60–70.

—— Castle, P., Held, R. (1964) 'Observations on the development of visually-directed reaching.' *Child Development*, **35**, 349–364.

Whyte, V.A., McDonald, P.V., Baillargeon, R., Newell, K.M. (1994) 'Mouthing and grasping of objects by young infants.' *Ecological Psychology*, **6**, 205–218.

Wohlwill, J.F. (1973) *The Study of Behavioral Development.* New York: Academic Press.

Zelazo, P.R., Zelazo, N.A., Kolb, S. (1972) 'Newborn walking.' *Science*, **177**, 1058–1059. *(Letter.)*

Zingg, R.M. (1940) 'Feral man and extreme cases of isolation.' *American Journal of Psychology*, **53**, 487–517.

13
PERCEPTION IN ACTION APPROACH TO CEREBRAL PALSY

David N. Lee, Claes von Hofsten and Ester Cotton

"Locomotion and manipulation are neither triggered nor commanded but *controlled*. They are constrained, guided, or steered, and only in this sense are they ruled or governed. And they are controlled not by the brain but by information, that is, by seeing oneself in the world. Control lies in the animal–environment system. Control is by the animal *in* its world, the animal itself having subsystems for perceiving the environment and concurrently for getting about in it and manipulating it." (Gibson 1979)

Basic nature of movement control

D. Claes, I would like you to meet these friends of mine, Fiona and Gordon. When I told them you were coming back to Edinburgh with me after the conference they said they'd like to meet you.

F. Hello. I hope the conference was stimulating. Gordon and I are particularly interested in cerebral palsy because we have a 4-year-old son who has hemiparetic problems.

G. Hi, Claes! I gather you and Dave were talking on related themes at the conference. About prospective control wasn't it? We were wondering whether there might be something there that could be helpful for Hamish.

C. I am very pleased to meet you both but sorry to hear about Hamish. I would be happy to talk about our ideas.

D. Since it's such a lovely day, how would you fancy going for a walk? Claes and I were thinking of going up Arthur's Seat and meeting Ester Cotton over there. She's in Scotland for a few days visiting colleagues in Conductive Education, and we were going to talk about possible ways of diagnosing and improving movement control in cerebral palsy.

C. It's a year or so since I was last up there. It's a regular ideas stomping ground for Dave and me—and Tam, the dog.

F. That sounds very good. We'll drive you over there . . .

Oh, it's good to be out. I can see why you choose to come here. You know, one thing that has struck Gordon and me about cerebral palsy is the different ways the children are affected, even those who are classified as hemiparetic.

C. That is a very important point. The children do need to be helped individually. The way we control our actions is of necessity complicated. There are numerous ways in which the system could go wrong and they all express themselves differently. To be able to treat the patient with cerebral palsy, one therefore has to be able to evaluate the different possible malfunctions of the system, and that, in turn, has to be based on ideas about how perception–action systems are constructed.

D. That's right. To help a child we need to understand what that child's basic movement problems are. But first we need to recognize that perception is inextricably linked with movement. To move purposefully we need perceptual information for controlling the movement, and to gain perceptual information we need to move. Perception and movement are two sides of the coin of action.

G. What kind of perceptual control is involved?

D. First and foremost control has to be prospective. That is, all movements have to be controlled by anticipating—usually non-consciously—what is very likely to happen next. For example, when you were driving over here you had to slow down behind several cars and negotiate a number of bends. This meant you had to start braking and steering correctly ahead of time. It would have been no use your waiting until you were right on top of the other car or bend before starting to act.

G. Yes, I can see that must have been so, but as you say, I wasn't conscious of it.

C. Consciousness is rarely involved in action control. In the control of movements, deliberate thinking might even interfere with performance (Gallwey 1986). It is well known that when athletes start thinking about their movements, performance tends to deteriorate. Deliberate thinking takes time and that puts certain limitations on the tasks in which it could be involved. The closer one gets to the implementation of the action the more important timing becomes and the more crucial becomes direct access to information about the future without the involvement of consciousness. Recent research on neurologically impaired patients (Goodale and Milner 1992) and from electrophysiological and behavioural studies in monkeys (Ungenleider and Mishkin 1982) suggests that there are diffcrent systems for representing visual information used in gearing the motor system to the external world and in evaluating and thinking about it.

The difference between thinking about movements and acting can be experienced, for instance, when learning a new dance. Just being able to describe the rules of dancing is of little help when trying to dance. The rules must be incorporated with the dance itself and act as guidelines for what should be done next. Furthermore, the rules are by necessity global and sketchy and cannot guide actions by themselves. Perception of what is going to happen next is needed throughout the execution of any action in order to steer it adaptively. To dance skilfully, one must perceive what the partner is about to do, what is about to happen to the other dancing couples on the floor and, last but not least, what is about to happen to one's own movements.

Action knowledge and perception are equally important aspects of action control. We need both to plan upcoming actions and to perceive what is going to happen next. According to Kawato and Gomi (1992), the cerebellar symptoms of hypotonia, hypermetria and intentional tremor could be understood as a degraded performance when motor control is forced to rely solely on perception after the internal models are destroyed, cannot be updated, or both.

F. Obviously the same applies right now as we walk up this rocky path. I not only need to know how to walk but also I have to look ahead and adjust my steps.

C. In fact knowing how to walk has to include procedures for where to look and what to look for. For instance, the colour of the rock you are about to step on is less relevant than whether it is slippery or not. But having picked out the rock you still have to control the movement of your foot to it. And that requires prospective control too.

G. But if I can see my foot as it approaches the rock surely I can continuously guide it to the rock.

D. Sure you can, but that doesn't mean that the control isn't prospective. Consider the visual information you're using right now. It, in fact, reached your eye a short while ago and has taken some time to connect up with your muscles. Therefore, you are working with outdated information. How then are your movements so smooth and accurate? It must be because the outdated information is sufficiently predictive to be useable.

G. Well, that's true. But the neural delay is not that long. Maybe about 150 ms. So you don't need to predict that far in advance.

D. Yes. But there's another reason why control has to be prospective—and often over a longer period than 150 ms. It's because muscular power is limited, which means that it will always take a finite time to make any movement. For example, in order to land properly on the next stone your leg needs to have stopped swinging as your foot reaches the stone. Therefore you need to start slowing your leg down in advance and to do this properly requires predictive information. Obviously the same applies even more so to stopping a car, particularly at motorway speeds. In that case it's the power of the brakes and the grip on the road that are the limiting factors.

F. So, as I am walking from one rock to the next I am using my eyes to lead my steps.

D. In fact, if we were to measure where your eyes are pointing then we'd more than likely find that your line of gaze is acting like a third leg, being planted on each rock a pace or two before you put your foot on it. That's what has been found in experiments (Hollands *et al.* 1995, van Wijck 1995).

G. But when I'm fixing my eyes on a place ahead I'm not just seeing where I'm looking. For example, I can still see my feet in the periphery of my vision when I'm looking ahead. So does it really matter where I fix my eyes, as long as it's more or less in the right direction?

C. It obviously depends on how tricky the footing is. On flat grass you can quite easily look around at the scenery briefly while walking. But over difficult ground like this you probably place your eyes as accurately as your feet.

Active *vs* passive movement: learning *vs* being treated

D. In other words, although all your movements do need to be continuously prospectively controlled, you do not have to be continuously picking up visual information for the control. That can be done intermittently. This is because the information is predictive and so can carry you over for a while. . . As just now when I spotted Ester while I was negotiating this path. Hi, Ester! Isn't it a beautiful day?

E. Hello, Dave. Yes, it certainly is.

D. Meet Fiona, Gordon and Claes. We were just discussing prospective control. Fiona and Gordon are particularly interested because they have a 4-year-old son who is hemiparetic.

C. Very pleased to meet you, Ester. I gather you have been working on Conductive Education up here. At the conference, Dave and I were talking from a scientific point of view about cerebral palsy, but neither of us has your therapeutic experience. It would be very valuable to discuss these matters with you.

F. It certainly would. So far we have been talking about how essential perceptual information is in prospectively controlling purposeful movements. As I understand it, improving active purposeful movement is a central aim of Conductive Education (Hári and Ákos 1988).

E. That's right. If you look back on therapy for cerebral palsy, you will find a large number of different methods. In the main they are based either on neurophysiology, attempting to inhibit spasticity, or on using normal development as stepping stones for improvement. In all these methods the patient is handled by the therapist who is *initiating* all the action.

In Conductive Education, Peto suggested that it is essential that the child is *active*, which means that the child is preparing herself for the motor act and is *intending* instead of waiting for someone to do something to her. The important main point was that Peto switched from treating the child to *helping the child learn*.

D. I certainly agree with the emphasis on helping the child learn how to do meaningful things. Skills obviously have to be developed by the child herself. They cannot be manipulated into her. What a good teacher basically does is set up appropriate tasks for her and helps structure the environmental support for those tasks—as well as providing encouragement and broad verbal directives. But the main work in developing a skill is up to the child. And it requires much *creative* learning. The reason the learning has to be creative is that effective practice does *not* consist in trying to replicate standard movements, though this is a common view. Rather, as Bernstein (1967) pointed out, developing a skill requires the individual to explore different approaches to the perceptuo-motor problem in order to find a solution that is optimal for that individual.

E. Yes, learning skills involves a number of things. First of all the child has to be *motivated* to do the task. Then, once they've begun to learn, they need to *use the skill, practise the skill and generalize the skill*. This means that everybody involved must understand that they will not learn without using the skills. To get that across is by far the most complicated thing in Conductive Education. The other thing is that the child must understand *what* it is she's learnt, *how* she learnt it, and *who* taught her. Out of that you get a new relationship between teacher and child.

You also need to consider that children learn differently in the very early years to how they learn later when they have passed the early period of maturation. What they learn very early is, of course, the typical things that human beings need, such as getting up from the floor, standing up, sitting down and using their hands. Many cerebral palsied children, even after a lot of treatment, cannot do these things when they are out of this period of maturation. Peto suggested that stimulation and interaction with the child is no longer sufficient beyond the age of 2–3 years and we should then turn to skill acquisition.

D. Earlier we were arguing that children should be treated as individuals when it comes to devising therapy for them. But at the same time we were trying to draw out common principles of control which run across all children and which could be used in diagnosis and treatment. What do you think ?

E. I think each child has individual problems, but there are common denominators for all cerebral palsied children in the dysfunctioning motor patterns (Cotton 1994a). These are best dealt with by teaching rather than treating, setting functional tasks rather than exercises, and by learning in a group rather than alone, so the child can see how the other children are succeeding and is motivated by this. We had a group of children where one child was suddenly able to walk a little bit with his chair. The whole group had been trying to do this for a long time and suddenly set off because they realized what it's all about, and so they learnt from one another. I think a group is very, very helpful, but it's got to be run very well.

F. It seems clear that the ideas underlying Conductive Education fit well with the idea of prospective control. However, what I learnt as a student is that our purposeful movements originate in reflexes and that doesn't seem to fit with your ideas.

C. I think the reflex concept is a bit misleading, especially the way it has been used in the developmental literature. If it just denotes a low-level organized sensorimotor system it is not totally wrong, because sensorimotor systems may be rather primitively or incompletely organized early in life. However, there is also a connotation of a movement triggered by a specific stimulus in an automatic, stereotyped way, which is less true. I'm not denying that certain stimuli give rise to very automatic and stereotyped reactions, like the knee jerk reflex, but such reactions are clearly not confined to neonates and, I would claim, not even typical for neonates. However, most movements performed by newborn infants are purposeful, flexible, and controlled by the subject (see, for example, von Hofsten 1982). Developmental neurologists have also been struck by the variability of the reactions they elicit in neonates (Touwen 1976) and how dependent they are on the mood of the infant. In summary, although neonatal behaviour may have many limitations, it is not just a set of reflexes. Most behaviours have the basic characteristics of actions. Therefore, I would claim that *action originates in action* rather than in reflexes.

  However, some of the pathological movements and postures performed by cerebral palsied children show obvious similarities with some neonatal behaviours, for instance the asymmetric tonic neck reflex and the Moro response. The main difference is that while those movements and postures show variability (Rönnqvist 1995) and functionality (van der Meer *et al.* 1995a) in neonates, they are stereotyped and nonfunctional in the child with cerebral palsy.

E. In Conductive Education we don't talk a lot about reflexes, but there's no doubt that the children are influenced by their tonic neck reflex and their Moro response. These are enormously disturbing but they can learn to control them by fixing their body with their hands and moving their head in all directions without letting go with either hand. At a later stage they will learn to let go with one hand—one hand fixing and one hand moving, as in all functional activities. A profoundly disabled child must learn this but must also discover that, when learning to feed herself, she cannot bend her right elbow when looking to the right, so she must turn her head to the left, bend the right elbow and quickly return to midline to put the spoon in her mouth. In short, she will learn how to *control* not *cure* her tonic neck reflex.

261

C. So when you talk about reflex you are mainly referring to unwanted movements, as opposed to arguing that the reflex is a basis for purposeful movements?

E. Yes, that's right. At one time treatment was about inhibiting reflexes by manual facilitation. However, it was found that it didn't really work, because as soon as you stopped, the reflexes returned. That's why you need to help the children *control* the unwanted movements as opposed to trying to eradicate them.

Establishing an action-base

G. I think these general principles for therapy that you have been discussing are all very important. But how does one apply these ideas to diagnosis and therapy?

D. We need to consider further general principles of movement control. To start with, controlling movements, both purposeful movements and unwanted ones, requires setting up a physical and perceptual action-base. To give you an example, Gordon: Stop just before that rock and then step onto it. . . You will notice that you were careful not to step onto that patch of ice. If you had, then your foot would have slipped back when you tried to propel yourself toward the rock. By stepping on a non-slippery patch you were setting up the *physical* part of your action-base for stepping onto the rock.

You also looked at the rock and kept your eyes on it, at least for part of the time while stepping toward it. There you were establishing the *perceptual* component of your action-base. Try to imagine what it would be like if you couldn't control your gaze like that but instead your eyes wandered all over the place as you were trying to step forward.

G. It doesn't bear thinking about! I also noticed that I kept my head steady.

D. That's because the head is a central perceptual base for action. It houses the eyes, ears, nose and acceleration sensors in the vestibular system and so has very close perceptual links with the environment. Thus to sense properly where you are and how you are moving in relation to things you need to control the movement of your head relative to the environment. A striking example is spinning around. A few rapid turns is enough to make you dizzy and disoriented, unless you control your head movement properly.

F. Yes, I learnt that when dancing. You have to turn your head and eyes to keep your gaze on a point for as long as possible, and then swing your head and eyes rapidly round the other way to catch the point again.

D. There have, in fact, been a number of studies showing how precisely head movement is controlled in a variety of situations, from daily activities like stepping down and walking, through to gymnastic feats like aerial somersaults (Pozzo *et al.* 1989, 1991).

G. Going back to the *physical* base for action, there is surely more to it than establishing adequate contact with the ground or other surface. For example, when I was swinging my foot onto that rock I had to move other parts of my body properly, otherwise, as I swung my foot forward, by equal and opposite reaction I would have tended to fall over backwards.

C. That's correct. Gravity is a strong force that will pull the body out of control very quickly if not used properly. There is essentially no time to do this in reponse to the pull; it has to be done in advance in order to preserve the flow of action. When this is not possible, as when you unexpectedly step on a slippery patch, the ongoing activity is interrupted and all energy has to be devoted to regaining balance.

E. The idea of establishing an action-base fits well with Peto's ideas. First of all, as I've already mentioned, Peto didn't follow normal development but suggested that any work with the children should start with *what they can do* and not with what we would like them to do or with what they cannot do. We observe the children to see what they can do and what they can use to help themselves. In order to learn any form of motor task a child needs a base or a point of departure from which she can progress. If she can grasp and hold on she will stand a better chance of being able to control her reflexes when moving her head around. Once she is symmetrical the eye-hand coordination also will improve.

Controlling approach: a basic problem in movement control

F. Oops! I almost fell there. I wasn't looking where I was going.

D. Fixing your gaze on the next destination point for your foot helps you in controlling approach to the destination.

F. So how I move my gaze is an important part of the whole action. In fact, I basically have to do the same with my gaze as with my feet. I have to move it to destinations to enable me to move my feet and hands to destinations.

D. Yes, controlling approach to destinations is in large measure what movement control is all about. Moving the hand to an object to be grasped, the foot to a stepping place, and gaze to a new location are clear instances. There are many equally important but less obvious examples, like standing up from a chair. There you have to move your centre of weight forward and upward and make sure that the forward movement stops when your weight is over your feet—that is, unless you want to continue forward. Another example is shifting your weight from side to side over each foot in turn as you walk. If you don't stop the sideways movement when your weight is over your foot but instead carry on then you'll veer off or lose balance.

G. Actually, Hamish seems to have those balance problems. He also has difficulty moving his left hand to things. He doesn't seem to be able to stop it at the right time. So I can see that controlling approach is a general problem. But how is approach to these various types of destination controlled?

F. Maybe if we could understand that we would be over halfway to understanding how to help children like Hamish.

Perceptual control of approach

G. It would seem that controlling approach requires much detailed perceptual information, such as how far my foot is from its destination, how fast it's moving, and how quickly it's slowing down. Then I need to do complicated calculations in my head to work out what to do next.

C. That's possible but you must agree it doesn't seem that way. For example, look at Tam chasing through the gorse bushes after that rabbit. His action just flows. I cannot believe he's doing complex sums for every footfall. Besides, why should he need to do the sums at all except to end up with something simpler in the way of information that was directly usable. And if that's the case then why go about it in a roundabout way?

D. Tam doesn't need masses of information to get around, and neither do we. What we need are quantities in our perceptual field that covary with those aspects of movement that we need to control. For example, when you hit a tennis ball, you need to time the swing of the racket correctly. Therefore you need to see when the ball will reach you.

G. What is there in my visual field that tells me this?

D. As the ball comes nearer its image grows in your visual field, as when you move your hand toward your face its image grows. Now, suppose there is a soccer ball approaching alongside the tennis ball. At each moment the two balls will be the same distance away. But the soccer ball is bigger than the tennis ball and so both its image and rate of growth of image will be bigger. Therefore neither the *size* of the image alone nor the *rate of growth* of the image alone can tell you how long the balls will take to reach you.

F. So there must be some quality to the image which is not affected by extraneous things like the size of the object and which measures the time to reach me directly.

D. The *tau* of the image does this. It tells you what the tau of the gap between you and the ball is.

F. What is tau?

D. Tau is a measure of the image or of the physical gap, just like the distance across the gap is a measure. The difference is that tau measures the *temporal* width of the gap rather than its spatial width. Tau is the time it would take the gap to close if the rate of closing stayed constant.

F. But what if the rate of closing of the gap is not constant?

D. That doesn't matter, because in general tau of the gap always provides a *constant velocity or first order estimate* of the time it will take for the gap to close. And this has an interesting implication. The way tau is changing over time tells you whether the gap is closing at a constant rate, or at an accelerating rate, or at a decelerating rate. If the gap is shrinking at a constant rate then tau will be changing at the constant rate of 1 second every second. But if the gap is shrinking at a decelerating rate then tau will be changing at a slower rate.

G. So, going back to the problem of walking, as I swing my foot forward, tau of the gap to the next rock is continuously changing, and this is mirrored by the tau of the image of the gap in my visual field. Could I use the speed at which tau is changing to slow down my foot properly?

D. Yes you could. The rule is simple. Suppose you detect that the speed at which tau is changing is slower than the critical speed of half a second every second. It can be shown mathematically that this implies you are slowing your foot down too quickly. Thus, if you carry on slowing your foot down at the current rate it will stop short of the rock. You therefore need to slow it down less. On the other hand, if you detect that the speed at which tau is changing is *faster* than the critical speed of half a second every second then this means you are not slowing your foot down fast enough. Therefore you need to slow it down more (Lee 1976, 1993).

Shifting gaze to change the action base

F. Could this tau rule be used in controlling any kind of approach?

D. Yes. For instance, consider shifting gaze to establish a new action base or to visually inspect something. This is something we have to do accurately on average about two or three times a second in order to pick up detailed information with our foveas for controlling our movements. To make small gaze shifts, we move only our eyes. But in general most of the body is involved in the act of looking, as just then when you turned to watch Tam jumping that fence.

F. It sounds very complicated, what with the eye rotating and shifting in space at the same time, and the head, shoulders and hips doing the same sort of thing. Do you think all these movements are individually controlled?

D. No. I think control is focused on the angular gap between the gaze line and its target. Basically, you have to quickly and smoothly reduce this gap to zero, just as you have to reduce to zero the gap between your foot and the rock you're about to step on. In both cases you need a combination of body movements, but the combination you use is not fixed. It varies from one occasion to the next. What is quite constant, however, is the way *tau* of the angular gap between the gaze line and its target changes when gaze movement is slowing down We have measured this on adults for different sizes of gaze shift. Tau decreases to zero in a way which is very close to linear.

F. You mean that when you plot tau of the gaze gap against time the data points lie very close to a straight line ?

D. That's right. And this indicates that the rate of change of tau—what we call *tau-dot*—is being kept constant during the slowing down phase, as in these graphs (Fig. 13.1).

F. Why should tau-dot be kept constant?

D. Because it turns out from the mathematics that keeping tau-dot constant is a way of ensuring that you stop on the target. It's a way of prospectively controlling your approach to the target so that you do not stop short or go shooting past it but stop just on it (Lee 1976).

Holding gaze to stabilize the action base

F. So, going back to the idea of using gaze as a third leg when walking over rough ground, I can see how you might shift gaze onto the next rock using this constant tau-dot procedure. But then you have to *hold* your gaze on the rock to help guide your foot there.

D. That's right. Even when you've got your gaze onto the rock you can't rest because your head is moving forward and so you have to continue to control your gaze to hold it on target. This was found in laboratory-based experiments using stepping-stones (Hollands *et al.* 1995, van Wijck 1995). It has also been found in basketball shooting. Skilled players orient their gaze to the basket even before the ball passed to them has quite reached their hands (Ripoll *et al.* 1986). In both examples, the person first visually establishes a perceptual action-base by shifting gaze to the goal of the movement, and then maintains the perceptual action-base by holding gaze on the goal while visually guiding the movement toward it.

G. Intuitively, shifting gaze seems more demanding than just keeping it on the target of interest—unless the target moves, of course.

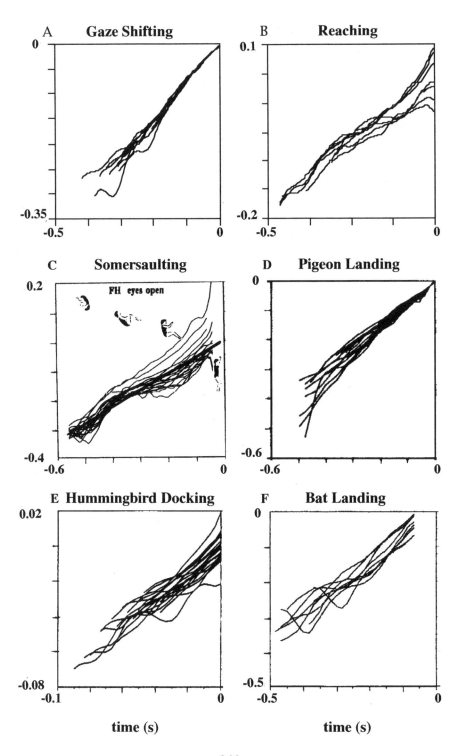

A **Gaze Shifting**

B **Reaching**

C **Somersaulting**

FH eyes open

D **Pigeon Landing**

E **Hummingbird Docking**

F **Bat Landing**

time (s)

time (s)

C. Keeping the eyes on target may actually be more difficult than just moving them there. One important reason is the high demand for gaze stability. Even the slightest slippage of the image on the retina will cause gross deterioration in acuity.

D. Keeping gaze on target is really not so different from shifting gaze to a target. Both involve controlling approach. Maintaining a particular goal state entails continually controlling approach to that goal state because of inevitable drifts away from it. This is as true for keeping balance, maintaining a steady direction of travel, maintaining steady body temperature, etc. Looking is especially demanding because it's so sensitive to drifts.

C. Gordon, you are right that a moving target introduces a complication, but even when the object we are looking at is stationary we are often moving ourselves, and this movement must to be compensated for as well. The adjustments must be predictive to avoid gaze drifts. Furthermore, if gaze is to stay on target, eye movements also have to compensate for head movements unrelated to the tracking of the target. Such head movements may arise as a result of more gross body movements like locomotion, from external perturbations of the head, or from the internal modulations of voluntary head movements. The eye movements must predict these modulations in head movement to be able to compensate for them.

G. Isn't this done as a fast reaction by the vestibulo-ocular reflex?

C. It is true that vestibular reactions are very fast. However, head acceleration is the stimulus for the vestibular system and that makes it possible to predict upcoming shifts of the head rather well. Quick head movements are well compensated for in adults and without a phase lag. Rosander and I (von Hofsten and Rosander 1996) recently found that this is also true for young infants (Fig. 13.2). We found that even in 1-month-old infants the compensatory eye movements were not systematically lagging the head

Fig. 13.1. *(Opposite)* Experimental results indicating that the tau theory of control of velocity of approach to a destination applies across different activities, different perceptual systems and different species. Plots of tau (τ) of the gap to the destination against time-to-contact with the destination are shown for individual trials during the deceleration phase of the approach. The theory predicts straight-line plots passing through the origin, which corresponds to keeping the rate of change of tau constant. Means (standard deviations) of the linear regression coefficients r^2 and slope for the plots are given below for each plot. r^2 measures the degree of linearity ($r^2 = 1$ corresponds to perfect linearity). Slope estimates the value of the constant rate of change of tau.

(A) Adult human gaze shifting using visual guidance; plots of tau of the changing *angular* gap between gaze and the destination direction [$r^2 = 0.997$ (0.003), slope = 0.782 (0.071)]. (B) Adult human reaching using visual guidance; plots of tau of the changing *distance* gap between the hand and the destination object [$r^2 = 0.959$ (0.014), slope = 0.525 (0.027)]. (C) Adult human trampolinist landing from an aerial somersault using visual and vestibular guidance; plots of tau of the changing *angular* gap between the head–toe axis and the just-off-vertical destination orientation of the axis at landing [$r^2 = 0.963$ (0.024), slope = 0.552 (0.071)] (Lee *et al.* 1992b). (D) Pigeon landing on a perch using visual guidance; plots of tau of the changing *distance* gap between the feet and the perch [$r^2 = 0.992$ (0.011), slope = 0.775 (0.109)] (Lee *et al.* 1993). (E) Hummingbird flying in to dock on a feeder tube [$r^2 = 0.975$ (0.036), slope = 0.710 (0.132)] (Lee *et al.* 1991). (F) Bat (*Eptesicus fuscus*) landing on a finger guiding by echolocation; plots of tau of the changing *distance* gap between the bat and the finger [$r^2 = 0.976$ (0.063), slope = 0.702 (0.052)] (Lee *et al.* 1995).

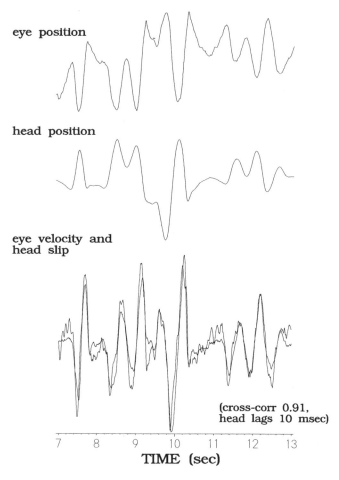

eye position

head position

eye velocity and
head slip

(cross-corr 0.91,
head lags 10 msec)

TIME (sec)

Fig. 13.2. Compensatory eye movements of a 2-month-old infant who is shaking her head with her eyes closed. Eye movements were recorded with electro-oculography and the head movements with an opto-electronic device (Selspot). The upper curve shows the head movements, the middle curve shows the compensatory eye movements, and the two lower curves show the eye velocity superimposed over the head slip. The head slip is the velocity gap that the compensatory eye movements have to make up in order to preserve a stable gaze. The cross-correlation showed a maximum value of $r = 0.91$ at an eye velocity lead of 10 ms.

movements. However, the precision improved considerably between 1 and 3 months of age.

G. One thing puzzles me. Earlier we talked about both head and eyes being involved in shifting gaze. How does the system know that the head movements, which are involved in the tracking, are not to be compensated for?

C. Good point! The fact is that the vestibular system is specialized to deal with fast changes. Head movements involved in tracking a target are generally much slower. That is why it is fairly easy to maintain fixation while you are shaking the head but almost impossible to keep fixation on a flying house-fly.

G. You mentioned that tracking must be predictive to avoid drifts. When do you observe such eye movements in children?

C. We have found that 1-month-olds substantially lag the target they are trying to track. However, already at 3 months of age they show good prospective control of their tracking movements (Aslin 1981, von Hofsten and Rosander 1996).

G. Do infants use the head at all when tracking a target?

C. Yes, they do and in a very flexible and useful way. Neonates don't use much head movement (Bloch and Carchon 1992), but 1-month-olds who cannot yet support their head in an upright position turn their head with a target they are tracking if given that possibility. We found that when infants were supported, head movements contributed significantly to tracking in 1-month-olds as well as 3-month-olds (von Hofsten and Rosander 1996). The amount of head movement increased with age. This was also found by Daniel and Lee (1990). They found that at 6 months of age, some infants even used predominantly head movements when tracking a target. Using both head and eye movements to stabilize gaze requires making certain demands on the system. These two component movements have to be timed and scaled to each other. This is only possible if each body part knows what the other body parts are going to do ahead of time.

G. I'm getting the idea that controlling gaze is rather a complicated business. It involves moving both the head and the eyes, and sensing the movements through the joints, muscles, vestibular system and eyes.

C. And it is extremely important that this system works properly because otherwise the child cannot extract the visual information she needs. Jacobsen (1996) at the University of Oslo studied multiply disabled children with severe eye movement problems who were diagnosed as 'cortically blind' and found that many of them had almost normal acuity. However, the fact that they could not control gaze made them unable to use the vision they had in a functional way. In other words, their movement disability created a perceptual disability.

D. Cerebral-palsied children also can have a similar problem. We measured eye–head co-ordination in 2- to 7-year-old hemiparetic children when they were trying to look at a small attractive object. In one experiment the object was moving from side to side in front of the child. In the other experiment the object was stationary and the child was oscillated on a swivel chair in front of it. The same experiments were also performed on normally developing 11- to 29-week-old babies, 3- to 4-year-old children and adults. Babies at 29 weeks of age coordinated the movement of their head with the movement of the object or chair very precisely and as accurately as the adults. However, none of the cerebral palsied children showed anywhere near the same head coordination. Their gaze error was also significantly greater than the error of even the 11-week-old babies (Lee *et al.* 1990).

Coupling seeing and feeling

F. With all this talk about holding gaze I cannot take my eyes off the ground in case I fall!

But the path's not so rough here that I should need to guide my feet very accurately onto the rocks.

C. In fact, if you hold your hands below your eyes so that you hide your feet but can still see the ground a pace or two ahead you will find that you don't actually need to see your feet.

F. That's true, though it is more jerky that way. Obviously seeing my feet helps, even on this easy ground. But when I can't see my feet does that mean that I am controlling the approach of my foot to the rock by *feel* in much the same way as I had been doing visually?

D. Controlling approach by feel is, in fact, something we do all the time—as when putting something to your mouth, for instance. It's easy to do this with the eyes closed, even if you put your head in an unusual position. So you can't be just using a memorized movement. We did the experiment recently, eating grapes. The movement of the hand to the mouth when the eyes were shut was not measurably different to when the eyes were open.

F. Was approach controlled by tau even when the eyes were shut?

D. Yes, the data indicated that both the speed and direction of approach of the hand to the mouth were controlled in terms of tau.

F. So tau is not restricted to vision?

D. No. It seems to apply generally. For example, two studies colleagues and I did with bats indicate that they use an acoustic version of tau when they are flying around using echolocation (Lee *et al.* 1992a, 1995). The same also appears true in human echolocation, from recent experiments in my lab.

G. To go back to stepping without seeing your feet: that's a bit different from moving your hand to your mouth, because you can presumably feel where both your hand and mouth are.

C. That's right, hand-to-mouth is matching felt position with felt position, whereas in the stepping example it is matching felt position to just-seen position.

D. In everyday life we constantly have to couple visual and non-visual information. We cannot keep an eye on every moving part of the body all at the same time. We therefore need to feel how our limbs are moving too. Coupling the visual and nonvisual information is crucial to developing and maintaining competent movement.

A little while ago we compared this coupling ability in children with hemiparetic cerebral palsy and normal children (Lee *et al.* 1990) by measuring how accurately they could locate three types of target with their hand when it was hidden from view. There was a *seen* target (a toy), a *felt* target (the child's other hand hidden from view) and a *seen-and-felt* target (the child's other hand in view). Here's a photograph of the set-up (Fig. 13.3).

The hemiparetic children performed less well than the normal children when localizing the targets, not only when using their affected hand but also when using their unaffected hand. Wann (1991) found similar visual/nonvisual proprioceptive coupling problems in children with cerebral palsy.

Examining the data further, we found that the hemiparetic children suffered distinct forms of disorder. In two, the felt position of the head/eyes was affected, which im-

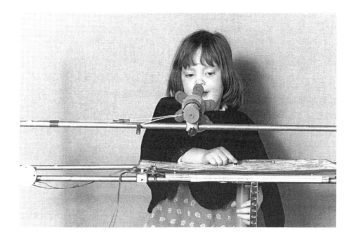

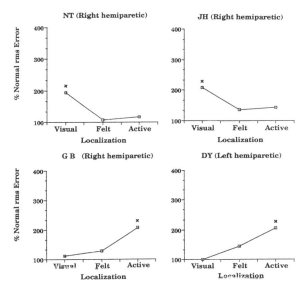

Fig. 13.3. *(Top)* Apparatus to measure ability to localize objects and one's own limbs. The child is wearing a cloak so that she cannot see her left hand and arm. With that hand she is moving a slider along a track, attempting to line it up beneath the *target* button on which her right finger rests. In this case, it is a *seen and felt target*. With her eyes closed, it would be a *felt target*. With her eyes open and finger not on the button, it would be a *seen target*. The three types of target were used in the experiment. The target was opposite either the child's left or right shoulder and the child used the left or right hand. Errors in positioning were read off the scale on the viewer's side of the apparatus. The toy in front of the child was rotated on 50% of trials on a random basis to keep up the child's interest.

(Bottom) Different error patterns of four hemiparetic children in: *visual localization* of targets (pointing with the unseen unaffected hand); *felt localization* of the affected limb (pointing to it with the unaffected hand with eyes covered); *active localization* with the affected limb (pointing with it, unseen, to a *seen* or *felt* target, whichever allowed the better performance). rms errors are plotted as a percentage of the mean rms error produced by 12 normal nursery school children. *Asterisks* indicate errors significantly (p<0.05, normal test) higher than those of the nursery school children (Lee *et al.* 1990).

271

paired their ability to visually localize objects with respect to the body. In two others, the ability to move their hemiparetic hand by feel to a seen position was impaired. This too would impair everyday actions.

C. Rösblad and I did a similar study with clumsy children (Rösblad and von Hofsten 1992). The task of the children was to point underneath a table top to targets either seen or felt on the table surface. We found a relatively strong dependence on vision in many of these children for localizing the targets correctly. It wasn't a problem with proprioception itself because they could guide their unseen hand to a seen target. The problem arose when they had to guide their unseen hand to a felt target. It was like the spatial frame of reference provided by vision was superior to the one provided by proprioception.

Ester, aren't there are a number of exercises used in Conductive Education that are directed at helping the child develop a good proprioceptive sense?

E. Yes, they move both hands together, holding a stick, first up above the head, then behind the neck and then to the chin and all the body parts. Everything we do is done in every position, in supine and prone, in sitting and standing and walking, and so on. The aim is to help them acquire a good body image as well as improve symmetry. It is their own correction that teaches them.

D. I remember you saying that children with cerebral palsy often have problems looking at their hands.

E. In the early period of life, many CP children do not see their hands enough. In fact some of them do not see them at all. It is very important that they play with their hands in this early period (Held and Bauer 1967). It has been suggested that the normal child is more interested in her hands than in the toys she has to play with (Elliott and Connolly 1973). In Conductive Education we do endless work with the hands, not only to teach the child functional skills but to develop the hands as the tool with which the child can change her dysfunctional motor patterns in general (Cotton 1994b).

We try to teach the children to look at their hands and, at the same time, express what they are doing in words—"I'm looking at my hands. I've got two hands. My hands are on the table"—and so on. However, if they didn't see their hands much when they were small then they seem reluctant to look at them.

D. Maybe this is because they developed some *feel* for their hands in their early months of life but, with not being able to see them much, they weren't able to couple the visual information with the information they got through the sensors in the joints and muscles. Thus, when confronted with the sight of something they have mainly only felt it is bewildering. I'm reminded of Oliver Sacks's book *A Leg to Stand On* where he describes what a disturbing and perplexing experience it was seeing his deafferented leg (Sacks 1984).

Reaching and catching

F. Don't reaching and catching involve both seeing and feeling in a very profound way? How early can you observe reaching in infants and how much does its early development rely on the infant seeing her hands?

C. Reaching can, in fact, be observed in neonates (von Hofsten 1982). I presented neonates with a distinct object moving with small jerky movements in front of them, and they made forward extended arm movements toward this object. The movements were never the same, but they did have something in common: they had a tendency to be directed toward the object, wherever it was positioned in the visual field. The reaches never resulted in grasping and rarely touching the object, but the hand emerged into the visual field towards the direction of gaze. In other words, the infants put their feelers towards where they were looking. It was like they were getting prepared to explore the environment. Dave has a similar story to tell.

D. Yes, these were experiments with 2-week-old babies (van der Meer *et al.* 1995a). Babies of that age when lying on their backs often wave their arms around with their head on one side. The behaviour appears meaningless but we suspect it is actually functional. It is an early stage of developing visual control of movement—they are exploring the visual correlates of self-produced and felt movement.

To test the idea, the babies had strings attached to their wrists which could be made to pull gently on their wrists in the direction of their feet (Fig. 13.4). With their head turned to one side they could see only one arm. What happened was that they resisted the pull of the string on that arm and moved it in much the same place and manner as when there was no string pulling at their wrist. On the other hand, the arm they could not see was pulled down by the string and moved less than before.

F. Mightn't this be due to the baby's asymmetrical posture?

D. A good question. However, the same result was obtained when the baby's arms were visually switched using video cameras and monitors. Thus, when the baby's head was turned to the right, for example, it saw not its right arm but its *left* arm, on a video monitor.

Taken together, the experiments showed that it was the *seen* arm that was kept up against the pull of the string, irrespective of whether the arm was on the same or opposite side as the head was turned. This is why we think the baby is engaged in important functional behaviour when waving its arms around. It is coupling the visual and non-visual proprioceptive systems in the business of guiding limb movement.

G. These movements are basically movements of the arms rather than manipulative movements. How do infants prepare for grasping an object?

C. The preparations are not always easy to detect with the naked eye. Things happen too fast and some of the preparations are rather subtle. One needs special equipment to get the required time–space resolution. There are many ways in which a reach is prepared. Take the opening and orientation of the hand, for instance. We found that 5-month-old infants adjust the orientation of the hand to the orientation of the object to be grasped (von Hofsten and Fazel-Zandy 1984) and that 9-month-olds adjust the opening of the hand to the size of the object to be grasped (von Hofsten and Rönnqvist 1988). Furthermore, at 5 months, infants prepare the grasp by starting to close the hand just before the object is encountered (von Hofsten and Rönnqvist 1988). So, when reaching for an object, the grasping is never accomplished by a grasp reflex. However, the most clear example of prospective control in reaching can be seen when infants reach for a moving object. They are quite clever at that. Reaches are aimed ahead of the target, towards a

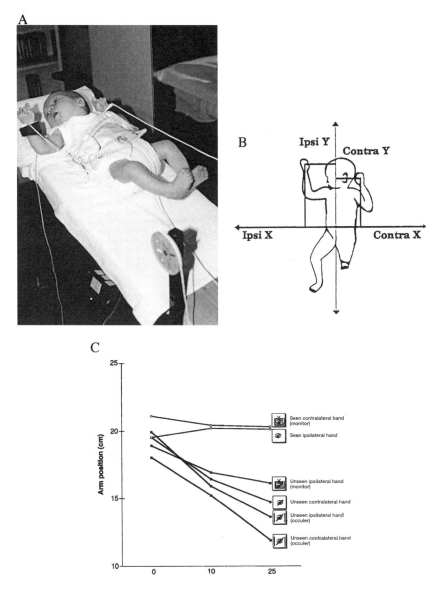

Fig. 13.4. (A) Neonatal arm waving experimental setup. The 18-day-old baby has strings attached to her wrists. The strings pass over pulleys and have weight pans (not shown) at their ends. When a small weight is put in a pan the string pulls on the baby's arm in the direction of its feet. If the baby does not resist the pull the arm would be drawn out of the baby's main field of view. The baby sees only the arm it is facing (as shown), *or* only the opposite arm (by means of a video monitor, not shown), *or* neither arm because they are occluded from view by screens. (B) The (*x*,*y*) coordinates of the images of the wrists were recorded at 62 Hz by means of an opto-electronic Selspot system. (C) Mean *y* coordinate of the wrists when weights of 0%, 10% or 25% of the baby's arm weight were attached to the strings. When a hand can be seen, either directly or on the video monitor, it is not pulled down toward the feet. Otherwise it is (van der Meer *et al.* 1995a).

274

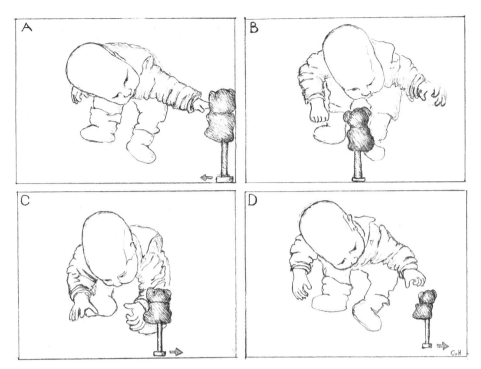

Fig. 13.5. A 6-month-old infant reaching for a teddy bear that moves diagonally down a screen at 40 cm/s. In the middle of the screen the teddy bear abruptly changes path and starts moving down the other diagonal. (A) The infant orients toward the moving object and starts preparing the reach. (B) The infant reaches for the object which is about to switch path. (C) The infant is still reaching for a position on the continuation of the original diagonal path while the object is moving on the other diagonal. (D) The infant is once more oriented towards the object.

future meeting point (von Hofsten 1980, 1983). I found that 8-month-old infants were quite capable of catching objects moving at 120 cm/s.

In another experiment (von Hofsten *et al.* 1993), we had objects move diagonally on a screen, coming within reach only for a fraction of a second (Fig. 13.5). The 6-month-old infants started to prepare the grasp already at the beginning of the target motion by activating the contralateral hand. On some trials we switched the motion paths at their intersection, so that the object would continue on the same side as it started. The subject would then continue reaching for the object on the contralateral side, in the continuation of its original path. No adjustments could be detected until at least a quarter of a second after the object had switched paths.

Finding out what is wrong

F. Mightn't a catching task be a useful diagnostic test?

D. Yes. Catching requires good control of gaze and hand and, as we've said, both abilities normally develop quite young. Since they are basic perceptuomotor abilities that are

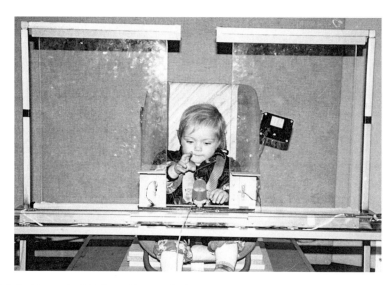

Fig. 13.6. An 11-month-old infant taking part in the toy-catching experiment (van der Meer *et al.* 1994).

needed for a wide range of activities in later life, if problems can be picked up early then therapeutic activities could be devised to try to help the children develop these basic abilities. I think most people would agree that the earlier you can find out what is wrong and start doing something about it the better for the child (Turnbull 1993).

At Edinburgh we have been comparing the catching performance of preterm neurologically at risk infants and normal infants (van der Meer *et al.* 1994, 1995b). The infants, 20 to 48 weeks old, sit facing the middle of a horizontal track that they can reach through a narrow gap in a transparent screen. A small attractive toy is moved along the track at four different speeds and the infant spontaneously tries to reach through the gap and catch the toy as it passes by. The last part of the toy's approach to the gap is screened from the infant's view (Fig. 13.6).

All but the youngest (20 week old) normal infant showed prospective control of gaze, by shifting gaze from the approaching toy to the catching place even before the toy had disappeared behind the screen. By the time the infants were 10 months old, the hand also started to move prospectively before the toy had disappeared. The neurologically at risk infants, however, were developmentally delayed in their prospective control of both gaze and hand.

The at risk infants were also developmentally delayed in the strategies they appeared to use to *time* their gaze shift and start the hand movement. The normal infants at about 8 months of age switched from timing based on the *distance gap* between toy and catching place to timing based on the tau gap. The distance gap strategy is, of course, less efficient than the tau gap strategy because it allows less time to act the faster the toy is moving.

Most of the at risk infants were delayed by about four months in when they switched

276

strategies. Two of the infants, however, still seemed to be using the less efficient distance gap strategy at 1 year of age. Interestingly, these were the only children in the at risk group who had neurologically abnormal scores, and at 18 and 21 months they were diagnosed as having mild and moderate cerebral palsy respectively.

G. Wouldn't catching tasks also be useful diagnostically for older children like Hamish?

C. Forsström and I studied catching in a group of neurologically impaired children aged 4 to 11 years (Forsström and von Hofsten 1982). The children had clear problems in carrying out the reaches, but we found that timing was actually the least affected aspect of the behavior. They reached further ahead of the target than a group of matched normal children, which gave them additional time to carry out their reaches. The result was that they essentially caught all the slow moving targets (50 cm/s) and 75% of the fast moving ones (100 cm/s). It was as if they took into account their movement impairments when planning their actions. In Dave's lab they have developed a catching task which is more adapted to children with cerebral palsy.

D. Up to now it has been used to measure interceptive timing skill in hemiparetic cerebral palsied children aged 4 to 8 years to try to find out where their basic movement problems lie (van der Weel *et al.* 1996).

The child sits on a chair close to a table facing up a sloping track with its bottom end at the table's edge (Fig. 13.7). A ball is rolled down the track at three different speeds past a bat hanging near the bottom of the track and the child has, by reaching forward, to strike the bat to knock the ball off the track as it passes. If it's done accurately the ball knocks over a stack of cans, which pleases the child no end! The track can be inclined at different angles to alter the speed at which the ball reaches the bat.

The aim was to find out about the basic control procedures being used in the game that might be defective in the children with cerebral palsy. Firstly, the results indicated that what governed the timing of the strike was the tau gap between ball and bat rather than the distance gap or the time gap. (The time gap was not the same as the tau gap because the ball was accelerating.) This applied whether the child struck with the affected or unaffected hand. Normal nursery school children behaved similarly. Thus, in using tau for timing the strike the cerebral palsied children were behaving with normal efficiency.

The children with cerebral palsy also used tau in an adaptive way. They used a *larger* tau value for timing the strike when striking with the *affected* hand than when striking with the unaffected hand. This meant they allowed themselves more time to strike with their less agile affected hand.

It was only when we examined how the children slowed down the forward movement of their hand to the bat that impairment in the children with cerebral palsy was revealed. Basically, both the cerebral palsied and the normal children appeared to be trying to follow the effective strategy of keeping the tau gap between hand and bat proportional to the tau gap between ball and bat (Fig. 13.7). The difference was that children with more severe cerebral palsy did this less accurately, apparently because of errors in perceiving the values of the taus. They did not appear to err so much on the movement side because their graphs were as straight as the nursery children's.

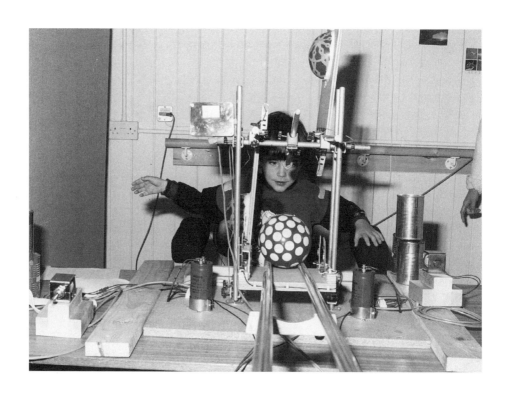

CP GR Affected hand

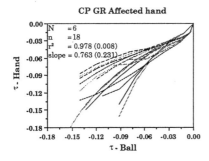

N = 6
n = 18
r² = 0.978 (0.008)
slope = 0.763 (0.231)

τ - Hand

τ - Ball

CP GR Non-affected hand

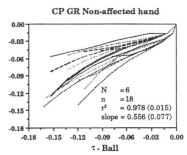

N = 6
n = 18
r² = 0.978 (0.015)
slope = 0.556 (0.077)

τ - Ball

Nurs. Lu Non-dominant hand

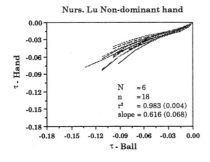

N = 6
n = 18
r² = 0.983 (0.004)
slope = 0.616 (0.068)

τ - Hand

τ - Ball

Nurs. Lu Dominant hand

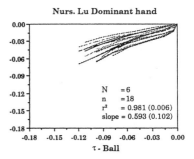

N = 6
n = 18
r² = 0.981 (0.006)
slope = 0.593 (0.102)

τ - Ball

E. I can see that both this game and the one for infants might be useful diagnostically. Do you think one needs to build up a whole battery of such tasks and test each child on all of them?

D. It is certainly essential to devise ways of assessing a child's perceptuomotor competence in detail in order to be able to develop appropriate therapeutic tasks for the child. But I don't think each child needs to be given the same battery of diagnostic tasks. Since children with cerebral palsy vary in their movement problems, they need to be assessed individually. Following the perception in action approach that we have been advocating, assessment might start off by seeking answers to four questions in sequence.

Question 1. If the child is unable to execute an action accurately, is this due to an inability to move as such, or to defective *control* of body movement? For example, if a particular body movement is poor in the context of one action but not in another then this would indicate defective control in the former action.

Question 2. If the child has difficulty *controlling* movement, as seems usually to be the case in cerebral palsy, then is the difficulty due to inadequate perceptual information for control or to *inadequate use* of the information? For example, if one action is performed poorly while another action requiring the same information for control is performed well, then this would indicate inadequate use of the information in the former action.

Question 3. If the child's difficulty is due, wholly or in part, to inadequate perceptual information for control, then at what level within the perceptual system does the defect lie? For example, in the case of vision, is there a problem in controlling movement of the head and eyes to direct gaze and/or does the problem lie in linking visual information to proprioceptive information obtained through the muscles?

Question 4. If part or all of the problem is due to inadequate use of perceptual information in control, then what particular control procedures are defective? For example, is control of *speed* of movement to a destination poor or does the problem lie with control of *direction* of movement?

Fig. 13.7. *(Opposite, top)* Child sitting in the ball hitting apparatus. Hand movements to the bat are recorded by an overhead Selspot camera. *(Bottom)* Tau of the gap between hand and bat (τ-Hand) is plotted against tau of the gap between ball and bat (τ-Ball). This was to test the hypothesis that the hand–bat tau is kept proportional to the ball–bat tau. This would be an effective strategy, ensuring that the hand reached the bat at the same time as the ball. If the strategy were followed precisely then plotting one tau against the other should result in a straight line through the origin. The cerebral palsied (CP) children and nursery (Nurs.) children all produced quite straight line results. The nursery children's lines go closely through the origin, indicating that they were keeping one tau proportional to the other. However, the most affected CP children's lines pass below the origin to varying degrees, which corresponds to them arriving late at the bat and being quite variable in this. The significant non-zero intercepts, together with the high r^2 values, indicate that the CP children were, like the nursery children, trying to keep τ-Hand proportional to τ-Ball, but on each trial there was an appreciable error on the perceptual side of their estimate of τ-Ball and/or τ-Hand, that error remaining constant during the trial. The CP children did not appear to err so much on the movement side because their r^2 values were as high as the nursery children's.

279

Improving movement control in children with cerebral palsy

F. Assuming these questions were answered, how then should we go about helping children with cerebral palsy?

C. To begin with, we can learn a useful general lesson from the early developing skills we have been discussing. Early behaviour is not elicited or driven by specific stimuli as a reflex notion suggests. It is driven by motives and controlled by perceptual information. This is especially apparent in infants who are learning new skills. It is most impressive to observe how they try to do things they have not yet mastered. Again we can take reaching as an example. Around 3 to 4 months of age, a normal infant will work systematically to get the hand to an object and grasp it. To start with, the attempts are not very successful but that doesn't seem to make much of a difference. The infants stubbornly continue. It is clear that it is the motive to grasp objects that gets the reaching system assembled. Motives decide what gets developed.

Motives also predict future goal states and are therefore an essential part of prospective control. Different things are prepared depending on what the child wants to do. When she wants to hit an object, a different goal-directed movement is prepared compared to when she wants to grasp it.

E. Yes, the important thing is to set goals, small and large. But it is important to bear in mind that normal movements are not often attainable in cerebral palsy. Although Peto was a high-flyer and, for example, wanted everybody to walk, he didn't expect them to walk normally. But he did expect them to walk well, to walk safely and to walk as far as was possible for them.

Goals are there to be reached. They motivate and create success.

G. I can certainly see that the motivation of the child and setting appropriate activities and goals are both extremely important. But how does one go about devising those activities?

D. We need to set up therapeutic activities tailored for each child individually, which require her to perform those actions that her assessment indicates she needs to practise in order to improve her basic perceptuomotor control. In general, the activities need to be chosen to improve the child's prospective control, as measured in her ability to control approach in various ways.

Since the child needs to be motivated to work on the activities, the activities would need to be fun and the child should not get bored with them. If that happened then related activities would need to be substituted.

The therapeutic activities would need to be directed towards both improving the everyday functional use of the body and improving the pick-up of perceptual information for controlling movement, when the assessment indicated this was causing the child a problem.

Suppose, for example, a child is hemiparetic like Hamish. One thing to concentrate on would be trying to improve functional use of the affected arm and hand *when it is used in conjunction with the unaffected limb*. This is because the affected hand is unlikely to become as dextrous as the unaffected hand and so the child is unlikely to use the affected hand for unimanual activities such as writing and drawing. The affected hand does, however, have an important role to play in bimanual actions. For example, it may often be needed to *support* the more dextrous actions of the unaffected hand, as when holding a Lego construction while adding another brick to it. A different but equally important type of bimanual activity is when *symmetrical* actions are required of the two limbs, as when carrying a tray. Sugden and Utley (1995) have recently found coupling, particularly of timing, between the hands in hemiparetic cerebral palsied children.

Commercially available toys, musical instruments and the like could be used straight off the shelf or modified to fulfil therapeutic requirements. Making music can both be a pleasurable interpersonal activity and exercise perceptuomotor control to varying degrees. It therefore offers a valuable therapeutic activity, which is recognized in many therapies, including of course Conductive Education and music therapy. For example, in music making one might work on improving a hemiparetic child's bimanual control of force—which translates into loudness—and timing. This could be done when they are playing along with a parent or other adult on a piano or percussion instrument. Lego, and its larger version Duplo, are examples of toys that offer valuable therapeutic activity since they pose a nicely graded series of problems for bimanual coordination.

F. What if the child had problems more on the perceptual side?

D. Then she should be helped to perceive more precisely. Learning applies to perceiving as well as to moving (Gibson and Gibson 1955, Gibson 1969). Suppose, for example, that the assessment indicated that the child could not visually locate an object accurately with respect to the body, so the hand could not be guided properly to the object unless it too could be seen. As I mentioned before, we have in fact found this problem of visual localization in some hemiparetic children. It would disturb performance of many everyday activities where the reaching hand or stepping foot isn't seen throughout the movement—which, of course, it doesn't normally need to be. A possible therapeutic activity in this case is drum-banging where the child's hand is kept out of sight under a cloth so she has to bang the drum, the edge of which she can see, without seeing the hand she bangs it with.

F. So the approach here is to *deprive* the child of one form of perceptual information (sight of the hand) in order to try to sharpen up sensitivity to another form of information (visual location of the drum relative to the body)?

D. That's right. But another approach to perceptual problems in movement control is to enhance the quality of the perceptual information. We have shown this to be effective, for example, in helping hemiparetic children extend the range of pronation–supination of the hand (van der Weel *et al.* 1991). The set-up was simple (Fig. 13.8). The child grasped a handle which was connected to a drum stick and could be turned like a door-handle by pronating and supinating the hand. They were given the task of turning the handle 'as far as possible' first one way and then the other. This is the kind of abstract task therapists often give, and the children's movement with the affected hand showed the typical limited range. However, when they were given the more concrete task of turning the handle so that the attached drumstick hit a drum on each side, their range of movement was significantly larger.

F. How do you think this difference in performance relates to the perceptual information that was available?

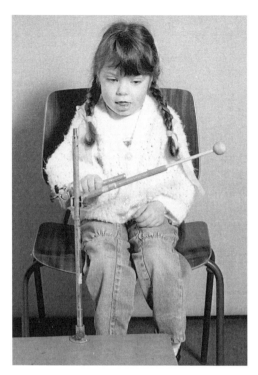

Fig. 13.8. A hemiparetic child taking part in the pronation–supination experiment.

D. In the bang-the-drums task, the child had visual, auditory and tactile information about the approach of the stick to the drum to control her movement to a well-specified destination—in addition to having muscle/joint proprioceptive information about her movement. In the more abstract move-as-far-as-you-can task, by contrast, the destination was less well defined—possibly only by a sense of muscular effort—and the perceptual information was more or less confined to muscle/joint proprioception. Providing extra perceptual information should not *necessarily* improve movement—in fact normal children performed equally well on the abstract and concrete tasks—but if the cerebral palsied child's muscle/joint proprioception is not up to par then the extra visual, auditory and tactile information should help, as indeed it appeared to. This result fits with the study I mentioned before (Lee *et al.* 1990) where we found proprioceptive deficiencies in hemiparetic children, some of whom also took part in this pronation/supination study.

There are other experiments which have a bearing on this issue of improving perceptual information. For example, Leont'ev and Zaporozhets (1960) found that patients with joint or peripheral nerve injury were able to reach higher when they were reaching to grasp an object than when they were simply trying to reach as high as they could. This could be explained by the patients having poor muscle/joint proprioception. Also, it has been found that both smoothness and coordination of movement can be improved by providing better perceptual information, both in hemiparetic stroke patients (Lough

282

1985—see also Lee and Young 1986) and in patients with Parkinson's disease (Frischer 1989).

C. Ester, don't the therapeutic musical activities Dave was talking about fit in well with *rhythmical intention* which, as I understand it, is a basic method in Conductive Education?

E. Yes. In Conductive Education we use language to express an intention, the goal. And the way to the goal is learnt rhythmically, which is important because of the poor rhythm due to spasticity or athetosis in our children. Thus the children might chant something like "My feet are on the floor; my feet are flat; I lean forward; I grasp the chair; I push the chair away; I stand up." Later it would just be "I put my feet on the floor; I stand up", and then just "I stand up." First we go through all the parts of the task, and in the end we can use the whole task.

It is for the conductor, as in an orchestra, to use the right tempo to reach the goal through her understanding of the task, the road to the task and the abilities of the group and each child. This is difficult to learn and needs musicality. Peto was ahead of his time, dealing with language and action.

D. I think the musical conductor analogy is a very good one. The rhythmical aspect of rhythmical intention seems to be important in the same way that it's important in music. When playing in a group or alone, rhythm is necessary to give you a means of prospectively controlling your actions. You can't go waiting to hear the drummer before coming in because if you did you would be a reaction time too late in entering. You need timing information, given by the beat of the music, to control your movements prospectively.

It seems that the essence of the rhythmical intention method is using words musically to specify concurrently the sequence of acts and the temporal structure of the sequence for the child to follow prospectively.

C. Would that be a good note to pause on? How about popping into the Sheep's Heid for some refreshment . . ?

ACKNOWLEDGEMENTS

The research reported was supported by grants to the first author from the Medical Research Council, the Science and Engineering Research Council, the European Office of Aerospace Research and Development, and the Scottish Office Home and Health Department; and by a grant to the second author from the Swedish Council for Social Research (project 92-0113:2C).

REFERENCES

Aslin, R.N. (1981) 'Development of smooth pursuit in human infants.' *In:* Fisher, D.F., Monty, R.A., Senders, J.W. (Eds.) *Eye Movements: Cognition and Visual Perception.* Hillsdale, NJ: Erlbaum, pp. 31–51.

Bernstein, N.A. (1967) *The Co-ordination and Regulation of Movements.* Oxford: Pergamon Press.

Bloch, H., Carchon, I. (1992) 'On the onset of eye–head coordination in infants.' *Behavioural Brain Research*, **49**, 85-90.

Cotton, E. (1994a) *The Basic Motor Pattern. 2nd Edn.* London: The Spastics Society.

—— (1994b) *The Hand as a Guide to Learning.* London: The Spastics Society.

Daniel, B.M., Lee, D.N. (1990) 'Development of looking with head and eyes.' *Journal of Experimental Child Psychology*, **50**, 200–216.

Elliott, J., Connolly, K. (1973) 'Hierarchical structure in skill development.' *In:* Connolly, K., Bruner, J. (Eds.) *The Growth of Competence.* London: Academic Press, pp. 135–168.

Forsström, A., von Hofsten, C. (1982) 'Visually directed reaching of children with motor impairments.' *Developmental Medicine and Child Neurology*, **24**, 653–661.

Frischer, M. (1989) 'Voluntary vs autonomous control of repetitive finger tapping in a patient with Parkinson's disease.' *Neuropsychologia*, **27**, 1261–1266.

Gallwey, W.T. (1986) *The Inner Game of Tennis*. London: Pan.

Gibson, E.J. (1969) *Principles of Perceptual Learning and Development*. New York: Appleton–Century–Crofts.

Gibson, J.J. (1979) *The Ecological Approach to Visual Perception*. Boston: Houghton–Mifflin.

—— Gibson, E.J. (1955) 'Perceptual learning: differentiation or enrichment?' *Psychological Review*, **62**, 32–41.

Goodale, M.A., Milner, A.D. (1992) 'Separate visual pathways for perception and action.' *Trends in Neurosciences*, **15**, 20–25.

Hári, M., Ákos, K. (1988) *Conductive Education*. London and New York: Routledge.

Held, R., Bauer, J.A. (1967) 'Visually guided reaching in monkeys after restricted rearing.' *Science*, **155**, 718–720.

Hollands, M.A., Marplehorvat, D.E., Henkes, S., Rowan, A.K. (1995) 'Human eye-movements during visually guided stepping.' *Journal of Motor Behaviour*, **27**, 155–163.

Jacobsen, K.H. (1996) 'Application of the preferential looking technique to vision testing in mentally retarded persons.' Doctoral dissertation, University of Oslo, Institute of Psychology.

Kawato, M., Gomi, H. (1992) 'The cerebellum and VOR/OKR learning models.' *Trends in Neurosciences*, **15**, 445–453.

Lee, D.N. (1976) 'A theory of visual control of braking based on information about time-to-collision.' *Perception*, **5**, 437–459.

—— (1993) 'Body–environment coupling.' *In:* Neiser, U. (Ed.) *Ecological and Interpersonal Knowledge of Self*. Cambridge: Cambridge University Press, pp. 43–67.

—— Young, D.S. (1986) 'Gearing action to the environment.' *In:* Heuer, H., Fromm, C. (Eds.) *Generation and Modulation of Action Patterns*. Heidelberg: Springer Verlag, pp. 217–230.

—— Daniel, B.M., Turnbull, J., Cook, M.L. (1990) 'Basic perceptuo-motor dysfunctions in cerebral palsy.' *In:* Jeannerod, M. (Ed.) *Attention and Performance. XIII: Motor Representation and Control*. Hillsdale, NJ: Erlbaum, pp. 583–603.

—— Reddish, P.E., Rand, D.T. (1991) 'Aerial docking by hummingbirds.' *Naturwissenschaften*, **78**, 526–527.

—— Van der Weel, F.R., Hitchcock, T., Matejowsky, E., Pettigrew, J.D. (1992a) 'Common principle of guidance by echolocation and vision.' *Journal of Comparative Physiology*, **A171**, 563–571.

—— Young, D.S., Rewt, D. (1992b) 'How do somersaulters land on their feet?' *Journal of Experimental Psychology: Human Perception and Performance*, **18**, 1195–1202.

—— Davies, M.N.O., Green, P.R., van der Weel, F.R. (1993) 'Visual control of velocity of approach by pigeons when landing.' *Journal of Experimental Biology*, **180**, 85–104.

—— Simmons, J.A., Saillant, P.A., Bouffard, F. (1995) 'Steering by echolocation: a paradigm of ecological acoustics.' *Journal of Comparative Physiology*, **A176**, 347–354.

Leont'ev, A.N., Zaporozhets, A.V. (1960) *Rehabilitation of Hand Function*. (Translated by B. Haigh; edited by W.R. Russell.) London: Pergamon Press.

Lough, S. (1985) 'Visuo-motor control following stroke: a motor skills perspective.' PhD thesis, University of Edinburgh.

Pozzo, T., Berthoz, A., Lefort, L. (1989) 'Head kinematic during various motor tasks in humans.' *In:* Allum, J.H.J., Hulliger, M. (Eds.) *Progress in Brain Research*. Amsterdam: Elsevier Science, pp. 377–383.

—— —— —— Vitte, E. (1991) 'Head stabilization during various locomotor tasks in humans. II. Patients with bilateral peripheral vestibular deficits.' *Experimental Brain Research*, **85**, 208–217.

Ripoll, H., Bard, C., Paillard, J. (1986) 'Stabilisation of head and eye on target as a factor in successful basketball shooting.' *Human Movement Science*, **5**, 47–58.

Rönnqvist, L. (1995) 'A critical examination of the Moro response in newborn infants—symmetry, state relation, underlying mechanisms.' *Neuropsychologia*, **33**, 713–726.

Rösblad, B., von Hofsten, C. (1992) 'Perceptual control of manual pointing in children with motor impairments.' *Physiotherapy, Theory and Practice*, **8**, 223–233.

Sacks, O. (1984) *A Leg to Stand On*. London: Pan.

Sugden, D., Utley, A. (1995) 'Interlimb coupling in children with hemiplegic cerebral palsy.' *Developmental Medicine and Child Neurology*, **37**, 293–309.

Touwen, B. (1976) *Neurological Development in Infancy. Clinics in Developmental Medicine No. 58*. London: Spastics International Medical Publications.

284

Turnbull, J.D. (1993) 'Early intervention for children with or at risk of cerebral palsy.' *American Journal of Diseases of Children*, **147**, 54–59.

Ungerleider, L.G., Mishkin, M. (1982) 'Two cortical visual systems.' *In:* Ingle, D.J., Goodale, M.A., Mansfield, R.J.W. (Eds.) *The Analysis of Visual Behaviour.* Cambridge: MIT Press, pp. 549–586.

van der Meer, A.L.H., van der Weel, F.R., Lee, D.N. (1994) 'Prospective control in catching by infants.' *Perception*, **23**, 287–302.

—— —— —— (1995a) 'The functional significance of arm movements in neonates.' *Science*, **267**, 693–695.

—— —— —— Laing, I.A., Lin, J-P. (1995b) 'Development of prospective control of catching moving objects in preterm at-risk infants.' *Developmental Medicine and Child Neurology*, **37**, 145–158.

van der Weel, F.R., van der Meer, A.L.H., Lee, D.N. (1991) 'Effect of task on movement control in cerebral palsy: implications for assessment and therapy.' *Developmental Medicine and Child Neurology*, **33**, 419–426.

—— —— —— (1996) 'Measuring dysfunction of basic movement control in cerebral palsy.' *Human Movement Science*, **15**, 253–283.

van Wijck, F. (1995) 'Watching your step: co-ordinating gaze and foot movements.' Dissertation, Edinburgh University, Department of Psychology.

von Hofsten, C. (1980) 'Predictive reaching for moving objects by human infants.' *Journal of Experimental Child Psychology*, **30**, 369–382.

—— (1982) 'Eye–hand co-ordination in newborns.' *Developmental Psychology*, **18**, 450–461.

—— (1983) 'Catching skills in infancy.' *Journal of Experimental Psychology: Human Perception and Performance*, **9**, 75–85.

—— Fazel-Zandy, S. (1984) 'Development of visually guided hand orientation in reaching.' *Journal of Experimental Child Psychology*, **38**, 208–219.

—— Rönnqvist, L. (1988) 'Preparation for grasping an object: a developmental study.' *Journal of Experimental Psychology: Human Perception and Performance*, **14**, 610–621.

—— Rosander, K. (1996) 'The development of gaze control and predictive tracking in young infants.' *Vision Research*, **36**, 81–96.

—— Vishton, P., Spelke, E.S., Rosander, K., Feng, Q. (1993) 'Principles of predictive action in 6-month-old infants.' *Paper presented at Psychonomics, Washington, DC, November 1993.*

Wann, J.P. (1991) 'The integrity of visual-proprioceptive mapping in cerebral palsy.' *Neuropsychologia*, **29**, 1095–1106.

14
VARIABILITY AND STABILITY IN THE DEVELOPMENT OF SKILLED ACTIONS

Edison de J. Manoel and Kevin J. Connolly

Our everyday behaviour consists largely of a wide range of skilled actions through which we operate on our environment to achieve a variety of goals. For example, we reach for and grasp objects such as cups and glasses; we manipulate tools like pens and cutlery; we move from location to location, and, of course, we engage in social acts such as talking, smiling and shaking hands. Our concern in this chapter is with how actions of this kind develop and how they are maintained and controlled.

Following the early and influential work of Gesell (1929, 1946), the prevailing theoretical framework for the study of motor development was the maturation hypothesis. Motor development was thought to be a consequence of unfolding structures in the nervous system, though McGraw (1945, 1946) recognized that the structure–function relationship could well be bidirectional. The process of maturation was judged to be essentially internally driven and was described by Gesell (1945, 1946) in a series of principles. After a period of vigorous activity the study of motor development lost momentum, in part because of the success of the early investigators in answering the questions of the day which were largely concerned with identifying the typical patterns of change.

Subsequently, the appearance of new ideas and theories such as cybernetics and information theory provided a framework within which the complexity of skilled action could be more satisfactorily considered (Craik 1947, 1948; Bartlett 1958; Welford 1958). This provided the background for what has become known as the information processing approach, which has exerted a great influence on the cognitive psychology of the second half of the 20th century. Although this approach did not emerge in response to questions about motor development, it came to dominate the direction of work in the 1960s and '70s. Basically, individuals, including children, were considered as systems that processed information. Various stages of processing were distinguished in which information is coded, transformed, decoded, stored, etc. The capacity to process information, as well as the strategies employed to do so, were the subject of study in individuals at different ages (*e.g.* Connolly 1970b, Thomas 1980). The control of movements was also treated from the point of view of information processing in which modes of control—open-loop, closed-loop and mixed control—were identified in children of different ages (Sugden 1980; McCracken 1983; Hay 1984, 1990; Kerr 1985). In more general terms the information processing approach regarded motor development as the building up of cognitive structures (subroutines, motor programmes, schema and so forth) which directed the organization and production of movement patterns of growing complexity. In contrast to the maturational hypothesis, the information processing approach put greater emphasis on the interaction of the individual with the environment and the significance of this interaction for the development of skilled action in children (Connolly 1970a, Kay 1970).

In spite of the progress which has been made we are still struggling with fundamental questions concerning the nature of skill development. More recently the emergence of a new framework, the dynamic systems approach (see Chapter 15) which is based on the work of Bernstein (1967) and Gibson (1966, 1979), has led to a radical change in the way in which the organization of skilled action is conceptualized. The formation of movement patterns is seen as a result of a self-organizing process among elements of the system. These elements include not only the central nervous system but also the peripheral nervous system, muscles, joints and limb systems as well as external forces (*e.g.* gravity) and perceptual information (*e.g.* optical flow). In this approach there is an emphasis on the description of changes in the physical dynamics and other elements of the action system that will interact in a nonlinear way leading to qualitative changes and hence changes in developmental status (Thelen 1986).

Though at present the dynamic systems approach is centre stage its importance and potential are the subject of debate (Aslin 1993). In applying the dynamic systems approach to the study of development we must avoid the basic mistake made with the information processing approach. Here the question of how cognitive processes emerge and develop became transformed into the issue of whether children at different ages could be shown to possess specific cognitive processes which could be activated in different situations (Valsiner 1992).

The information processing approach has its basis in concepts such as symbols and representation which organize the perceptions and actions of organisms. The dynamic systems approach, on the other hand, eschews representation altogether and is concerned with the dynamics of generating movement patterns in a self-organizing manner. Thus, how each of these approaches explains order in skilled actions is controversial (see Meijer and Roth 1988) and goes back to the philosophical roots of each. The nature of this controversy characterizes what Kuhn (1970) would call a crisis in the current scientific thinking regarding skilled actions (cf. Abernethy and Sparrow 1992). In such circumstances, it is necessary to reappraise the alternative paradigms and to reconsider the fundamental issue: what is the nature of motor skill development? Our primary purpose is to discuss some aspects of these issues and offer a perspective for the investigation of the development of skilled actions.

In particular, we are interested in variability and stability as features of the development of skilled actions. Among individuals of the same species the pattern of developmental change is similar. However, there is significant variation in the precise process by which individuals achieve the same developmental outcomes (Connolly 1986). The behaviour acquired is stable in the sense that an individual can perform the same action even though the context is changed. This means that the behaviour which comprises the action is variable, while the goal or purpose is constant. The behaviour itself has certain general features that are invariant from one attempt to another. Other features are driven by the environment and are never the same from one occurrence to another. Variability of this kind is necessary; it is functional because it enables the individual to adapt to continuously changing circumstances. Variability cannot simply be regarded as a nuisance which limits the organism. Its source and nature are important because variability is essential for development to take place. In what follows we shall attempt an explanation of skill development which takes proper account of this.

Skilled actions and development

Individuals interact with their environment primarily through skilled actions. It is through skilled actions that they overcome the many variable requirements imposed by the environment and it is a consequence of skilled action that they are able to modify and control it in some respects and to some degree. Understanding how skilled motor actions are organized is thus a general and important matter.

Skilled actions are goal-directed and the performer exhibits great flexibility in order to reach a particular goal. To act in the environment it is necessary to move, and the production of movements is associated with various action systems: posture, locomotion, manipulation, nonverbal communication, speech, etc. (Reed 1982, Rosenbaum 1991). An important feature of skilled actions is that although movements are necessary for their realization they are not of themselves sufficient explanation for the action (Connolly 1975, Newell 1978). Different means can be deployed to achieve the specified end, and the same means can also be used to realize different ends (Bruner and Bruner 1968, Elliott and Connolly 1974). Furthermore, a skilled individual can also produce movement patterns that are unique to a given occasion (Turvey 1977, Glencross 1980). A fundamental feature of skilled action is the intention to achieve a particular goal. The intention is translated into behaviour by an action programme, that is a programme of events directed at achieving the goal. How detailed such a programme is and whether it is necessary for the patterning and ordering of movements is the subject of controversy between the information processing and dynamic systems approaches.

Once an individual becomes skilled, her actions show stability. In the face of any perturbation, behaviour is changed in order to permit the realization of the goal. To understand this stability it is important to consider two features of actions, namely motor equivalence and motor constancy (Berkinblit *et al.* 1986). Motor equivalence refers to spontaneous variations between means and ends in an action. Motor constancy refers to the ability to make adjustments in movement patterns to accommodate environmental variations and demands. Motor equivalence and constancy are products of a process in which the system becomes stable. In this process the pattern of interaction among the system's components becomes well defined and a given action is established. In the study of how skilled actions are stabilized it has become customary to emphasize invariance (*e.g.* Schmidt 1985). However, stability is a dynamic state which is maintained by changes. Which components of an action are varied and how they are varied also merits careful attention.

There are many problems involved in organizing a highly complex dynamic system of the kind exemplified by a young child. Two problems that have frequently been emphasized in the literature are those of controlling degrees of freedom and context conditioned variability (Bernstein 1967, Turvey *et al.* 1978). The system has many degrees of freedom (anatomical, neural and energetic) that have to be controlled and this represents an enormous task for a single controller to perform. Furthermore, there is no isomorphic mapping between the neural and the muscular systems. This is complicated even further by variations in the physical interaction between the muscular system and the environment. The puzzle that remains is how motor equivalence and constancy are achieved in the action, bearing in mind the number of degrees of freedom to be controlled and the nonlinearity between neural and motor systems.

The concept of development also has implications that must be taken into account. Development implies changes which involve the orderly appearance of new structures and processes. Implicit is the idea of emergence, that is to say there exists a nonlinear relationship between past and present states in the individual. There are various factors acting on behaviour as it changes over time which make development a very complex process. Neurological maturation and biomechanical changes accompanying growth imply hardware changes affecting performance (Connolly 1970a), or even acting as leading promoters of change as shown by Thelen (1986) in her studies of the emergence of locomotion. Similarly, cognitive changes involving more complex action programmes are changes of a software kind (Connolly 1970a). How these two kinds of change interact is a problem that goes back to the issue of how structure and function are related in biological systems. To draw a line between these two levels is difficult; furthermore, there is no necessary dominance of one over the other (Connolly and Manoel 1991). These factors act also in different time scales and come from different sources. Traditionally, distinctions have been made by attributing changes to innate patterns or to acquired, *i.e.* learned, patterns. Innate patterns were considered to be a consequence of the evolutionary history of the species and they constituted the main focus of studies of motor development. Learned patterns on the other hand were considered to be a function of experience and culture and were the subject of study in the domain of motor learning. This dichotomy gave rise to misconceptions about how skilled actions develop (Connolly 1981). On the one hand, innate behaviour was thought to be fixed and genetically determined, while on the other, learned behaviour was assumed to be acquired by an organism without a history and subject to no constraints. Recently, there have been attempts to go beyond such a dichotomy because of the misleading simplicity entailed in attributing causal roles in the emergence of behaviour to either maturation or external stimulation. Behaviour patterns are assumed to emerge from an organism–environment coaction (Oyama 1985, Gottlieb 1992).

How processes with such different timescales as evolution, development and learning relate to and influence each other is an issue which is yet to be properly addressed in the study of motor behaviour. Nevertheless, motor development can be considered a process of acquiring skilled actions over an individual's lifetime. In this process, stability is temporary, and as such, it must be considered in dynamic terms. This dynamic feature also leads to an apparent paradox which is the occurrence at the same time of marked similarities and marked variations between individuals.

The relativity of stability in the development of skilled actions

The issue of stability and its role in development is a point of contention among developmentalists (*e.g.* Piaget 1960, von Bertalanffy 1960). Considering both skilled actions and their development it is clear that process (development) and product (the skilled action itself)

289

share an important property, namely nonlinearity. In the organization of a skill and in the process by which this organization changes over time, the whole is more than the sum of the parts. Put another way, it is not a trivial matter to infer the properties of the whole from a knowledge of the properties of the parts and the laws governing their interaction (Simon 1981). Both skilled actions and their development are governed by the basic properties of open systems (von Bertalanffy 1952). Open systems are constantly engaged in transactions with the environment and movements are of central importance to this. The dynamics of the process mean that skilled actions reflect a flux of changes which vary in their timescale. For instance, motor skills show changes on a short timescale which are essential in order for an individual to adjust to quite minor environmental variations. Movements have to be modified continually because the spatio-temporal configuration of the individual with respect to salient features in the environment continually varies—for example, the changing position of the hand and arm as they move across a sheet of paper in writing. Thus, there are transient changes in the way in which actions are organized. Skilled actions also show long-term changes in their pattern of organization. These changes are usually called development; they are more permanent and they are characterized by an increase in the diversity and complexity of behaviour. The main characteristic of open systems is the spontaneous shifts they make toward more complex states of organization (von Bertalanffy 1952). These shifts imply that development is a process leading to nonequilibrium states rather than simply states characterized by greater stability (von Bertalanffy 1960). Stability is but a temporary state in a course marked by changes and transitions. Development implies novelty and complexity, which in turn lead the system to more unstable, uncertain and improbable states.

The application of control theories to investigate developing systems has many pitfalls. Specifically, control theories are concerned with how structures may be stabilized and maintained. To this end, control relies heavily on negative feedback. Any perturbation is counteracted by processes whose function is to return and maintain the system in a given state. In biological and social systems, though, negative feedback is only one of the means of control. There is also positive feedback, when the system searches for new states after it has been perturbed. This will lead to the destabilization of the system, but in combination with negative feedback new patterns may emerge; that is to say, development takes place (Maruyama 1963, 1982; Milsum 1968; Jantsch 1980).

The emphasis on negative feedback has been a major characteristic of theories of skill acquisition—e.g. Adams's (1971) closed-loop theory and Schmidt's (1975) schema theory. In theories of this kind the interest is largely on how the performance becomes stable, whereas how the stable structure, once acquired, is modified and reorganized into a new one has been of little concern (Choshi and Tani 1983). This is a fundamental problem if a closer link between motor learning and motor development studies is to be achieved. As Connolly and Bruner (1974) pointed out, the essential feature of competence in skilled action is the continuous reorganization and recombination of action programmes to meet new and often more complex requirements. Hence motor skill acquisition is best conceptualized as a continuous process, with change as its main feature.

A further consequence of the emphasis on negative feedback and stability led to certain basic aspects of biological regulation, which are reflected in the dynamic interactions within a system, being overlooked. The components of a system maintain their capacity to regulate as demonstrated by their equipotentiality, called by von Bertalanffy (1952) 'primary regulation'. Another important set of regulations are the so-called 'secondary regulations'. The progressive differentiation of components leads to the more fixed structures loosing their power for regulation, or having it reduced (low equipotentiality). These regulations are based on structural arrangements of the kind central to cybernetics, that is, negative feedback. Secondary regulations have an important role in maintaining homeostasis in physiological systems. Yet, as far as development is concerned primary regulations appear to be the principal factor giving rise to the increasing complexity of skilled actions.

In order to fully appreciate how such primary regulations can act it is necessary to consider the temporal dimension of open systems. According to the second law of thermodynamics, order should decrease and entropy increase. However, open systems constitute an exception to this law. They are characterized by states which are far from equilibrium, and hence they often shift towards higher order states. Prigogine (1961) established a distinction between states that is fundamental for the understanding of dynamic regulations in open systems. Some systems show stationary states which are characterized by the stability of parameters in the pattern of interaction between components within the system. Prigogine considered these systems to have time-independent states because with the passage of time there is no change in order, *i.e.* in entropy. However, there are other systems that show steady states. These systems are in a time-dependent state because there are changes in their components; entropy as well as order can increase or decrease. Systems showing steady states are marked by fluctuations in their components, which makes stability an artefact arising from our tendency to measure the system's product rather than its process. These fluctuations can reach levels that lead to a breakdown of the system's structure and hence the generation of spontaneous shifts towards new states of organization.

Goal-directed systems present steady states in which stability is relative. A system is stable with respect to achieving a particular goal which is part of its past experiences and this implies that the system is in a time-independent state. However, the same system is unstable with respect to achieving goals that are possible consequences of future experiences. The acquisition of new action programmes is possible because the individual is in a time-dependent state. This will lead to the continuous reorganization of simpler programmes into new and more complex ones. The relativity of steady states is a condition for the spontaneous shifts toward more organized complexity (von Bertalanffy 1952, Prigogine and Stengers 1984).

The internal fluctuations which generate entropy guarantee that the system's behaviour is guided not only to immediate goals but also to possible future ones. The system is then in a dual state which entails stability as well as instability. The system is not static over time, but rather fluctuates within certain limits. Random behaviour, noise, variation and inconsistency are all features that can be related to the process of increasing fluctuations, thereby leading to new levels of organization (Maruyama 1963, 1982; Klingsporn 1973; Conrad 1983; Prigogine and Stengers 1984; Yates 1984). The problem with the cybernetic or negative feedback model is that only the stable side of a system's state is emphasized, thus noise, randomness, variation and so on come to be regarded as factors which must be eliminated. In one sense, skilled motor actions are such dynamic open systems. They provide the means by which organisms interact with their environment. This interaction may be characterized by the goals an organism chooses. If the means available to an individual at a given time (her behavioural repertoire) are not appropriate, a succession of changes takes place as the individual goes through a series of transitions characteristic of the shift from an immature to a mature state. For example, an infant of 12 months who is taking her first steps in independent upright locomotion typically shows a much more unstable performance than she will two years later. As a consequence of the transitions that have occurred the 3-year-old child shows a more refined walking pattern that can be described as mature compared with her early efforts. A similar example is provided by an adult who is not familiar with a particular motor task and does not know a satisfactory method of achieving the relevant goal. In this case, the novice will go through a series of transitions marking the passage to becoming a skilled operator.

Studies of motor development have described these transitions as a succession of events from a state of low organization or relatively great disorder to a state of higher organization or greater order and stability (*e.g.* Kugler 1986). In a broad sense, the mature individual is able to master the many degrees of freedom in her motor system (Bernstein 1967). In relation to short timescale changes these transitions are described as phases or stages of learning. For example, Fitts and Posner (1967) suggested three phases: the cognitive, the associative and the autonomous. In the cognitive phase the learner must come to understand the goal and find a method of reaching it. In the associative phase the learner reduces response errors by improving the selection and execution of the action programme. Augmented feedback from an external source is essential during this stage. Finally, in the autonomous phase the performer is able to monitor her own responses and augmented feedback is no longer needed. There is a shift in the attentional demand from components of the programme to the programme as a whole and to the environment in which the action is performed. This permits great stability in execution because errors are corrected quickly, and quite often they are even anticipated (Schmidt 1988a). Another interpretation of this process, more in line with Bernstein's ideas, is offered by Vereijken *et al.* (1992b) who found evidence for the three stages of learning proposed by Bernstein (1967). They investigated the acquisition of a cyclical skill (ski slalom) and showed that individuals went through the following stages: (i) constraining degrees of freedom, (ii) relaxing constraints on degrees of freedom, and (iii) exploiting active and passive forces (gravity, inertial forces) in improving performance. In both cases these three stages entail the formation of a self-regulating process. As Adams (1971) pointed out, the individual will acquire a frame of reference, that is a perceptual trace, that will act as a comparator for commands issued in the programme, desired outcomes, and actual results. Once the perceptual trace is formed, the performer can monitor her own responses using negative feedback to reach and maintain a desired state.

The main feature of this conception is the gradual decrease of entropy so that the system becomes stable. However, taking Prigogine's notion of steady state, skill would be in a time-dependent state and thus marked by stability as well as instability (Fig. 14.1). Indeed, once a goal is achieved, *e.g.* being able to walk or reaching the autonomous stage in a particular task, the configuration of the organism–environment interaction changes. The environmental context may also change as well as the consequences of an action. In one

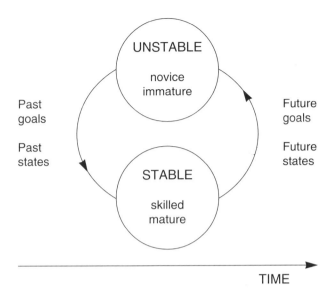

Fig. 14.1. The relativity of steady states in skilled action.

sense, there is a hierarchy of environments and goals (Koestler 1967, Sommerhoff 1974, Tani 1987) in which as one goal is reached, other possible ones can be tried, or a skill having been performed in one context, other broader contexts arise. Elliott and Connolly (1974) distinguished two main elements in the organization of manipulative hand movements. The first set they called anatomical subroutines, which should be viewed more as hardware factors exerting influences on motor responses. In the case of manipulative hand movements they can be seen as postures in which behaviour is definable in anatomical terms, like pronation of the hand. These postures afford certain hand movements. For instance, grasping a pen using the distal phalanges of the index finger and thumb and supporting it on the lateral surface of the second finger (an adult tripod grip) allows movements of the pen quite different from those which are possible when the pen is held between the ventral surfaces of the fingers and the palm. The second set they called operational subroutines, which are definable in relation to a particular effect in the environment. *e.g.* opening a door or hitting a ball.

The anatomical constraints ease the demands on the programme in terms of the specification of details about how the object will be grasped. On the other hand, the effects which movements can cause in the environment need to be understood and incorporated into the programme. Once a child has mastered the use of a particular subroutine to produce a given environmental outcome, it can be used in attaining other goals in different contexts. It will define new operational subroutines for which control may not be stable—for example, a young child might adopt a digital grip that permits different patterns of digit movement, but the control over these movements is still rudimentary. Under these circumstances, an individual will become a novice again. Time, as Prigogine pointed out (Prigogine 1978, Prigogine and Stengers 1984), is a fundamental element in this process. Stability, in a sense, refers to past events, hence the internal models regulating the actions are a reflection of the organism's history. Instability which refers to future events means that internal models must change as time passes. As in the case of walking, the 3-year-old's performance reflects a more mature state than the same behaviour in the same infant 18 months earlier. Still, in relation to future and possible contexts, *e.g.* walking on different surfaces, at different speeds, and while doing other things, the child's behaviour is immature. The relative state of a skill in time means that the stability–instability duality implies constant fluctuations or variability in behaviour which can lead to the emergence of a new pattern (Prigogine and Stengers 1984). The significance of this duality for the experimental investigation of skilled action (Kelso 1992) and, in particular, its development, is only now being appreciated (Thelen 1989, Thelen *et al.* 1992, Zanone *et al.* 1993).

The stability–instability duality is important in relation to a fundamental problem in motor skill development, that of understanding how the transitions from simpler patterns to more complex ones take place. In motor skill development such transitions are not only about the refinement of an action programme, but mostly about the integration of existing programmes into more complex ones. This is a difficult matter to investigate experimentally since it assumes that we can identify in some objective fashion action programmes and their components, components which were once simple programmes in their own right. In order to do this a taxonomy dealing with the natural history of skilled actions is needed but such a taxonomy is not yet available.

Hierarchy and complementarity in motor skill development
In the study of the development of skilled actions at least two fundamental changes must be considered, those involving increases in the diversity and in the complexity of motor behaviour (Connolly 1986, Tani *et al.* 1988). Motor behaviour gradually becomes more differentiated, *e.g.* walking starts to be varied in terms of speed, form, direction, and so on. This leads to an increase in the individual's repertoire, that is to increased diversity. New behaviours and new properties build on earlier changes leading to the formation of integrated hierarchies which provide increasing complexity. For instance, running and jumping can be combined in a single programme for the long jump. One important issue is to understand these processes, the increase in diversity followed by, or coupled with, an increase in the complexity of the individual's behavioural repertoire. A further challenge is to investigate the extent to which these two processes interact in development. Indeed, one of the questions raised by the study of motor development is how a child changes from a state characterized by a very limited repertoire of actions to a subsequent state in which actions can be performed in various ways. The means–end relationships become flexible, and diversity in skilled action increases, giving rise to motor equivalence and to constancy in motor behaviour (Glencross 1980, Keogh and Sugden 1985, Connolly and Dalgleish 1989).

Over the past 30 years these problems have been considered by a number of authors. The issue of diversity was addressed by assuming the existence of a generalized motor programme which could be instantiated by a schema to fit different situations for a given class of movements (Schmidt 1975, Shapiro and Schmidt 1982). A different approach was employed by Turvey and his colleagues who argued that the matter was not dealt with by a central programme but by the assembly of simpler elements into synergies or coordinative structures (Turvey 1977, Turvey *et al.* 1978). Following the intention to achieve a particular goal, action is geared to the environment, and consequently the assembly of components will result in unique patterns fitted to each occasion. The pattern of acquisition proposed by each of these approaches is concerned primarily with the achievement of stability. In the schema theory the process is marked by a refinement of the generalized motor programme and the strengthening of schema to instantiate it (van Rossum 1987). In the coordinative structure model, the individual changes from a state where degrees of freedom are frozen to a subsequent state in which constraints on them are relaxed and the performer becomes able to exploit active and passive forces to optimize performance and apply it to different situations (Bernstein 1967; Turvey *et al.* 1982; Vereijken *et al.* 1992a,b; Woollacott and Sveistrup 1992).

From a developmental point of view a fundamental problem is how a child who is able to perform a number of simple actions becomes able to integrate these simpler actions into new and more complex patterns. The problem of how complexity is brought about has so far attracted comparatively little attention. Its importance lies in the fact that development refers to the appearance of new and more complex structures from earlier and simpler ones. One line of investigation was established by the proposition that skills are modular (Bruner 1970, 1973; Connolly 1970a, 1973). Basically, the idea is that there exists a process called modularization whereby a simple action programme gradually with use becomes more consistent and predictable. When this reaches a certain level the action can be decontextualized—that is to say it is no longer tied to a specific context but can be performed in other contexts and deployed as a component of other larger and more complex action programmes. To accomplish this process, Bruner (1970) argued that it was first necessary to reduce the degrees of freedom in the system being regulated. This is then followed by the consolidation and mastery of these degrees of freedom. This process, whereby an act becomes more automatic, is characterized by a decrease in variability and a more predictable spatiotemporal patterning. Connolly (1973) suggested that with modularization there is also the formation of rules of transformation whereby skill constituents or subroutines are combined into different and more complex programmes. Elliott and Connolly (1974) argued that the subroutine was a basic unit in the development of a hierarchical structure.

Two problems arise with the idea proposed by Bruner and Connolly. First, it is assumed that the stability of units will lead to reorganization, but how this change is accomplished is not specified. Stabilization alone is unlikely to promote hierarchical restructuring. There must be important modifications to the structure of a subroutine before it can become part of a new act. Second, the emphasis on the stability of the subroutine plays down the role of fluctuations in the structure of the action programme. These fluctuations are essential for the organization and reorganization of skilled actions. The stability–instability duality which characterizes skilled actions was not considered in the theory, making it inadequate to explain development and particularly to deal with some anomalous results produced by experiments designed to test the modularization hypothesis (Moss and Hogg 1983).

A radically different line of enquiry is that originating from Haken's (1983) synergetics where skilled action is defined by order or collective variables resulting from the interaction of a number of elements, many of which are nonspecific to the action system (Thelen 1989). The elements change at different rates and some of these changes, the so called rate-limiting or control parameters, cause radical shifts in the interaction of elements and hence generate an emergent and new mode of behaviour. In these circumstances the system is said to undergo a phase transition which is characterized by the emergence of new properties, *i.e.* new actions emerge.

The dynamic systems approach (see Chapter 15), in particular, puts great emphasis on the role of exploration in the promotion of transitions in skilled actions (Thelen 1990, Vereijken and Whiting 1990, Thelen *et al.* 1992). Development is seen as a process of exploring the dynamics of action which leads to the discovery of regions of stability (Warren 1990). This process has been called *exploration search strategies* corresponding to the continual exploration of body and task spaces (Newell *et al.* 1989a, Newell 1991, Newell and McDonald 1992). The role of exploration is advocated in the idea of neuronal group selection (Edelman 1987). Exploration is vital for the selection of neural networks that will in turn guide behaviour in the discovery of optimal motor solutions to problems presented in the environment (Sporns and Edelman 1993). From a developmental point of view, an important question is where the capacity to explore the environment comes from. Furthermore, there is a need for some criteria by which to judge what should be selected and what should not. An answer to the first problem has been offered on the grounds that the infant is already equipped with a rich repertoire of movement patterns that goes back to the prenatal period (Prechtl 1986; see Chapter 2). There is indeed a continuity between fetal movement patterns and those of newborn infants (Prechtl 1984). Dynamic patterns have also been found to be similar in the case of spontaneous movements and goal-directed behaviour (Thelen 1979). In relation to the second problem, it is assumed that there are evolutionary constraints that provide the system with a set of values against which movement outcomes can be judged (Edelman 1987). However, the change in complexity which is reflected in the appearance of skilled actions requires an explanation in terms of which structure or control element was acquired to permit such a pattern of complexity. Although invariances found between the intrinsic dynamics of spontaneous and instrumental behaviour are important in clarifying the organization of motor behaviour they do not explain development, which is about change, transition and adaptation. In this sense, an important theoretical consideration is how the notion of exploration search strategy is linked with the idea of stability–instability–stability proposed by Kelso and his colleagues (Kelso 1990, Schoner *et al.* 1992, Zanone and Kelso 1992). The emergence, breakdown and reorganization of structures characterize a basic process by which complexity increases in skilled action. Neuronal group selection might act in this process by shaping and forming networks according to a particular set of constraints which follow the emergence of a structure. Thus a more fundamental process is due to the dynamic interaction of the system's components, *i.e.* adaptation and self-organization. Attention has been drawn to this view in regard to evolution theory with its emphasis on the role of natural selection (von Bertalanffy 1969, Waddington 1969, Kauffman 1991).

The impression that emerges from this brief consideration of theories of motor skill development is one of fragmentation, with different frameworks dealing with different aspects of the phenomenon of development. Thelen and colleagues have tried to deal with the gaps by incorporating aspects of the synergetic approach with features of a neural theory based on Edelman's propositions (Thelen and Ulrich 1991, Thelen *et al.* 1993). However, the rejection of the notion of representation and its role in the organization of action presents difficulties with respect to extending the theoretical model into a more robust theory of motor skill development (for example, see criticisms by Pew 1984, Requin *et al.* 1984, Pew and Rosenbaum 1988, Schmidt 1988b, Rosenbaum 1991, Shaffer 1992). The investigation of very young infants introduces the prospect of dealing with a number of prestructured patterns (*e.g.* Prechtl 1986) characterized by Edelman (1987) as a primary repertoire of behaviour, or by Kelso (1990) as intrinsic dynamics. Thus, it is quite logical to explain the early organization of behaviour on the basis of an exploration of the intrinsic dynamics. However, further development implies changes in the intrinsic dynamics. In that sense what constraints act upon later in the exploration is less clear. Assuming movement coordination to be determined solely by a self-organizing process begs the question about what it is that guarantees that a particular goal will be reliably attained (see also Aslin 1993). Freedom of interaction among constituent elements is a necessary but not a sufficient condition for organization (Weiss 1967).

The principal problem may be the neglect of a basic systems principle, that of hierarchical order. This principle highlights the multilevel organization in which a system branches into subsystems which, in turn, branch into subsystems of a lower order (Koestler 1969). The unities might be independent or they may originate from the same unity as is most common in the biological realm (von Bertalanffy 1969). There are many kinds of hierarchies (Scholz 1982, Zylstra 1992). Control hierarchies (von Bertalanffy 1952, 1968; Koestler 1967, 1969; Weiss 1969, 1971) are particularly interesting in connection with motor skill development. A basic feature of this kind of hierarchy is the balance which exists between autonomy and constraint in all levels of the hierarchy (Koestler 1967, Gatlin 1972, Salthe 1985). A control hierarchy restrains the degrees of freedom of the parts in a subordinate level. At the same time, paradoxically, constraints permit a greater level of freedom. As Allen and Starr (1982) point out, constraints give freedom from an infinite and unmanageable set of choices. They quote an example from the world of music: the fugue form has in its rules powerful constraints, but within them Bach was free to write any fugue he wanted to. In chess, too, there are very clear constraints on how each piece can be moved, but from these constraints the number of possible ways to conduct the game is extraordinarily large. In fact, the organization of living systems is possible because constraints function as boundary conditions for one level upon its subordinate levels (Pattee 1973, Allen and Starr 1982).

The evolution of a complex system always implies a hierarchical development leading to a two-level organization; at the higher level, the informational or symbolic mode, and at a lower level, the dynamic or energetic mode (Nicolis 1986). This is a very important notion because, in one sense, it suggests a flow of information up and down the hierarchy. In another sense, it indicates that the interface between levels is one of the major problems in understanding complexity. Most of the criticisms made of the use of the hierarchy concept refer to the authoritative character of the controller and the passive role of the controlled apparatus. Particularly in relation to motor control and development, this kind of criticism has been made in the dynamic systems approach. Several authors have argued that there is no need to invoke concepts of control, hierarchical levels or representation to explain the organization of motor behaviour, which can be solved by the structure of the motor apparatus itself (Kelso 1981, Kelso and Tuller 1984, Kugler and Turvey 1987, Thelen *et al.* 1987). However, Pattee (1972) argues that this view is a form of naive realism, because if concepts of hierarchical levels, function and constraint are seen only as a useful way of speaking about the underlying physics of phenomena, then there is no objective difference between living and non-living matter. In evolution, Pattee argues that an integrated set of rules or grammar gives physical structures their symbolic attributes.

The problem of complexity in biological systems cannot be solved solely by looking at the molecular level or solely by the application of non-equilibrium thermodynamics (Pattee 1973). This is because there is a hierarchical control operating between levels of organization. As Pattee points out, hierarchical control is a problem of the interface between levels. The organization of motor behaviour can be seen as based in the dynamic properties of the motor apparatus and the oscillatory properties of the nervous system (*e.g.* Kelso 1984, Kugler and Turvey 1987). However, the system must have a control element which assigns operations in the brain (Kohout 1976). This control may be seen as a hierarchy composed by unities acting with relative autonomy and integration (Koestler 1969).

The principle of hierarchical order leads to another principle important in understanding complex systems, namely that of complementarity. To express this simply one can say that there are multiple ways to describe systems events. In fact, a single description cannot capture the nature of complexity in living systems (Pattee 1977). The complementarity is most important in regard to two contradictory modes of description in biological systems, dynamic and symbolic. Pattee (1987) argues that an adequate description cannot be made solely in terms of rate-dependent factors, *i.e.* the system's dynamics, rather it must also include a rate-independent factor, *i.e.* information.

In the development of biological systems the dynamic interaction between elements leads to the emergence of constraints which in turn condition the elements into a collective behaviour (Pattee 1973). Thus, an authority relation of the upper level over the lower level is established. There are two ways in which coordinate sets of constraints can arise spontaneously from more or less chaotic beginnings (Pattee 1972). The first involves the assembly of elementary units into larger ones. Pattee calls this the formation of complexity from simplicity. The second involves chaotic aggregations of extreme complexity within which there arise persistent regularities, which condense out simple behaviour. Pattee calls this the formation of simplicity from complexity arguing that it is this second way of spontaneous organization that accounts for the origin of new hierarchical levels of control. Weiss (1967) points out a similar kind of change leading to the emergence and increase of complexity in open systems.

Two particular issues challenge researchers in the study of motor skill development. First, there is a need to consider the principle of complementarity to link and integrate what have been seen as rival and sometimes exclusive modes of description, the symbolic and the dynamic (Pattee 1977, 1982, 1987). Second, there is a question of hierarchical development in which information or the symbolic mode, harnesses and is harnessed by the dynamic

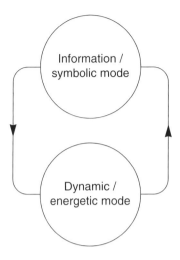

Fig. 14.2. Hierarchical development and complementarity.

or energetic mode (Weiss 1967, 1969; Pattee 1973, 1976, 1987; Nicolis 1986). In both cases, a new theoretical framework is necessary when the process of development is assumed to be a hierarchical one. Information is thus seen as an emergent property from dynamic or rate-dependent processes (Pattee 1977) and a complementarity is established between them, rather than a reduction of one mode to the other (Fig. 14.2).

Perspectives on the study of motor skill development
The issue of complementarity has been considered by Beek (1989). He investigated the acquisition of a juggling skill, and came to the conclusion that it could not be explained solely on the basis of autonomous, dynamic or rate-dependent processes. Beek and Beek (1988) proposed that apart from dynamic processes acting to produce movement patterns, there exists what they called external forcing which exerts a form of control on the system's intrinsic dynamics This external forcing can be seen as a form of programme or also as a result of the social interactions through which parents establish constraints on aspects of their infant's behaviour (Valsiner 1987). From this position a two-step research strategy was proposed. The first step involved analysing movements to identify the system's intrinsic dynamics (Zanone *et al.* 1993). The second step is to assume that what cannot be explained on the basis of intrinsic dynamics arises from external forcing. Thus, external forcing is defined in close relation to the system's own dynamics. Hopkins *et al.* (1993) advocate such a strategy in developmental research. They suggest that in the course of motor development autonomous processes can be progressively tuned to external forcing, *i.e.* to the symbolic mode. However, questions remain: for example, how does external forcing develop and what are its origins?

The problems of how dynamic and symbolic modes change and how they interact are major issues for a theory of motor skill development. Development is about change in the

299

state of the system. However, intrinsic dynamics are always seen as an invariant or stable feature of the system, and how it changes is a problem yet to be properly addressed.

Another important issue is intention. In the dynamic systems approach intention has been considered as one of the factors constraining the degrees of freedom. In this sense, intention is seen as a rate-independent process by Turvey (1990), while Thelen *et al.* (1993) see it as a rate-limiting factor in the emergence of voluntary reaching. Schoner and Kelso (1988) see intention as leading the system to achieve an environmental goal. In fact, intention is seen to create a competition between the system's intrinsic dynamics and the task dynamics that will result in the achievement of the specified goal. From a developmental perspective, an important question concerns what is formed in this competition between different dynamics. According to Bruner (1973) intention involves (i) anticipation of the outcome of an act, (ii) selection among appropriate means for achieving a particular end, and (iii) the sustained direction of behaviour during the development of means. It is also reflected neurophysiologically in the corollary discharge or efferent copy (Sperry 1950, von Holst 1954) or the image of achievement (Pribram 1971). This implies that intention is part of a process in which a programme is formed to direct the sequence of events toward achieving a goal (Connolly 1977). The process may also be a hierarchical one (Miller *et al.* 1960). Thus, one alternative to the proposition put forward by Hopkins *et al.* (1993) is to consider the action programme in a more dynamic way.

We propose that determinacy and indeterminacy, though opposites, can be considered complementary features of an action programme. This involves the application of Weiss's (1969) macro- and micro-determinacy notion in the organization of systems. From this point of view action programmes are considered as structures having two levels, the macroscopic and the microscopic (Fig. 14.3). At the macroscopic level, the programme is defined by an overall pattern related to the intention and to environmental outcomes. This pattern is invariant and well-defined. At the microscopic level, the movement pattern is ill-defined, and it can assume different forms because of the interactions between the components of the programme. Such a programme has flexible strategies (Koestler 1967) guided to accommodate particular arrangements in the environment. In writing the letter A, an individual will show a particular sequence of strokes that does not vary in its timing (Viviani and Terzuolo 1980). This reflects the macroscopic level of the programme. However, the time taken to write the letter, or its size, can vary without affecting the product. This corresponds to the microscopic level of the programme. Another example is provided by the routines performed by a gymnast. They may appear highly consistent in terms of the movement patterns, but the details of ballistic movements are varied from occasion to occasion. As Welford *et al.* (1969) demonstrated, ballistic movements have two phases: the first phase, distance-covering movements, tends to be quite consistent, but the second, homing phase is variable and ill-defined and this is what allows fine adjustments to be made.

Since skilled actions are structured at both the macroscopic and microscopic levels, they can be repeated over and over again without losing their identity, though the movements employed are different on each occasion. In one sense, the structure of skill shows determinacy at the macroscopic level, while simultaneously showing indeterminacy at the microscopic level (Weiss 1969). The macroscopic level imposes constraints on the micro-

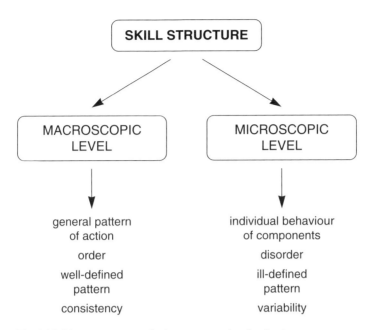

Fig. 14.3. Macro-structure and micro-structure levels of action programmes.

scopic level. This means that the macroscopic level broadly shapes or conditions rather than controls the microscopic level (Pattee 1973). At the microscopic level, the elements retain certain degrees of freedom which are fundamental for their reorganization into new patterns (Weiss 1967).

One hypothesis that stems from this view is that initially both the macroscopic and microscopic levels of an action programme will be marked by disorder. This disorder will be reflected by great variability in both the macrostructure and microstructure of the programme. The macrostructure then gradually becomes stable while variability remains in the microstructure. This variability in the microstructure is essential for the reorganization of the programme into a new and more complex one. The hypothesis was tested by Manoel and Connolly (1995) in an investigation of serial coincident timing in children. The performance of 9-year-old children was marked by stability at the macrostructure level indicated by consistency in the overall timing of the action. At the same time, variability was maintained at the microstructure level as indicated by variations in the absolute timing of the components. In contrast, 6-year-old children showed marked variability in both the macro- and microstructures of the action programme.

Macroscopic and microscopic levels of action programmes and the natural history of skilled actions

How the macroscopic and microscopic levels of action programmes are formed and reorganized into new and more complex programmes is fundamental to understanding skill development. Observations on the performance of simple manipulative skills in preschool children showed that the number of grip patterns used reduced as they got older (Connolly and Elliott 1972, Connolly 1973). This observation was interpreted as variability giving way to consistency as skill was acquired and appears to be at odds with the argument presented here. However, we now believe such an interpretation is incorrect. Certain grips permit the manipulation of an object within the hand by intrinsic movements, others do not (see Elliott and Connolly 1984). The use of grips which permit intrinsic movements in fact increases available variability; what we see developmentally is not a reduction in variability but a shift in its locus.

The flux of events which accompanies the emergence of the macroscopic and microscopic levels of an action programme has been described by Connolly and Dalgleish (1989, 1993). In their analysis of the development of a tool-using skill by infants, in this case the use of a spoon in feeding, they found a general trend in which there was evident differentiation between the components of the action. Four principal stages in the development of the skill were identified: (1) the appearance of simple repetitive actions with the spoon; (2) the outline construction of the action sequence, namely spoon-to-dish-to-mouth; (3) the incorporation of function, that is the transfer of food from dish to mouth; and (4) the incorporation of correction routines, which makes the action much more flexible. Variability in behaviour is seen from the outset but certain consistencies appear—for example, there is increased consistency in the hand used to grasp the spoon. However, what a detailed, fine-grained analysis reveals is that the locus of variability shifts and the means by which variability is maintained, and indeed much increased, also changes. For example, a small number of grip patterns come to be preferred and used most of the time. At first sight this appears to be a reduction in variability, but it is not, because the grip patterns which become preferentially used are those which permit manipulation of the spoon by intrinsic movements. These grips were classed as flexible and distinguished from rigid patterns which do not allow the spoon to be manipulated within the hand. As skill in using the tool is acquired the variability available to the infant is increased greatly in a number of ways. In fact, development serves to increase the degrees of freedom available to the infant as means for managing them become available.

The capacity to reach for and grasp objects is fundamentally important for man, the great apes and primates generally. The actions involve the properties of the motor apparatus and imply knowledge about the environment. Knowledge of the operations necessary to accomplish the task (such as positioning the body appropriately to approach the object, followed by a reach which brings the hand to an appropriate position and a grasp which is such that the object is held in a stable and secure way, appropriate to the individual's intention) is also entailed. A number of constraints can be identified in these activities. There are anatomical constraints such as the posture which the hand adopts. There are also task constraints linked to the object such as its size, shape and weight. These will interact in various ways, but a central consideration is the purpose, or the end to be achieved by the action. There is a relative independence between anatomy and function since the same anatomical configuration can serve different functional ends (Connolly and Elliott 1972, Elliott and Connolly 1974). Connolly (1973) found that preschool children changed their

MACRO-STRUCTURE

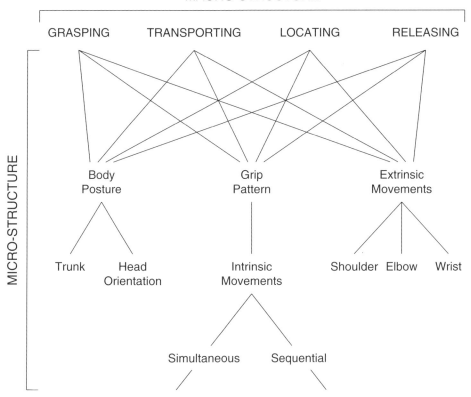

Fig. 14.4. The hierarchical organization of an action programme for inserting a rod into a hole.

grip on a rod as the diameter increased, in order to better achieve the goal of the task. It was argued that the nature of the grip pattern was determined by the functional properties of the hand and the demands imposed by the task. By changing the requirements imposed by a task we can investigate how grips are employed to achieve a given goal.

An action which young children commonly perform is to place one object inside another larger one. A toy which makes use of this predilection is the 'posting box', the lid of which has various shaped holes cut into it through which the child inserts appropriately shaped blocks. The action of inserting blocks through appropriately shaped holes can be analysed at its macro- and microstructure levels. At the level of the macrostructure the operations and their sequence is fixed, while at the microstructure level which components are used and how they are deployed is variable (Fig. 14.4). An important question, therefore, is what are the developmental features of the microstructure level of the action programme?

Important elements in the action programme relate to how the object is grasped, that is the configuration of the object and the hand, and how the object is manipulated to complete the task. This may involve movements of the digits, provided that the grip pattern employed

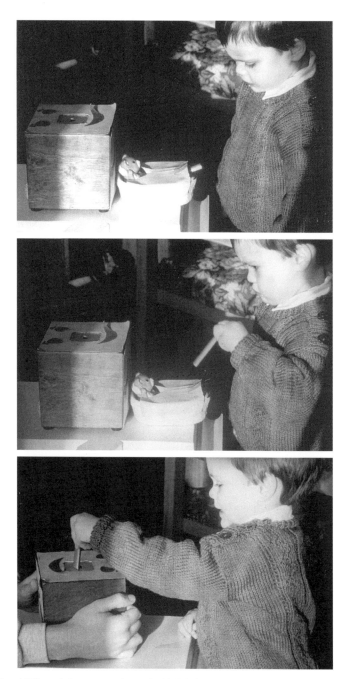

Fig. 14.5. The child's task is to grasp the rod which is just sticking out from the bottom of the teddy bear's bed *(top)* and then to transport the rod *(centre)* to the hole in the lid of the box and insert it there *(bottom)*. The rod sticks out approximately 1 cm from the 'bed' and must therefore be grasped by the fingertips.

is flexible (see Connolly and Elliott 1972, Connolly and Dalgleish 1989). Intrinsic movements are not possible when the object is held between flexed fingers and the palm of the hand. In this case the grip is rigid.

To explore the relationship between the macro- and microstructure of a skill we observed three groups of children performing a task which involved inserting a rod through a hole in the lid of a box. The task entailed (1) grasping and holding the rod in a stable configuration, (2) transporting the rod to the target hole, (3) locating the rod into the hole, and (4) releasing the rod once located (Fig. 14.5). The rod was approximately 5 cm long, about as thick as a pencil and made from aluminium. The hole in the box had the same cross-sectional shape as the rod but was slightly larger in order that the rod might readily be inserted. Rods of two different cross-sectional shapes, circular and semicircular, were used. The rod having the circular cross-section could be inserted in any orientation and this was therefore called the *low constraint* (LC) condition. To insert the rod with the semicircular cross-section required that it be quite precisely aligned with the semicircular hole otherwise insertion was impossible. This more difficult condition was called the *high constraint* (HC) condition. Three groups of children, with mean ages of 31, 48 and 63 months, were observed performing the task.

The children sat or stood before a small table on which the box was placed. They were asked to pick up the rod and place it in the box through the hole in the top. The observer demonstrated the task and invited the child to do it. The nature of the task was clear and no child showed any sign of failing to understand what was required. Each child was asked to perform the task first ten times in the LC condition then ten times in the HC condition. The children were videotaped performing the trials. The tape was subsequently viewed and the occurrence of a number of behaviour categories was recorded. These included the number (range) of different grips and intrinsic movements (movement of the object within the hand) and the proportion of flexible and rigid grips. These data were collected separately for the three phases of the task, Grasping, Approach and Location, which correspond to the task components (1), (2) and (3) above. As a measure of stability the number of times a grip was modified after the initial grasping phase was also noted.

Comparing the children's performance in the two conditions revealed a shift in the variable features of the programme's microstructure among the age groups. The older children showed more flexible grips and used more intrinsic movements. The 31 months group showed greater variation in grip patterns (Fig. 14.6) but these were predominantly rigid grips (Fig. 14.7). The two older groups used fewer grip patterns (Fig. 14.6) but they tended to be flexible. Consequently, older children tended to show more variation in the use of intrinsic movements (Fig. 14.8). From 31 to 48 to 63 months there appears to be a qualitative shift in the way macro- and microstructures are linked in the action programme. Grips tend to become more consistent, and variability becomes available via the increased degrees of freedom afforded by flexible grips and the use of different extrinsic movements, mostly simple and reciprocal synergies (see Elliott and Connolly 1984). The shift from the LC to the HC condition led to increases in variability in the two behaviour categories (grip configuration and intrinsic movements) in all three age groups. Evidence of group differences remained, however, because the young children showed more variation in grip patterns while the two older groups showed more variation in intrinsic movements.

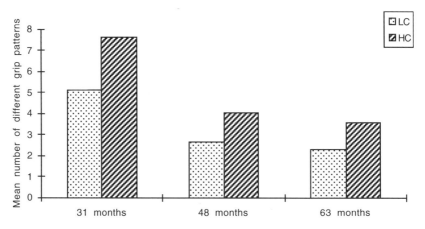

Fig. 14.6. Number of grips shown by three groups of children in low (LC) and high (HC) constraint conditions.

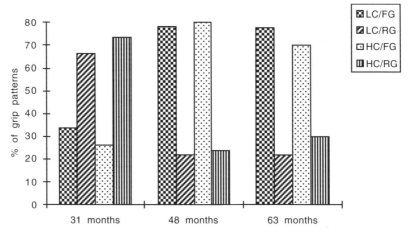

Fig. 14.7. Rigid (RG) and flexible (FG) grips used by the three groups of children in the low (LC) and high (HC) constraint conditions.

These results suggest that change in the microstructure is taking place as development proceeds. Their main feature is not an increase in consistency as the data on grips seems to suggest but principally a shift in the locus of variability following the use of flexible grips. Variability is not now seen in the range of grips so much as in the appearance of various forms of intrinsic movements.

As mentioned above, one view of development is that the organization of behaviour is due not only to an action programme but to the interplay of organismic, environmental and task constraints (Newell 1986). In this context we might ask whether the age differences

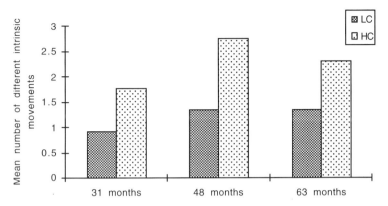

Fig. 14.8. Use of intrinsic movements in low (LC) and high (HC) constraint conditions by the three groups of children.

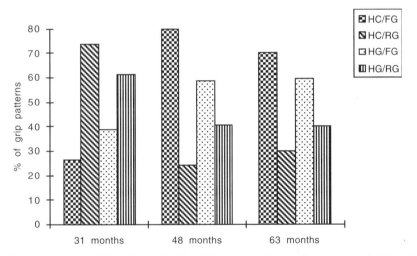

Fig. 14.9. Proportion of rigid (RG) and flexible (FG) grips used by the three groups of children in the high grasp (HG) and high constraint (HC) conditions.

observed in the ranges of grips and intrinsic movements are due only to the way macroscopic and microscopic levels of the programme are established. To examine this question, the same three groups of children were asked to repeat the HC condition and a variant where access to the rod was restricted in the grasping phase. This new condition was called *high grasping* (HG). The child was led to use the fingertips to grasp the rod, and hence encouraged to adopt a flexible grip (see Fig. 14.5). In these circumstances the younger group showed a relationship between grips and intrinsic movements similar to those shown by the older groups.

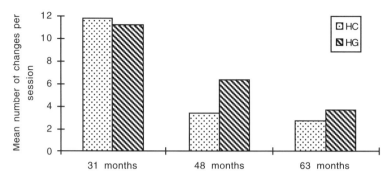

Fig. 14.10. Changes in grip pattern produced by the three groups of children in the high constraint (HC) and high grasp (HG) conditions.

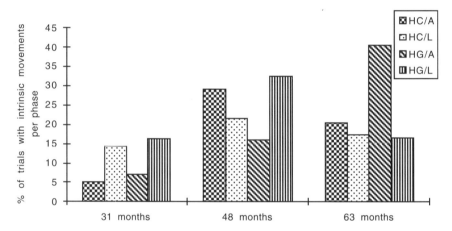

Fig. 14.11. Proportion of trials with intrinsic movements in the approach (A) and locating (L) phases in the high constraint (HC) and high grasp (HG) conditions for the three groups of children.

Looking at the proportion of rigid and flexible grips (Fig. 14.9) it is evident that the youngest group (31 months) show an increase in the use of flexible grips. However, the two older groups had a higher percentage of flexible grips in the HG condition. A question which comes to mind is whether the stability of behaviour is increased by this new task constraint. If this were so it would imply that the action programme is not the main determinant of the organization of an action. To examine this the number of changes in the grip patterns were noted in the HC and HG conditions. In spite of adopting more flexible grips, the 31 months group changed grip many times after the grasping phase in the HG condition (Fig. 14.10). The older groups also showed a slight increase in the frequency of grip changes, perhaps in an attempt to counteract the decrease in the use of flexible grips. Although the task constraint in the grasping phase led to more flexible grips, an increase in intrinsic movements was observed only for the two older groups, in particular the 48 months group in the location phase and the 63 months group in the approach phase (Fig. 14.11).

Thus there is evidence that task constraints can exert an influence on the programme's microstructure which leads to a change in the components of the action programme. However, when it comes to the actual operation of the programme the presence of a new or modified component can make the system more unstable. Task and anatomical constraints interacted and led to the use of more flexible grips in the youngest group but this did not improve their stability since fluctuations in grips were maintained at a level similar to those in the HC condition. Children in the two older groups responded by increasing their use of intrinsic movements in either the approach or location phase. The fluctuations generated in the HG condition may have affected the boundary conditions of the programme so that the children, particularly the two older groups, resorted to changing grips in the search for hand configurations which afforded greater stability. Intrinsic movements may play a central role in this search.

In recent years there has been a claim that children can demonstrate well-coordinated behaviour provided that their interaction with the task and the environment is properly arranged. These claims, stemming from the dynamic systems approach, have been used to dismiss the idea of programmes controlling behaviour (Newell *et al.* 1989b,c, 1993). In the task described here there was certainly an interaction between the object and the anatomical configuration of the hand but the problem is still with the degrees of freedom in the elaboration of the action programme. Being led to adopt a grip with more degrees of freedom (a flexible grip) seems to have resulted in increased instability. However, young children repeatedly showed a predominance of rigid grips even after four months of systematically repeating the HG condition (Manoel 1993). Our assumption is that this is a matter of hierarchical development and not simply perceiving affordances and having a good match between body scale and the object's physical properties.

In the study of development, it is necessary to consider the interplay between fluctuations and instabilities (Zanone *et al.* 1993). In our model, the relation between the macro- and microscopic levels is one in which the micro- is not controlled in a strict sense by the macro-, rather, the macroscopic level conditions the microscopic level (Weiss 1969). In hierarchical development, fluctuations in the microstructure are supposed to have an important role in breaking the existing stability and leading the system to search for a new order (Prigogine and Stengers 1984). To understand this process it is necessary to analyse how far the system's stability can be pushed. Thus, an important question is how environmental variations are matched by the variability of the action programme. To explore this question, we again asked the same children to repeat the HC condition but with the addition of a further modification; the orientation of the box, and consequently the target hole, was changed after the child had grasped the rod and begun the action. In this condition, called *high location* (HL), turning the box 90° to the right or the left, or even through 180°, required that the child adjust the orientation of the rod in the approach and location phases. This unpredictable change in the orientation of the box produced a large effect on the children's performance. There were changes in different features of the programme due to increases in the range of both grip patterns and intrinsic movements. Although all three groups of children tended

309

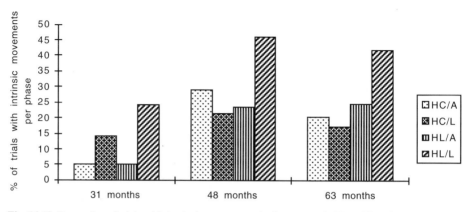

Fig. 14.12. Proportion of trials with intrinsic movements in the approach (A) and locating (L) phases in the high constraint (HC) and high location (HL) conditions.

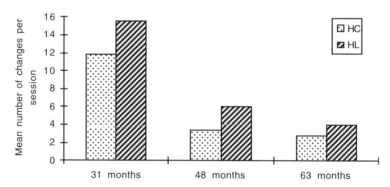

Fig. 14.13. Changes in grip position made by the three groups of children in the high constraint (HC) and high location (HL) conditions.

to show changes in the same direction, the two older groups responded by much greater increases in the use of intrinsic movements, particularly in the location phase (Fig. 14.12). The 31 and 48 months groups showed fluctuations mainly in terms of grips. They changed grip patterns more often after the grasping phase (Fig. 14.13). The 63 months group was evidently less perturbed as they showed fewer changes in grip patterns in the HL condition. Nevertheless, these older children revealed that they still have some way to go in their development because the instability caused in the HL condition led to increases in the percentage of rigid grips (Fig. 14.14).

These observations help to identify some examples of the changes possible in the programme's microstructure. The main feature of the model outlined here is the consideration of opposites, determinacy and indeterminacy, as complementary features of action programmes. The modular theory proposed in the early 1970s (Bruner 1970; Connolly 1970a, 1973) is not adequate for understanding development. The findings presented here

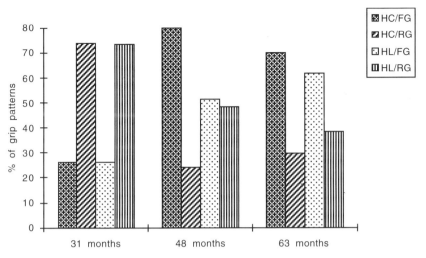

Fig. 14.14. Proportion of rigid (RG) and flexible (FG) grips produced by the three groups of children under the high constraint (HC) and high location (HL) conditions.

indicate that the unit of action went through a flux of changes in its components. Contrary to the prediction from the modular hypothesis variability did not decrease, rather it changed its locus, as the data on the development of spoon use suggested (Connolly and Dalgleish 1989, 1993). This might reflect a shift in the constraints imposed by the macrostructure on the microstructure. In the same vein, the idea that development is accomplished by constraining and then relaxing degrees of freedom also needs attention. The main feature of the younger group was variability in action rather than constraint. There was indeed restriction in how the rod was grasped, since most grips were rigid. However, the children changed grips quite often within a trial and between trials, not to mention the variability observed in the combinations of arm joints, *i.e.* extrinsic movements, used particularly in the location of the rod into the target hole. The idea of a programme with macro- and microstructures shifts the focus away from invariances in motor behaviour to a more balanced view in which variability has an essential role in motor development (Manoel and Connolly 1995) This idea might be particularly useful in the treatment of disabled children. Touwen (1978) has argued that an essential feature of normal development is behavioural variability. It would be interesting to examine the acquisition of a motor skill by disabled children in terms of macro- and microstructure change. Following Touwen's ideas one would expect greater consistency at the microstructure level. This would result in impairment in the capacity of these children to reorganize their action programmes.

Final remarks
Skilled action, like other complex systems, cannot be explained in terms of either symbolic or dynamic modes of description alone, rather the problem lies in how the two modes are related (Pattee 1982). Indeed, a fundamental feature of the principle of complementarity is

to articulate two modes of description that are opposites (Pattee 1978). Hierarchy theory is a framework in which this paradoxical articulation has been attempted. Koestler (1967, 1969) argued that the essence of open systems is that they entail two trends, autonomy and integration. Weiss (1967, 1969) and Pattee (1973) also pointed to an apparent paradox of living systems in which determinacy and indeterminacy coexist. In fact, the major feature of complex systems is the balance between autonomy and control among the different levels in the system's organization (von Bertalanffy 1952), and in developmental terms the balance between maintaining and breaking down structures (Lorenz 1974, 1977).

Given these considerations, the principles of complementarity and hierarchical order are important for a theory of the development of skilled action. The attempt outlined here is still rudimentary; nevertheless, the notions of macrostructure and microstructure in the organization of actions constitutes an important starting point. We have provided also some empirical evidence to support this way of considering development. The process we are dealing with is certainly complex. Concepts such as development, acquisition, learning and evolution are sometimes used as if they were synonymous, sometimes as if they were complementary. However, they refer to processes in which changes in the system take place on different timescales and are very likely influenced by different sets of variables. In terms of timescale, learning involves changes over a comparatively short period. In this sense, learning is encapsulated within development which involves changes over much longer periods and even throughout the lifespan. Accordingly, evolution encompasses development and learning, since it implies changes in the history of a species or population rather than an individual. How these three processes are linked, whether they can be explained by the same concepts and, if not, how different concepts and timescales can be related, are questions which still have to be addressed. It is not a new problem. More than 30 years ago Tinbergen (1963) identified four classes of explanation for behaviour. These were explanations in terms of proximate cause, function, development and evolution. No single explanation is better because a complete picture of behaviour will be produced only by the complementarity (Pattee 1978) and interdependence between them (Hinde 1990).

ACKNOWLEDGEMENTS

We are grateful to Professors Herbert Pick, Jr and Go Tani for their helpful comments on earlier versions of this chapter. The work was largely undertaken while the first author was on leave from the School of Physical Education and Sport, University of São Paulo and in receipt of a scholarship from the CAPES—Ministry of Education, Brazil.

REFERENCES

Abernethy, B., Sparrow, W. A. (1992) 'The rise and fall of dominant paradigms in motor behaviour research.' *In:* Summers, J.J. (Ed.) *Approaches to the Study of Motor Control and Learning.* Amsterdam: North Holland, pp. 3–45.

Adams, J. (1971) 'A closed loop theory of motor learning.' *Journal of Motor Behavior*, **3**, 111–150.

Allen, T.F.H., Starr, T.B. (1982) *Hierarchy: Perspectives for Ecological Complexity.* Chicago: Chicago University Press.

Aslin, R.N. (1993) 'Commentary. The strange attractiveness of dynamic systems to development.' *In:* Smith, L., Thelen, E. (Eds.) *A Dynamic Systems Approach to Development.* London: Bradford Books, pp. 385–399.

Bartlett, F. C. (1958) *Thinking: An Experimental and Social Study.* London: George Allen & Unwin.

Beek, P.J. (1989) *Juggling Dynamics.* Amsterdam: Free University Press.

—— Beek, W.J. (1988) 'Tools for constructing dynamical models of rhythmic movements.' *Human Movement Science,* **7**, 301–342.

Berkinblit, M.B., Feldman, A.G., Fukson, O.I. (1986) 'Adaptability of innate motor patterns and motor control mechanisms.' *Behavioral and Brain Sciences,* **9**, 585–638.

Bernstein, N. (1967) *The Co-ordination and Regulation of Movements.* Oxford: Pergamon Press.

Bruner, J.S. (1970) 'The growth and structure of skill.' *In:* Connolly, K.J. (Ed.) *Mechanisms of Motor Skill Development.* London: Academic Press, pp. 63–92.

—— (1973) 'Organization of early skilled action.' *Child Development,* **44**, 1–11.

—— Bruner, B.M. (1968) 'On voluntary action and its hierarchical structure.' *International Journal of Psychology,* **3**, 239–255.

Choshi, K., Tani, G. (1983) 'Stable systems and adaptive systems in motor learning.' *In: The Science of Movement V.* Tokyo: Japanese Association of Biomechanics, Kyorin, pp. 346–351.

Connolly, K.J. (1970a) 'Skill development: problems and plans.' *In:* Connolly, K. J. (Ed.) *Mechanisms of Motor Skill Development.* London: Academic Press, pp. 3–17.

—— (1970b) 'Response speed, temporal sequencing and information processing in children.' *In:* Connolly, K. J. (Ed.) *Mechanisms of Motor Skill Development.* London: Academic Press, pp. 161–188.

—— (1973) 'Factors influencing the learning of manual skills by young children.' *In:* Hinde, R., Stevenson-Hinde, J. (Eds.) *Constraints on Learning.* London: Academic Press, pp. 337–363.

—— (1975) 'Movement, action and skill.' *In:* Holt, K.S. (Ed.) *Movement and Child Development. Clinics in Developmental Medicine No. 55.* London: Spastics International Medical Publications, pp. 102–110.

—— (1977) 'The nature of motor skill development.' *Journal of Human Movement Studies,* **3**, 128–143.

—— (1981) 'Maturation and the ontogeny of motor skills.' *In:* Connolly K.J., Prechtl, H.F.R. (Eds.) *Maturation and Development: Biological and Psychological Perspectives. Clinics in Developmental Medicine No. 77/78.* London: Spastics International Medical Publications, pp. 216–230.

—— (1986) 'A perspective on motor development.' *In:* Wade, M. G., Whiting, H. T. A. (Eds.) *Motor Development in Children: Aspects of Coordination and Control.* Dordrecht: Martinus Nijhoff, pp. 3–22.

—— Bruner, J.S. (1974) 'Competence: its nature and nurture.' *In:* Connolly, K.J., Bruner, J.S. (Eds.) *The Growth of Competence.* London: Academic Press, pp. 3–7.

—— Dalgleish, M. (1989) 'The emergence of a tool-using skill in infancy.' *Developmental Psychology,* **25**, 894–912.

—— —— (1993) 'Individual patterns of tool use by infants.' *In:* Kalverboer, A.F., Hopkins, B., Geuze, R. (Eds.) *Motor Development in Early and Later Childhood: Longitudinal Approaches.* Cambridge: Cambridge University Press, pp. 174–204.

—— Elliott, J.M. (1972) 'Evolution and ontogeny of hand function.' *In:* Blurton-Jones, N. (Ed.) *Ethological Studies of Child Behaviour.* Cambridge: Cambridge University Press, pp. 329–383.

—— Manoel, E.deJ. (1991) 'Hierarchies and tool-use strategies.' *Behavioral and Brain Sciences,* **14**, 554–555.

Conrad, M. (1983) *Adaptability: The Significance of Variability from Molecule to Ecosystem.* New York: Plenum Press.

Craik, K.J.W. (1947) 'Theory of the human operator in control systems. I. The operator as an engineering system.' *British Journal of Psychology,* **38**, 56–61.

—— (1948) 'Theory of the human operator in control systems. II. Man as an element in a control system.' *British Journal of Psychology,* **38**, 142–148.

Edelman, G.E. (1987) *Neural Darwinism.* New York: Basic Books.

Elliott, J.M., Connolly, K.J. (1974) 'Hierarchical structure in skill development.' *In:* Connolly, K.J., Bruner, J.S. (Eds.) *The Growth of Competence.* London: Academic Press, pp. 135–168.

—— —— (1984) 'A classification of manipulative hand movements.' *Developmental Medicine and Child Neurology,* **26**, 283–296.

Fitts, P.M., Posner, M.I. (1967) *Human Performance.* Belmont, CA: Brooks Cole.

Gatlin, L.L. (1972) *Information Theory and the Living System.* New York: Columbia University Press.

Gesell, A. (1929) 'Maturation and infant behavior pattern.' *Psychological Review,* **36**, 307–319.

—— (1945) *The Embryology of Behavior.* (Reprinted 1988 as *Classics in Developmental Medicine No. 3.* London: Mac Keith Press.)

—— (1946) 'The ontogenesis of infant behavior.' *In:* Carmichael, L. (Ed.) *Manual of Child Psychology.* New York: Wiley, pp. 295–331.

Gibson, J.J. (1966) *The Senses Considered as Perceptual Systems.* Boston: Houghton–Mifflin.

313

—— (1979) *The Ecological Approach to Visual Perception*. Boston: Houghton–Mifflin.

Glencross, D.J. (1980) 'Levels and strategies of response organisation.' *In:* Stelmach, G.E., Requin, J. (Eds.) *Tutorials in Motor Behavior*. Amsterdam: North Holland, pp. 551–566.

Gottlieb, G. (1992) *Individual Development and Evolution*. New York: Oxford University Press.

Haken, H. (1983) *Synergetics: an Introduction*. Berlin: Springer Verlag.

Hay, L. (1984) 'A discontinuity in the development of motor control in children.' *In:* Prinz, W., Sanders, A.F. (Eds.) *Cognition and Motor Processes*. Berlin: Springer Verlag, pp. 351–359.

—— (1990) 'Developmental changes in eye–hand coordination behaviors: preprogramming versus feedback control.' *In:* Bard, C., Fleury, M., Hay, L. (Eds.) *Development of Eye–hand Coordination Across the Life Span*. Columbia: University of South Carolina Press, pp. 217–244.

Hinde, R. A. (1990) 'The Croonian Lecture, 1990. The interdependence of the behavioural sciences.' *Philosophical Transactions of the Royal Society of London, Series B: Biological Sciences*, **329**, 217–227.

Hopkins, B., Beek, P.J., Kalverboer, A.F. (1993) 'Theoretical issues in the longitudinal study of motor development.' *In:* Kalverboer, A.F., Hopkins, B., Geuze, R. (Eds.) *Motor Development in Early and Later Childhood: Longitudinal Approaches*. Cambridge: Cambridge University Press, pp. 343–371.

Jantsch, E. (1980) *The Self-Organizing Universe: Scientific and Human Implications of an Emerging Paradigm of Evolution*. Oxford: Pergamon Press.

Kauffman, S.A. (1991) 'Antichaos and adaptation.' *Scientific American*, **265** (2), 78–84.

Kay, H. (1970) 'Analysing motor skill performance.' *In:* Connolly, K.J. (Ed.) *Mechanisms of Motor Skill Development*. London: Academic Press, pp. 139–151.

Kelso, J.A.S. (1981) 'Contrasting perspectives on order and regulation in movement.' *In:* Long, J., Baddeley, A. (Eds.) *Attention and Performance, IX*. Hillsdale, NJ: Lawrence Erlbaum, pp. 437–457.

—— (1984) 'Phase transitions and critical behavior in human bimanual coordination.' *American Journal of Physiology*, **246**, R1000–R1004.

—— (1990) 'Phase transitions: foundations of behavior.' *In:* Haken, H., Stadler, M. (Eds.) *Synergetics of Cognition*. Berlin: Springer Verlag, pp. 249–268.

—— (1992) 'Theoretical concepts and strategies for understanding perceptual-motor skill: from information capacity in closed systems to self-organization in open, nonequilibrium systems.' *Journal of Experimental Psychology: General*, **121**, 260–261.

—— Tuller, B. (1984) 'A dynamical basis for action systems.' *In:* Gazzaniga, M.S. (Ed.) *Handbook of Cognitive Neuroscience*. New York: Plenum Press, pp. 321–356.

Keogh, J.F., Sugden, D. (1985) *Movement Skill Development*. New York: Macmillan.

Kerr, R. (1985) 'Fitt's law and motor control in children.' *In:* Clark, J.E., Humphrey, J.H. (Eds.) *Motor Development: Current Selected Research. Vol. 1*. Princeton, NJ: Princeton Book Company, pp. 45–33.

Klingsporn, M.J. (1973) 'The significance of variability.' *Behavioral Science*, **18**, 441–447.

Koestler, A. (1967) *The Ghost in the Machine*. London: Hutchinson.

Koestler, A. (1969) 'Beyond atomism and holism—the concept of holon.' *In:* Koestler, A., Smythies, J.R. (Eds.) *Beyond Reductionism*. London: Hutchinson, pp. 192–232.

Kohout, L.J. (1976) 'Representation of functional hierarchies of movement in the brain.' *International Journal of Man–Machine Studies*, **8**, 699–709.

Kugler, P.N. (1986) 'A morphological perspective on the origin and evolution of movement patterns.' *In:* Wade, MG, Whiting, H.T.A. (Eds.) *Motor Development in Children: Aspects of Coordination and Control*. Dordrecht: Martinus Nijhoff, pp. 459–525.

—— Turvey, M.T. (1987) *Information, Natural Law and the Self Assembly of Rhythmic Movements*. Hillsdale, NJ: Erlbaum.

Kuhn, T.S. (1970) *The Structure of Scientific Revolutions*. Chicago: Chicago University Press.

Lorenz, K.Z. (1974) 'Analogy as a source of knowledge.' *Science*, **185**, 229–234.

—— (1977) *Behind the Mirror*. London: Methuen.

Manoel, E.deJ. (1993) 'Adaptive control and variablity in the development of skilled actions.' PhD thesis, University of Sheffield.

—— Connolly, K.J. (1995) 'Variability and the development of skilled actions.' *International Journal of Psychophysiology*, **19**, 129–147.

Maruyama, M. (1963) 'The second cybernetics: deviation-amplifying mutual causal processes.' *American Scientist*, **51**, 164–179.

—— (1982) 'Four different causal metatypes in biological and social sciences.' *In:* Schieve, W.C., Allen, P.M. (Eds.) *Self-Organization and Dissipative Structures*. Austin: University of Texas Press, pp. 354–361.

McCracken, H.D. (1983) 'Movement control in a reciprocal tapping task: a developmental study.' *Journal of Motor Behavior*, **15**, 262–279.

McGraw, M.B. (1945) *The Neuromuscular Maturation of the Human Infant*. (Reprinted 1989 as *Classics in Developmental Medicine No. 4*. London: Mac Keith Press.)

—— (1946) 'Maturation of behaviour.' *In:* Carmichael, L. (Ed.) *Manual of Child Psychology*. New York: Wiley, pp. 332–369.

Meijer, O., Roth, K. (Eds.) (1988) *Complex Movement Behaviour: The Motor–Action Controversy*. Amsterdam: North Holland.

Miller, G.A., Galanter, E., Pribram, K.A. (1960) *Plans and the Structure of Behavior*. New York: Holt.

Milsum, J.H. (Ed.) (1968) *Positive Feedback*. London: Pergamon Press.

Moss, S.C., Hogg, J. (1983) 'The development and integration of fine motor sequences in 12- to 18-month-old children: a test of the modular theory of motor skill acquisition.' *Genetic Psychology Monographs*, **107**, 145–187.

Newell, K.M. (1978) 'Some issues on action plans.' *In:* Stelmach, G.E. (Ed.) *Information Processing in Motor Control and Learning*. New York: Academic Press, pp. 41–54.

—— (1986) 'Constraints on the development of coordination.' *In:* Wade, M.G., Whiting, H.T.A. (Eds.) *Motor Development in Children: Aspects of Coordination and Control*. Dordrecht: Martinus Nijhoff, pp. 341–360.

—— (1991) 'Motor skill acquisition.' *Annual Review of Psychology*, **42**, 213–237.

—— McDonald, P.V. (1992) 'Searching for solutions to the coordination function: learning as exploratory behavior.' *In:* Stelmach G.E., Requin, R. (Eds.) *Tutorials in Motor Behaviour, II*. Amsterdam: North Holland, pp. 517–532.

—— Kugler, P.N., van Emmerik, R.E.A., McDonald, P.V. (1989a) 'Search strategies and the acquisition of coordination.' *In:* Wallace, S.A. (Ed.) *Perspectives on the Coordination of Movement*. Amsterdam: North Holland, pp. 85–122.

—— Scully, D.M., McDonald, P.V., Baillargeon, R. (1989b) 'Task constraints and infant grip configurations.' *Developmental Psychobiology*, **22**, 817–831.

—— —— Tenenbaum, F., Hardiman, S. (1989c) 'Body scale and the development of prehension.' *Developmental Psychobiology*, **22**, 1–13.

—— McDonald, P.V., Baillargeon, R. (1993) 'Body scale and infant grip configurations.' *Developmental Psychobiology*, **26**, 195–205.

Nicolis, J.S. (1986) *Dynamics of Hierarchical Systems: an Evolutionary Approach*. Berlin: Springer Verlag.

Oyama, S. (1985) *The Ontogeny of Information: Developmental Systems and Evolution*. Cambridge: Cambridge University Press.

Pattee, H.H. (1972) 'Laws and constraints, symbols and languages.' *In:* Waddington, C.H. (Ed.) *Towards a Theoretical Biology. Vol. 4. Essays*. Edinburgh: Edinburgh University Press, pp. 248–258.

—— (1973) 'The physical basis and origin of hierarchical control.' *In:* Pattee, H.H. (Ed.) *Hierarchy Theory: The Challenge of Complex Systems*. New York: George Braziller, pp. 71–108.

—— (1976) 'The role of instabilities in the evolution of control hierarchies.' *In:* Burns, T.R., Buckley, W. (Eds.) *Power and Control*. London: Sage, pp. 171–184.

—— (1977) 'Dynamic and linguistic modes of complex systems.' *International Journal of General Systems*, **3**, 259–266.

—— (1978) 'The complementarity principle in biological and social structures.' *Journal of Social and Biological Structures*, **1**, 191–200.

—— (1982) 'The need for complementarity in models of cognitive behavior: a response to Fowler and Turvey.' *In:* Weimer, W.B., Palermo, D.S. (Eds.) *Cognition and the Symbolic Processes. Vol. 2*. Hillsdale, NJ: Erlbaum, pp. 21–30.

—— (1987) 'Instabilities and information in biological self-organization.' *In:* Yates, F.E. (Ed.) *The Self-Organizing Systems: the Emergence of Order*. New York: Plenum Press, pp. 325–338.

Pew, R.W. (1984) 'A distributed processing view of human motor control.' *In:* Prinz, W, Sanders, A.F. (Eds.) *Cognition and Motor Processes*. Heidelberg: Springer Verlag, pp. 19–27.

—— Rosenbaum, D.A. (1988) 'Human movement control: computation, representation and implementation.' *In:* Atkinson, R.C., Herrnstein, R.J., Lindzey, G., Duncan Luce, R. (Eds.) *Steven's Handbook of Experimental Psychology. Vol. 2. Learning and Cognition*. New York: Wiley, pp. 473–509.

Piaget, J. (1960) 'Reply to comments concerning the part played by equilibrium processes in the psychobiological development of the child.' *In:* Tanner, J.M., Inhelder, B. (Eds.) *Discussions on Child Development. Vol. 4*. London: Tavistock, pp. 77–83.

315

Prechtl, H.F.R. (1984) 'Continuity and change in early neural development.' *In:* Prechtl, H.F.R. (Ed.) *Continuity of Neural Functions from Prenatal to Postnatal Life. Clinics in Developmental Medicine No. 94.* London: Spastics International Medical Publications, pp. 1–15.

—— (1986) 'Prenatal motor development.' *In:* Wade, M.G., Whiting, H.T.A. (Eds.) *Motor Development in Children: Aspects of Coordination and Control.* Dordrecht: Martinus Nijhoff, pp. 53–64.

Pribram, K. (1971) *Languages of the Brain.* Englewood Cliffs, NJ: Prentice Hall.

Prigogine, I. (1961) *Introduction to Thermodynamics of Irreversible Processes.* New York: Interscience.

—— (1978) 'Time, structure, and fluctuations.' *Science,* **201,** 777–785.

—— Stengers, I. (1984) *Order out of Chaos.* New York: Bantam.

Reed, E.S. (1982) 'An outline of a theory of action systems.' *Journal of Motor Behavior,* **14,** 98–134.

Requin, J., Semjem, A., Bonnet, M. (1984) 'Bernstein's purposeful brain.' *In:* Whiting, H.T.A. (Ed.) *Human Motor Actions: Bernstein Reassessed.* Amsterdam: North Holland, pp. 467–504.

Rosenbaum, D. (1991) *Human Motor Control.* London: Academic Press.

Salthe, S.N. (1985) *Evolving Hierarchical Systems.* Columbia: Columbia University Press.

Schmidt, R.A. (1975) 'A schema theory of discrete motor skill learning.' *Psychological Review,* **82,** 225–260.

—— (1985) 'The search for invariance in skilled movement behavior.' *Research Quarterly for Exercise and Sport,* **56,** 188–200.

—— (1988a) *Motor Control and Learning. 2nd Edn.* Champaign, IL: Human Kinetics Publishers.

—— (1988b) 'Motor and action perspectives on motor behaviour.' *In:* Meijer, O., Roth, K. (Eds.) *Complex Movement Behaviour: the Motor–Action Controversy.* Amsterdam: North Holland, pp. 3–44.

Scholz, C. (1982) 'The architecture of hierarchy.' *General Systems,* **27,** 283–289.

Schoner, G., Kelso, J.A.S. (1988) 'Dynamic patterns of biological coordination: theoretical strategies and new results.' *In:* Kelso, J.A.S., Mandell, A.J., Schlesinger, M.F. (Eds.) *Dynamic Patterns in Complex Systems.* Singapore: World Scientific Publications, pp. 77–102.

—— Zanone, P.G., Kelso, J.A.S. (1992) 'Learning as change of coordination dynamics: theory and experiment.' *Journal of Motor Behavior,* **24,** 29–48.

Shaffer, L.H. (1992) 'Motor programming and control.' *In:* Stelmach, G.E., Requin, J. (Eds.) *Tutorials in Motor Behaviour. II.* Amsterdam: North Holland, pp. 371–383.

Shapiro, D.C., Schmidt, R.A. (1982) 'The schema theory: recent evidence and development implications.' *In:* Kelso, J.A., Clark, J. (Eds.) *The Development of Movement Control and Coordination.* Chichester: Wiley, pp. 113–150.

Simon, H.A. (1981) *The Sciences of the Artificial. 2nd Edn.* Cambridge: MIT Press.

Sommerhoff, G. (1974) *Logic of the Living Brain.* London: Wiley.

Sperry, R.W. (1950) 'Neural basis of the spontaneous optokinetic responses produced by visual inversion.' *Journal of Comparative and Physiological Psychology,* **43,** 482–489.

Sporns, O., Edelman, G.M. (1993) 'Solving Bernstein's problem: a proposal for the development of coordinated movement by selection.' *Child Development,* **64,** 960–981.

Sugden, D.A. (1980) 'Movement speed in children.' *Journal of Motor Behavior,* **12,** 125–132.

Tani, G. (1987) 'Educação Física na pré-escola e nas quatro primeiras séries do primeiro grau: um abordagem desenvolvimentista I.' *Kinesis,* **3,** 19–41.

—— Manoel, E.deJ., Kokubun, E., Proenca, J.E. (1988) *Educação Fisica Escolar: Fundamentos para uma Abordagem Desenvolvimentista.* São Paulo: EPU/Editora da Universidade de São Paulo.

Thelen, E. (1979) 'Rhythmical stereotypes in normal infants.' *Animal Behaviour,* **27,** 699–715.

—— (1986) 'Development of coordinated movement: Implications for early human development.' *In:* Wade, M.G., Whiting, H.T.A. (Eds.) *Motor Development: Aspects of Coordination and Control.* Dordrecht: Martinus Nijhoff, pp. 107–124.

—— (1989) 'Self-organization in developmental processes: can systems approaches work?' *In:* Gunnar, M., Thelen, E. (Eds.) *Systems in Development. Minnesota Symposium on Child Psychology, Vol. 24.* Hillsdale, NJ: Erlbaum, pp. 77–117.

—— (1990) 'Coupling perception and action in the development of skill: a dynamic approach.' *In:* Block, H., Bertenthal, B.I. (Eds.) *Sensory-motor Organizations and Development in Infancy and Early Childhood.* Dordrecht: Kluwer, pp. 39–56.

—— Ulrich, B.D. (1991) 'Hidden skills: a dynamic systems analysis of treadmill stepping during the first year.' *Monographs of the Society for Research in Child Development,* **56,** 1–104.

—— Kelso, J.A.S., Fogel, A. (1987) 'Self-organizing systems and infant motor development.' *Developmental Review,* **7,** 739–765.

316

—— Zernicke, R., Schneider, K., Jensen, J., Kamm, K., Corbetta, D. (1992) 'The role of intersegmental dynamics in infant neuromotor development.' *In:* Stelmach, G. E., Requin, J. (Eds.) *Tutorials in Motor Behavior. II.* Amsterdam: North Holland, pp. 533–548.

—— Corbetta, D., Kamm, K., Spencer, J.P, Schneider, K., Zernicke, R. F. (1993) 'The transition to reaching: mapping intention and intrinsic dynamics.' *Child Development*, **64**, 1058–1098.

Thomas, J. R. (1980) 'Acquisition of motor skills: information processing differences between children and adults.' *Research Quarterly for Exercise and Sport*, **51**, 158–173.

Tinbergen, N. (1963) 'On aims and methods of ethology.' *Zeitschrift für Tierpsychologie*, **20**, 410–433.

Touwen, B. (1978) 'Variablity and stereotypy in normal and deviant development. *In:* Apley, J. (Ed.) *Care of the Handicapped Child. Clinics in Developmental Medicine No. 67.* London: Spastics International Medical Publications, pp. 99–110.

Turvey, M.T. (1977) 'Preliminaries to theory of action with reference to vision.' *In:* Shaw, R., Brandford, J. (Eds.) *Perceiving, Acting and Knowing.* Hillsdale, NJ: Erlbaum, pp. 211–265.

—— (1990) 'The challenge of a physical account of action: a personal view.' *In:* Whiting, H.T.A., Meijer, O.G., van Wieingen, P.C.W. (Eds.) *The Natural–Physical Approach to Movement Control.* Amsterdam: Free University Press, pp. 57–93.

—— Fitch, H.L., Tuller, B. (1982) 'The Bernstein perspective: I. The problems of degrees of freedom and context-conditioned variability.' *In:* Kelso, J.A.S. (Ed.) *Human Motor Behavior: an Introduction.* Hillsdale, NJ: Erlbaum, pp. 239–252

—— Shaw, R.E., Mace, W. (1978) 'Issues in the theory of action: degrees of freedom, coordinative structure and coalitions.' *In:* Requin, J. (Ed.) *Attention and Performance. VII.* Hillsdale, NJ: Erlbaum, pp. 557–595.

Valsiner, J. (1987) *Culture and the Development of Children's Actions.* Chichester: Wiley.

—— (1992) 'Social development of human cognitive processes and its study.' *Estudos Avançados. Coleção Documentos. CiÍnciaCognitiva*, **10**. Universidade de São Paulo.

Vereijken, B., Whiting, H. T. A. (1990) 'In defence of discovery learning.' *Canadian Journal of Sport Sciences*, **15**, 99–106.

—— van Emmerik, R.E.A., Whiting, H.T.A., Newell, K.M. (1992a) 'Free(z)ing degrees of freedom in skill acquisition.' *Journal of Motor Behavior*, **24**, 133–142.

—— Whiting, H.T.A., Beek, W.J. (1992b) 'A dynamical systems approach to skill acquisition.' *Quarterly Journal of Experimental Psychology*, **45A**, 323–344.

Viviani, P., Terzuolo, C. (1980) 'Space–time invariance in learned motor skills.' *In:* Stelmach, G.E., Requin, J. (Eds.) *Tutorials in Motor Behavior.* Amsterdam: North Holland, pp. 525–536.

von Bertalanffy, L. (1952) *Problems of Life.* London: Watts.

—— (1960) 'Comments on Professor Piaget's paper.' *In:* Tanner, J.M., Inhelder, B. (Eds.) *Discussions on Child Development, Vol. 4.* London: Tavistock, pp. 56–84.

—— (1968) *General Systems Theory.* New York: George Braziller.

—— (1969) 'Chance and law.' *In:* Koestler, A., Smythies, J. (Eds.) *Beyond Reductionism.* London: Hutchinson, pp. 56–84.

von Holst, E. (1954) 'Relations between the central nervous system and peripheral organs.' *British Journal of Animal Behaviour*, **2**, 89–94.

van Rossum, J.H.A. (1987) *Motor Development and Practice: the Variability of Practice Hypothesis in Perspective.* Amsterdam: Free University Press.

Waddington, C.H. (1969) 'The theory of evolution today.' *In:* Koestler, A., Smythies, J.F. (Eds.) *Beyond Reductionism.* London: Hutchinson, pp. 357–395.

Warren, W. (1990) 'The perception–action coupling.' *In:* Block, H., Bertenthal, B.I. (Eds.) *Sensory-motor Organizations and Development in Infancy and Early Childhood.* Dordrecht: Kluwer, pp. 23–38.

Weiss, P.A. (1967) 'One plus one does not equal two.' *In:* Quarton, G., Melnechuk, T., Schmidt, F.O. (Eds.) *The Neurosciences: a Study Program.* New York: Rockefeller University Press, pp. 801–821.

—— (1969) 'Living systems: determinism stratified.' *In:* Koestler, A., Smythies, J.R. (Eds.) *Beyond Reductionism.* London: Hutchinson, pp. 3–55.

—— (1971) 'The basic concept of hierarchical systems.' *In:* Weiss, P.A. (Ed.) *Hierarchically Organized Systems in Theory and Practice.* New York: Hafner, pp. 1–44.

Welford, A.T. (1958) *Ageing and Human Skill.* London: Oxford University Press.

—— Norris, A. H., Shock, N. W. (1969) 'Speed and accuracy of movement and their changes with age.' *Acta Psychologica*, **30**, 3–15.

317

Woollacott, M., Sveistrup, H. (1992) 'Changes in the sequencing and timing of muscle response coordination associated with development transitions in balance abilities.' *Human Movement Science*, **11**, 23–36.

Yates, F.E. (1984) 'The dynamics of adaptation in living systems.' *In:* Selfridge, O.G., Rissland, E.W., Arbib, M.A. (Eds.) *Adaptive Control of Ill-Defined Systems.* New York: Plenum Press, pp. 89–113.

Zanone, P.G., Kelso, J.A.S. (1992) 'Learning and transfer as dynamical paradigms for behavioral changes.' *In:* Stelmach, G.E., Requin, J. (Eds.) *Tutorials in Motor Behavior. II.* Amsterdam: North Holland, pp. 563–582.

—— —— Jeka, J. J. (1993) 'Concepts and methods for a dynamical approach to behavioral coordination and change.' *In:* Savelsbergh, G.J.P. (Ed.) *The Development of Coordination in Infancy.* Amsterdam: North Holland, pp. 89–135.

Zylstra, U. (1992) 'Living things as hierarchically organized structures.' *Synthese*, **91**, 111–133.

15
DYNAMIC SYSTEMS THEORY AND SKILL DEVELOPMENT IN INFANTS AND CHILDREN

Beverly D. Ulrich

Early attempts to explain skill development

Researchers have been studying motor development since the early part of this century and they have left us with voluminous descriptions of how motor skills change with age. For example, we know that infants usually creep before they walk, display stable postural control while sitting before they control their posture when standing upright, and begin to utter their first words at about the same time as they produce their first independent steps. At another level, we know that myelination (and thus the speed of neural transmission) increases, visual acuity and depth perception improve, and flexor and extensor dominance of antagonist and agonist muscle groups shift over the first year of life. What scientists have done less well is explain the origins of new behaviors. We know little of how the mechanisms and behaviors are linked to form the *process* that drives change. Several theories have been proposed to explain change, but until recently none has proved adequate for understanding the overall behavior of the human organism.

Neural-based approaches

The most widely accepted theory of motor development, maturation theory, dates from the first half of this century, with the work of Arnold Gesell, Myrtle McGraw and their contemporaries (Gesell 1928; Shirley 1931; McGraw 1932, 1943; Bayley 1935). These investigators used longitudinal observations to document the sequence of motor behaviors displayed by infants and young children. They attributed the relatively uniform sequence and universality of patterns displayed largely to the autonomous unfolding of the central nervous system (CNS). They correlated over time the observed changes in movement form with more indirectly observed changes in neural mechanisms and searched for rules governing the order of change. One rule, for instance, was that motor development always proceeded in a cephalocaudal and proximal–distal direction. They assumed that changes in neural organization were programmed into the system; over time the nervous system inevitably matured, engendering new behaviors.

Contemporary motor development researchers have long abandoned the maturationist program of detailing the sequence and order of motor milestones. Nonetheless, many textbooks continue to follow a maturationist position by presenting motor milestone sequences with little discussion of the processes underlying their appearance, which suggests that development simply happens. While most developmentalists at least acknowledge the duality of nature and nurture influences on behavior, the underlying maturationist theme continues to dominate in the work in behavioral genetics and some neurally based research models. For example, Konner (1991) recently stated that "Motor development sequences are largely genetically programmed." Forssberg (1985) attributed the disappearance of neonatal stepping and the reappearance of stepping in the service of locomotion (two motor milestones) to the maturation of supraspinal neural centers. He also proposed that when infants begin to walk they first make contact at touchdown with the front part of the foot because humans retain the neural code for this gait pattern from earlier evolutionary periods. He claimed that "neural circuits specific for humans develop late in ontogeny and transform the original, non-plantigrade motor activity to a plantigrade locomotor pattern." In a similar vein the emergence of early reaching behaviors has been attributed to the maturation of appropriate pathways in the brain (von Hofsten 1984, Jeannerod 1988).

Cognitive approaches
Piagetian theory and information processing theory are two further approaches that have been used to explain aspects of motor development. Both have been described as cognitive theories because there is an emphasis on the formation of plans for behavior, variously called 'schemata' (Piaget 1952), 'representations' (Mounoud and Vinter 1981) and 'generalized motor programs' (Schmidt 1975). The aspect of Piaget's work that received most attention from students of motor development was his concept of stages. According to Piaget (1952; see Beilin 1989), stages are qualitatively different ways of thinking or behaving that reflect underlying structural changes. They occur in a fixed order and none can be skipped. Further, shifts in behavior and their cognitive representations arise from the interaction of the organism with its environment. Qualitative shifts in the patterns children use to perform simple motor tasks, such as throwing and jumping, have been described since the 1930s (Wild 1938, Zimmerman 1956, Hellebrandt *et al.* 1961, Roberton 1978, Seefeldt and Haubenstricker 1982). The parallels between Piaget's notion of cognitive sequences and observed sequences in motor development led to the suggestion that motor patterns emerged from processes similar to those described by Piaget. A few investigators have tested whether motor sequences met Piaget's sequence criteria, such as invariant order and universality (*e.g.* Roberton 1977, Williams 1980, Langendorfer 1987) but none have tested the validity of the underlying theory, that is, why pattern shifts occur.

More has been done experimentally from an information processing perspective. Models devised by experimental psychologists were first used for studies of adult motor performance and subsequently applied in studies of development. The underlying notion of the information processing approach is that a motor act arises from a sequence of cognitive processes, starting at the level of information input to sensory receptors and ending with the initiation of muscle activity. Mechanisms such as sensory perception, encoding, storage, response selection, retrieval, the assembly of schemata or rules, knowledge of results, and error correction have been proposed and experiments designed to investigate their impact on motor performance (*e.g.* Barclay and Newell 1980, Clark 1982, Gallagher and Thomas 1984). Performance was measured most often in terms of time taken (*e.g.* lag between stimulus presentation and response initiation) and accuracy (errors in distance and direction from target). We have learned from information processing studies that as children become older they respond faster and more accurately, and that mechanisms, such as memory strategies, change over time and this in turn affects behavioral outcome.

Some limitations of previous approaches
While research grounded in maturationist and cognitive approaches added to our information base, it has not explained the richness, diversity, and dynamic nature of motor skill acquisition. For several reasons, these approaches fall short of explaining both *behavior* in real time and the *process of change*.

Maturationists assume that because people progress through relatively uniform sequences and patterns of behavior over developmental time that instructions for each of these behaviors must be encoded in the CNS in advance. Many problems are inherent in such an assumption. First, innate plans for motor outputs require that all of the information needed to define each pattern used over the lifespan be anticipated and encoded in the genetic material. But it is not at all clear how genetic codes can be translated into even simple patterned neural organization, much less complex three-dimensional movements. Second, dedicating sets of neurons to the status of directing and controlling unique patterns of movement would require an extremely large storage capacity. It would have to accommodate an almost infinite number of possibilities for human movement. Lastly, behavior is much more than a simple neural pattern. Movement form derives from multiple convergent sources, including, but not limited to, the elastic properties of muscles, absolute and relative segmental masses and lengths, posture, initial conditions, the integrity of sensory systems, and intention.

Information processing models, like maturationist approaches, are essentially prescriptive in nature. They rely on the pre-existence of generalized motor programs but do not specify their origin. The focus in these models has been on the construction of general purpose rules and instructions that exist generally before, and separate from, the functional behavior itself. Clearly an individual's history of movement experience influences the information stored in the CNS, and that information in turn affects behavior. But these models ignore the movement itself, the actual coordination of body movements through space. By assuming that the representation of the movement *is* the movement, such approaches ignore the complexity of behavior and the dynamic involvement of peripheral influences.

Those who followed Piaget's stage theory approach limited their scope to describing the patterns which infants and children displayed and to verifying their invariant order. They described the product of development, but not the process (Connolly 1970). They left many important questions unanswered, such as, what causes transitions from one pattern to another, how do performers adapt their patterns to varied goals, and, the most basic question, what is the origin of patterned behaviors?

So, where does this leave us?
If neural structures, cognitive constructs, and anatomical and physiological mechanisms contribute to behavior but do not explain it, what does? If detailed plans do not exist in advance, how do we acquire generic locomotor skills, specialized tool use, and the ability to improvise movements like reaching for the telephone while shifting the position of one's

chair as one opens a drawer to find the telephone directory? For this we must look to models that incorporate properties of complex systems, ones in which behaviors arise from the cooperation of many individual parts, and in which development is a process to which mechanisms provide descriptive detail but not an explanation at the macroscopic level. Such an approach is offered by dynamic systems theory. Dynamic systems approaches 'seek to understand the overall behavior of a system, not by dissecting it into parts, but by asking how and under what circumstances the parts cooperate to produce a whole pattern' (Thelen 1996).

Where does dynamic systems theory come from and what is it?

The first principle of a dynamic approach is that behavior arises from the interaction of multiple subsystems. But multicausality is not a novel idea. Systems approaches have been elaborated for many years (*e.g.* Waddington 1966, von Bertalanffy 1968, Lerner 1978) and this single characteristic is not sufficient to explain the scope of dynamic systems theory. In the following sections I will outline the rich set of concepts, principles and analytical techniques that comprise dynamic systems theory. Only by recognizing the breadth of this perspective can we realize how and why dynamic systems theory offers a significant step forward in understanding the process of behavioral change.

For those concerned with development, dynamic(al) systems theory has emerged as the most commonly used name for an approach that has variously been labeled the study of dynamic pattern formation, synergetics, nonlinear systems, complex systems, and chaos, or chaotic patterns. The different terms reflect convergent approaches to the study of change and complexity in diverse disciplines. Synergetics, for example, originated as a theory of the spontaneous formation of structure in open physical systems, such as lasers, hydrodynamics, and chemical instabilities (Haken 1983). Chaos theorists have focused on the behaviors of complex systems that appear random, including weather patterns, economic behavior, normal EEG and abnormal ECG rhythms (for compilations of diverse examples see, for example, Glass and Mackey 1988, Waldrop 1992).

Fundamental to all of these approaches is an interest in change in the patterns of behavior of complex systems, regardless of the material substrates involved. By the early 1980s investigators began to recognize that human organisms demonstrate the basic properties common to dynamic systems (Kelso *et al.* 1980, Kugler *et al.* 1980). The basic criterion for a dynamic system is that it changes over time; this clearly fits human behavior. In addition, change often occurs as a nonlinear shift from one pattern of organization to another; many sets of descriptive data attest to qualitative shifts in patterned movement. Dynamic systems are also complex, but their behavioral patterns can be characterized by relatively simple mathematical formulations, such as equations of motion (Thelen and Ulrich 1991).

The work of the Soviet physiologist Nicolai Bernstein (1967; see also Whiting 1984) provided a cornerstone in the theoretical foundation for the study of skills as motor behaviorists shifted from neural and cognitive based approaches to a dynamic systems approach. Bernstein was the first to argue that motor acts cannot be controlled by explicit one-to-one mappings between neural commands and movement trajectories. He recognized that controlling each body component (muscles or joints) separately could very quickly become an impossibly unwieldy endeavor. Consider, for example, that over 700 muscles and 100 joints comprise the human walking system. He referred to this complexity and redundancy of possible movement coordinations as the degrees of freedom problem. His solution was that we learn to constrain muscle groupings to act as interactive units, which he called coordinative structures.

Further, Bernstein proposed that explanations for movement must go beyond simply describing muscle function, for several reasons. First, many additional sources contribute significantly to motor output, including inertia and reactive forces. Second, the contributions of active and passive forces are ever changing. In real-world repetitions of the same task, contexts and postures vary and perturbations must be accommodated. These contextual variations require that the muscle activation patterns be flexible and assembled to match functional needs.

Thus, many of Bernstein's ideas link quite well with principles emanating from studies of dynamic systems and seem to have melded into the theoretical approach taken at present by many investigating motor development. In this chapter I shall focus largely on principles specific to dynamic systems theory although Bernstein's influence is also recognized.

Mapping dynamic systems principles to data
Dynamic systems theory has been applied to a wide range of motor behaviors, from locomotion, to bouncing, to reaching and grasping, finger and wrist flexions and extensions, and cardiac activity. Individual researchers, however, often focus on selected constructs rather than testing the theory in its entirety. For this reason, and with the goal of sampling a broad array of work in dynamic systems, I will present a variety of studies as I refer to each principle in the sections that follow. I will also limit the examples almost exclusively to studies involving human development. One point bears repeating: although I refer to the dynamic systems theory in the singular, the nature of its origins in several disciplines is reflected in variations in the terminology preferred by individual researchers (*e.g.* order parameter *vs* collective variable) as well as in the principles on which they focus. It would be more accurate to think of the following principles as concepts from dynamic systems *theories* that have proven to be particularly relevant or useful to the study of developmental issues.

Self-organization in complex systems
Perhaps the most fundamental principle of dynamic systems theory is that patterns of behavior can emerge spontaneously from the cooperation of multiple subsystems or components. Detailed plans for new behaviors, therefore, are not represented *a priori* in the brain, nor do movement patterns, such as walking or talking, arise from the inevitable maturation of neural centers or fixed central pattern generators. Human systems belong to the broad category of open, nonequilibrium thermodynamic systems. That is, they are complex, open to information flow, and they both dissipate and take in energy. Studies of nonliving members of this category have clearly shown that under certain conditions such systems are capable of self-organizing into new patterns of behavior. A system such as the atmosphere, with its changing weather patterns, presents an example in which self-organization seems logical.

It is also a system with which almost everyone is familiar. For instance, funnel clouds appear in the skies quite spontaneously. No one feels compelled to search for 'plans of action' that guide this pattern formation. Simply, under certain conditions (*e.g.* a sufficient temperature differential between the earth and the atmosphere, and appropriate barometric pressure and humidity), the collective interplay of multiple factors results in the emergence of a distinctly recognizable pattern, a funnel cloud. Each of the relevant subsystems is dynamic and critical to the outcome but none embodies instructions for the pattern that emerges.

From a dynamic systems view the emergence of patterned human movement is self-organizing as well, just as in other complex, thermodynamic systems. Multiple subsystems, intrinsic and extrinsic, contribute to behavioral outcomes. These include, for example, neuronal organization, muscle strength, joint structures and ranges of motion, motivational and arousal levels, the support surface, and the task. As an heuristic, consider how normal infants shift posture from prone to seated when they accomplish this for the first time. Typically, they push their trunks upward, then lean slightly to one side as they bring their legs forward, together, on the opposite side of their bodies via hip and knee flexion, until both legs are in front of the trunk and extended. Infants with Down syndrome begin the task in a similar way, pushing up with their arms. Thereafter, the similarity ends. The patterns diverge as infants with Down syndrome abduct at both hip joints, bring each leg forward on opposite sides of the body until they meet in front (Lydic and Steele 1979). For both groups of infants the coordination pattern emerges spontaneously, and is self-organized and opportunistic. The kinematics and kinetics are different, simply because infants with Down syndrome possess a significantly greater range of hip motion than normally developing infants, making hip abduction the 'path of least resistance' for their leg movements in this context. When their hip abduction is restricted by elastic leg bands, as are sometimes prescribed by therapists, infants with Down syndrome display a pattern similar to nondisabled infants in performing this task.

Several studies provide experimental evidence for the view that motor behavior is self-organized rather than prescribed. Esther Thelen's (1986) discovery, that when 7-month-old infants were supported upright on a motor-driven treadmill they responded immediately to the dynamics of this context by producing alternating steps, provides a classic example of self-organization. These infants were not yet voluntarily attempting to step or pulling themselves upright. Further, they appeared to be oblivious to the actions of their legs, yet across a range of treadmill belt speeds their responses remained stable. In subsequent studies the flexible nature of this neuromuscular cooperation was demonstrated (Thelen *et al.* 1987b, Thelen and Ulrich 1991). When the treadmill belt was split so that one leg was moved backwards twice as fast as the other, a shift in the cycle durations of each leg occurred immediately, and infants thereby maintained alternation in the lower limb system. In that context, discrepant peripheral sensory input to the legs was compensated for by both legs. To use Bernstein's (1967) terminology, the infant's legs behaved as a bilateral coordinative structure, or synergy.

Treadmill steps clearly arise from the confluence of multiple subsystems. The sensory receptors that detect the dynamics of the context, neurons that activate leg muscle synergies, and the extensor dominance of leg muscles when infants are supported upright comprise some of the intrinsic subsystems that contribute to this behavior. The mechanical action of the treadmill belt, supplemental postural control and weight support provided by an experimenter are extrinsic. All are required. The subsystems necessary for new behaviors to emerge may seem quite obvious, but too great a concentration on a single subsystem or mechanism sometimes leads us to underestimate the contribution of other critical factors and so miss what drives the process of behavioral change.

An example of how identifying nonobvious factors that affect behavior can inform our understanding of the process of development is provided by Benson (1993). She examined the impact of season of birth on the onset of locomotion. Her results showed that babies born in the winter and spring, in a region with significant seasonal weather changes, crawled three weeks earlier than babies born in the summer and fall. She argued that experience is a critical subsystem involved in the onset of locomotion. Parents may be more likely in warm weather to provide babies with opportunities to be on the floor in less restrictive clothing, which encourages exploration and motivates them to move. As infants attempt to explore their environment they develop strength and discover patterns of limb coordination that 'work'. When these opportunities occur at the developmentally appropriate point (when infants are ready to benefit from them), change may occur more rapidly. Infants' activity and exploration, therefore, drive the process of change, while the timing of the change may be paced by their environment.

Further evidence supports the role of experience not only in the emergence of locomotion, but also in the qualitative patterns produced, thus strengthening the argument that self-organization, rather than prescription, underlies patterned behavior. When infants begin to walk they always contact the floor first with the front part of their foot or flat-footed; the adult-like heel strike appears several months later (Sutherland *et al.* 1980; Forssberg 1985). Neural maturationists have argued that the shift to heel strike awaits the development of neural circuits in the spinal cord (Forssberg 1985). An alternative proposal, from a dynamic systems perspective, is that the heel strike coordination pattern is available but not functional until strength and balance control allow a prolonged single leg stance, which allows time for ankle dorsiflexion before foot contact (Thelen and Cooke 1987). Thelen *et al.* (1992) presented data to support this argument. They found that the proportion of steps with heel strike increased during infants' first year of walking, and that the increase in heel strike paralleled the decrease in step width and increase in step length and velocity. They concluded that "heel strike requires a swing of sufficient duration and amplitude to allow the additional joint rotation, and that this, in turn, depends upon a strong and stable period of single leg support." They argued that as infants practice walking they increase leg strength and control, which results in longer steps, and enables the infant to discover a pattern of coordination in which the heel absorbs the impact when the foot contacts the floor.

If the emergence of heel strike patterns were prescribed by maturational processes then a link between a shift into demonstrating this pattern and functional control, *i.e.* balance and stance duration, would not be necessary. Furthermore it should not be possible for prewalking infants to produce stepping patterns that show heel strike coordination. However, when prewalking infants produced alternating steps on a treadmill, while foot contact occurred most frequently via toe-first and flat-footed, heel strike patterns appeared as well

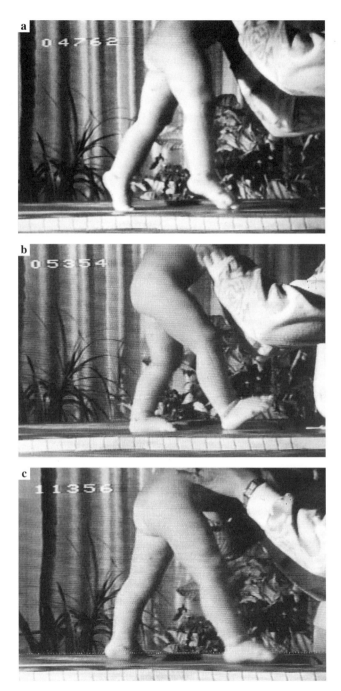

Fig. 15.1. Foot contact patterns produced at touchdown by a prewalking infant stepping on a motorized treadmill. All three coordination patterns—toe first *(a)*, heel strike *(b)*, and flat footed *(c)*—were demonstrated during the same test session on the same day.

326

(Fig. 15.1) (Thelen and Ulrich 1991, Ulrich *et al.* 1992). The experimenter's support, movement of the belt, the infant's current level of neuromuscular organization, leg strength and postural control converged to enable the infant system to coordinate limb patterns in multiple ways, including a pattern not normally seen in prewalkers or new walkers. This suggests that the constraints of independent walking, particularly instability, rather than neural maturation, initially limit the coordination patterns that infants can use in walking.

The significant impact that multiple subsystems have on patterns of behavior and their emergence, and the self-organizing and flexible nature of coordination patterns, do not support traditional explanations for the development of actions such as crawling, walking and reaching. Although critics have maintained that dynamic systems theorists minimize the role of the CNS and place greater emphasis on peripheral and mechanical properties (von Hofsten 1989), this is not correct. A systems view recognizes the mutual importance of subsystems; however, no subsystem, including the nervous system, has logical priority. The complementarity of dynamic systems with CNS development is discussed below.

Context and task
The principle that the context and task share in determining behavioral patterns is implicitly expressed by the concept that behaviors emerge from the confluence of multiple subsystems. Subsystems include both intrinsic and extrinsic factors. An important point about their contribution is that both context and task drive the particular pattern which is assembled. For example, when neonates are held upright they produce alternating steps (Peiper 1963). By 6–8 weeks of age infants fail to step when held in this way but when held upright and partially submerged in warm water they will (Thelen *et al.* 1984). Prior to the discovery that submersion 'worked', conventional wisdom held that the 'disappearance' of newborn stepping occurred because supraspinal centers matured and inhibited the spinal cord pattern generators. In 1982, Thelen and Fisher argued for an alternative explanation. They had discovered a parallel between the disappearance of stepping and increases in body weight and changes in body composition. Because the weight gained was largely subcutaneous fat, they argued that this nonmuscle tissue created a load that the relatively weak muscles of infants had difficulty lifting in the upright posture. The submersion experiment (Thelen *et al.* 1984) supported their claims. By changing the context from out of water to underwater, which made the legs more bouyant and easier to lift, the infant system was again able to produce alternating steps.

That task variations can also drive behavior was illustrated in a pair of studies conducted by Newell, Scully and colleagues (Newell *et al.* 1989a,b). They showed that the grip pattern produced when one reaches for an object is an emergent property of the organism (size and structure of body segments) and task constraints (object size). In their first study, Newell *et al.* (1989b) compared the grip patterns of preschoolers and adults as they reached for cubes of various sizes. Although the number of joint coordination patterns possible for two hands is over 1000, both young children and adults used the same five basic grip configurations. Shifts from one pattern to another occurred at the same ratio of hand size to cube size for both groups. Thus, the interaction between organismic and task constraints predicted the pattern produced.

In a subsequent study, Newell *et al.* (1989a) demonstrated that task constraints affected the grip configuration of infants and challenged the traditional explanation for age-related changes in infants' grip patterns. In the 1930s, Halverson (1931, 1937) described an orderly sequence of change in patterns used by infants to grasp a small cube, from initially encircling the cube with the hand to using a fine pincer grasp. Halverson attributed these shifts to neural maturation, and this explanation has, traditionally, been accepted. Newell and colleagues argued that the narrow task constraints Halverson used (a 2.5 cm cube) affected both the observed behavior and the interpretation of the results. To demonstrate this point they presented infants with objects of varied sizes and in varied orientations. They also extended their analyses of hand configurations to pre- and post-contact portions of the reach. Results showed that infants who had just learned to reach, 4-month-olds, systematically differentiated their hand configurations as a function of the properties of the object in essentially the same way as 8-month-olds. However, while older infants used visual information regarding object size and shape to modulate finger and hand coordination prior to touching the object, younger infants required additional haptic cues and modulated their grips after initial contact (Newell *et al.* 1989a). The researchers concluded that task-relevant information caused even very young infants to shift their grasping patterns. Nevertheless, some aspects of behavioral outcome, for instance the timing of grip pattern adjustments within the reaching behavior, changed with age as a consequence of changes in infants' sensorimotor subsystems, that is, their ability to use visual cues alone to adjust their grip.

Attractors—stable and unstable
In dynamic systems terminology attractor states are preferred patterns of behavior. Some patterns are preferred under certain circumstances in that the system 'wants' to perform them. For instance, adults typically pick up a small cube with their thumb and index finger. Other patterns could be used but they are performed with more difficulty and are more easily disrupted. A stable attractor has a high probability of occurring, and when perturbed the system returns quickly to that pattern—that is, the time it takes for the system to recover from the interruption (relaxation time) is minimal. Further, newly emergent behaviors tend to be more variable than previously performed stable patterns (Schöner and Kelso 1988).

The stability of an attractor is a function of the system's history, the current status of its subsystems, the context and the goal. Thus, over developmental time, anatomical and physiological changes, coupled with experience and intentions, may cause shifts in attractors. In order for one attractor to be replaced by another, some component of the system must disrupt the current stability, induce variability, or make other solutions possible so that the system can explore alternatives.

The dynamic nature of attractors is illustrated by the distinct shifts in the preferred patterns of locomotion that occur during the first year of life (Fig. 15.2). One early solution for moving through space emerges when infants develop sufficient trunk strength to roll over. With this strategy babies move from one location to another, but distance traversed is limited, as is their control of the pathway. Later, crawling forward on hands and knees emerges, displacing rolling as the locomotor attractor. Several subsystems have been linked to the onset of this locomotor pattern (Goldfield 1989). These include: sufficient strength

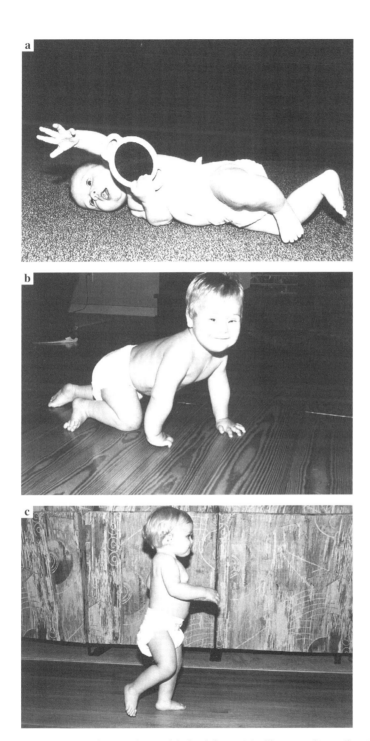

Fig. 15.2. Examples of patterns of locomotion used during infancy: *(a)* rolling over, *(b)* crawling, *(c)* walking.

329

for bearing weight in 'tripod' stance; control of head orientation during shifting gaze; unimanual hand preference for reaching; and leg kicks that are contralateral to arm movements. Thus, the combination of these new capabilities enables a new locomotor pattern to emerge. Subsequently, when leg strength and upright postural control increase sufficiently to enable infants to shift their weight from one limb to another, walking replaces crawling as the stable attractor. However, the behavior of new walkers is relatively unstable and easily disrupted, leading to stumbles and falls. When stressed, infants often revert to crawling as they attempt to increase their velocity. With experience, the walking attractor becomes more stable and crawling virtually disappears as a means of locomotion.

Clark *et al.* (1988) examined the impact of experience on the stability of stepping patterns in infants. They found that infants who had just begun to walk demonstrated an interlimb phasing of 0.5 (*i.e.* halfway through the cycle of one limb the other limb began its cycle), just like more experienced infants and adults. But the standard deviations of interlimb phasing were high. Variability reduced gradually with experience, and by the time infants had three months experience their interlimb phasing exhibited adult-like stability. When experimenters held infants' hands to help them walk, infants' interlimb coupling became less variable. Holding hands provides infants with increased postural support. Therefore, it is likely that postural stability gained through experience works to improve interlimb coupling.

Other locomotor attractors emerge over developmental time in a predictable sequence, including running, galloping, jumping, hopping and skipping. Humans have an enormous number of degrees of freedom making all of these patterns, and more, possible in the service of locomotion. Yet, we tend to demonstrate a limited subset of these, to which we are attracted. We walk rather than gallop or jump across the room because, from a strictly mechanical perspective, the 0.5 interlimb phasing is the most stable and efficient form of bipedal locomotion (Raibert 1986). Throughout most of our lives we alternate our steps as we climb stairs, yet at developmentally young and old stages of life we mark time, placing both feet on each step before moving onto the next one. These varied patterns emerge in the service of this task, not because of genetically coded information that prescribes and turns on and off various coordination patterns, but because the patterns fit the current status of the performer and the task. The degree to which all humans are attracted to the same patterns of coordination reflects the degree to which their intrinsic constraints (*e.g.* physical and physiological structures) and extrinsic constraints (task and context) converge.

Nonlinear phase shifts, control parameters
Over time, as one or more underlying subsystems of a complex system gradually change, their impact may become sufficient to incur a relatively abrupt reorganization of the system into a new pattern. This reorganization is referred to as a nonlinear phase shift. As systems approach a transition, stability of the pattern, or attractor, decreases. For example, in the previous paragraph I described the shift from alternating steps when climbing stairs to marking time. As strength, balance, or confidence in one's ability to raise one's body on a set of risers diminishes, theoretically we would predict an increase in instability (more variability between the interlimb phasings) and that it would take longer to recover from a perturbation, such as a stumble. When this instability reaches sufficient proportions, a shift

to a new interlimb phasing should occur. In the laboratory we could induce such shifts extrinsically by inducing vibrations in the stairs (as one might experience in an earthquake) and a similar behavioral transition should emerge.

The components of the system that engender phase shifts in coordination patterns are called control parameters. The term is somewhat misleading because these components do not control by containing the details of the new behavior or expressing new rules for action. Control parameters simply, by their own gradual change, cause the system to reach a point where the 'current' pattern fails to work as well as it did. Behavior becomes unstable for a period of time, the system explores new possibilities, and ultimately it discovers a new, more effective pattern. Control parameters are variables to which the system is sensitive; they may be internal or external to the system.

Changes over time in infants' pre-speech vocalizations provide an example of phase shifts caused by changes in internal control parameters. Like many other motor behaviors, infants' vocalizations during the first year of life demonstrate a relatively universal sequence of qualitative shifts (Oller 1980, 1986). These changes in the sounds produced have been attributed to underlying changes in the articulators (*e.g.* gradual changes in the relative size and shape of the oral cavity, tongue and lips, and relative location of the soft palate to the nasal cavity) and infants' increasing control over them (Oller 1980, Stark 1980). Therefore, changes in both anatomy and motor control act as control parameters. Further, most of the anatomical remodeling that occurs during infancy is believed to be due to infants' own movements. Behaviors such as sucking, crying and vocalizing exert mechanical stresses that mould the orofacial structure and strengthen muscles (Bosma 1972, Fletcher 1973). Therefore, shifts in an infant's pre-speech vocalizations arise from a dynamic cycle in which her actions affect underlying structures, which in turn create new possibilities for action.

External factors can act as control parameters as well. As I mentioned previously, Thelen (1986) experimentally manipulated the context for 7-month-old infants to bring about a nonlinear shift in lower limb patterns. She supported infants upright, first on a stationary treadmill belt, then on a moving belt. In the stationary condition—as in their normal environment—infants rarely stepped, but when the belt began to move their legs backward they responded with consistent alternating stepping patterns. By supporting the infants upright, Thelen provided a posture that facilitated stepping. Along with intrinsic subsystems, the moving belt acted as the control parameter, providing dynamic information to the leg muscles and joints sufficient to cause a shift into alternating stepping.

The control parameter(s) for the emergence of a particular pattern may vary over time and across populations. By studying infants' responses to the treadmill longitudinally, Thelen and Ulrich (1991) found that subsystems within the infant must progress sufficiently to enable the movements of the treadmill belt to elicit alternating steps. That is, the treadmill was not equally effective across all ages. Between ages 1 and 3 months some infants responded with a few steps while others produced no alternating steps. Between 3 and 5 months of age all infants shifted into increasingly stable alternating stepping patterns in response to stimulation on the treadmill. The ages at which infants began to respond reflected individual differences in when leg postures shifted sufficiently from the highly flexed neonatal configuration to more extended hip and knee joints, thus allowing the legs to be

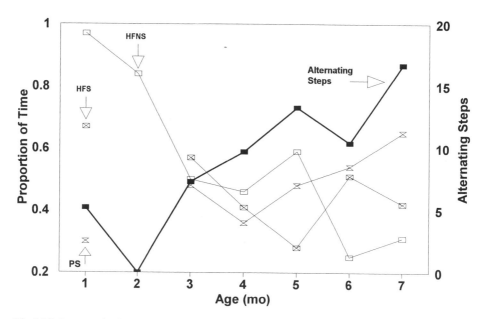

Fig. 15.3. An example of data collected from an infant showing the relation between changes in the control parameter (leg posture displayed on the treadmill) and the alternating steps produced. Leg posture variables plotted include: highly flexed (*vs* extended) when not stepping (HFNS), highly flexed during the swing phase when stepping (HFS), and forward movement of foot during swing was planar (*vs* rotated medially) (PS).

stretched back by the belt movement. Leg posture, therefore, is a control parameter early in life; until the frequency with which infants extended, rather than flexed, their legs increased sufficiently the treadmill was relatively ineffective in driving the infant interlimb system to produce alternating steps (Fig. 15.3).

Results from a subsequent study by Ulrich *et al.* (1995) illustrated that for the same behavior, different variables can act as control parameters in different populations. They examined the emergence of treadmill stepping over time in infants with Down syndrome (DS). Infants with DS shifted into stable responsiveness to the treadmill, as did nondisabled infants, but at older ages (median age was 14 months). Further, the ability of infants with DS to respond to the treadmill was not related to leg posture, the control parameter for nondisabled infants. Long before infants with DS began to step consistently on the treadmill they extended their legs when held upright. Instead, the onset of stable alternating steps appeared coincident with sufficient improvement in leg strength and hip control (Fig. 15.4). This difference occurred because of underlying differences in the subsystems of these two groups. For example, infants with DS have less stable hip and knee joints (*i.e.* a greater range of motion), lower muscle tone and poorer postural control. While extended leg postures may have been dominant early in life for both groups, infants with DS required more time to acquire sufficient control over their hip girdles and legs to allow the treadmill to shift their behavior into alternating stepping.

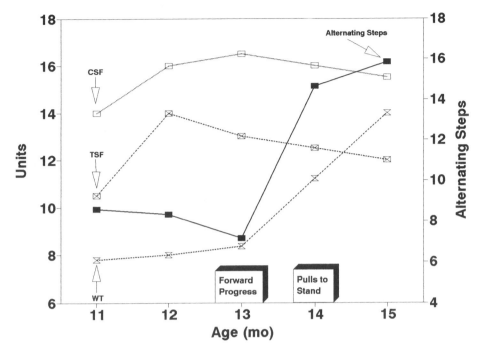

Fig. 15.4. An example of data collected from an infant with Down syndrome showing the relation between changes in the control parameters and alternating steps produced on a treadmill. Variables plotted include: calf skinfold (CSF); thigh skinfold (TSF); body weight (WT); and age when infant was first able to (i) make forward progress when prone, and (ii) pull to standing upright. Change in these variables converged with the shift into alternating stepping consistently across subjects, and suggested that leg strength and hip control were the control parameters for treadmill stepping.

Intrinsic dynamics

Although behavioral outcomes are self-organized, the behaviors that result are not always effective or efficient. When infants and children set goals for themselves and attempt to produce novel behaviors such as crawling over objects in their path, learning to propel themselves on a swing or whistling to signal a friend, success is achieved by a process of problem solving. They must discover solutions by exploring their own intrinsic dynamics relative to the context in which they exist and to the task demands. Intrinsic dynamics may be defined as the collective behavior of the system that occurs in the absence of specific task requirements (Zanone *et al.* 1993). This collective behavior arises from the interactions of one's history of movement experiences, biomechanical properties (*e.g.* body mass, joint ranges of motion) and neurophysiological properties (*e.g.* viscoelastic properties of muscle, sensory thresholds, energy levels, etc.). Therefore, what each performer brings to the movement context, what he or she 'comes with', is unique.

Thelen *et al.* (1993) examined how intrinsic dynamics affect skill acquisition. They studied four infants throughout their first year of life, and focused on how each one learned to reach. The study design included richly detailed profiles and multiple levels of kinematic and kinetic analysis. They proposed that infants' intrinsic dynamics "act as both constraints on the reaching problem and the physical and informational raw materials from which each infant must assemble an action to fit the specified goal—get the hand to the toy." The results showed that the first successful reaches occurred at differing ages and emerged from a variety of possible solutions, but that each solution reflected the infant's individual intrinsic movement characteristics. Briefly, two infants' spontaneous arm movements tended to be large and quite forceful. At the point of transition to first successful reaches their spontaneous behaviors showed large coactive phasic bursts of muscle activity, often rhythmical in nature. Limb movements were large, cyclical and coupled. When presented with a toy, they damped their oscillatory behavior by increasing muscle stiffness. With their elbows held rigid, their forearms and hands were less subject to uncontrolled torques produced at the trunk and shoulders, enabling them to orient their hands to the target. The other two infants were generally less vigorous and produced slower spontaneous movements. Their solutions required scaling up on muscle torques to lift their arms farther away from their bodies than usual and toward the goal. They produced reaches that were relatively slow, with minimal perturbations caused by uncontrolled trunk and shoulder torques because the overall muscle torque generated was small. It should be noted that, although the kinematics of the 'slower' infants looked smoother, successive reaches were no less variable in accuracy of contact and ability subsequently to grasp the object than those of the 'faster' movers.

Details of infants' kinematic and kinetic data illustrated the diversity of early reaches. The only consistent element was contact with the toy. Thelen *et al.* (1993) concluded that when infants reached they were not expressing a fixed program of muscle activation patterns but rather they were discovering how to adjust their ongoing dynamics to produce adequate force and stiffness to meet the goal.

If discovering how to adjust one's intrinsic dynamics to task demands is part of the process of skill acquisition then difficulty in adapting limb movements may contribute to delayed motor skill development. Ulrich *et al.* (in press) tested this proposition by comparing the spontaneous behaviors of normally developing infants and infants with DS. Previously it had been found that when the spontaneous leg movements of normal infants were perturbed by attaching a weight to one leg, the motor output of both legs changed, but changed differentially (Thelen *et al.* 1987a). That is, the movement frequency of the weighted leg decreased relative to when neither leg was weighted, while the unweighted leg increased its frequency. This suggests that one aspect of the intrinsic dynamics of normal infants is a bilateral sensitivity and adaptability to unilateral sensory information. Ulrich *et al.* extended the work to include infants with DS because these infants (a) have been characterized as less sensitive to sensory information (Lewis and Bryant 1982, Cunningham 1988) and (b) acquire functional skills much more slowly than nondisabled infants (Dyer *et al.* 1990, Ulrich *et al.* 1995). To examine thresholds of sensitivity to the perturbation the paradigm was also modified to include three different weights as the perturbation.

The results of the experiment showed that both groups of infants adapted their movements by increasing activity levels of the unweighted leg relative to the weighted leg, particularly when the heavier weights were added. However, thresholds varied between infants in both groups and across repeated presentations of the perturbation. Nevertheless, more infants with DS than nondisabled infants demonstrated minimal overt adaptation. Follow-up data indicated that the infants who were most responsive to perturbations tended also to be among the earliest to learn to crawl, pull to standing, and walk. Conversely, infants who were least responsive tended to be among the last to acquire these skills. These data appear to support the notion that difficulty in adapting one's intrinsic dynamics to changes in the context or the task can constrain the rate of skill acquisition.

Collective variables

One further tenet of dynamic systems theory that must be considered relates to describing and defining the behavior (or the attractor) itself. In dynamic systems terms, when the many degrees of freedom of a complex system self-organize and the result is a patterned output, the behavior can be characterized by one or more collective variables. These collective variables are also called order parameters (Haken 1983, Jeka and Kelso 1989). A collective variable is a low-dimensional descriptor of a complex system's behavior, often expressed as an equation of motion. An extension of this is to define the behavior more narrowly as the coupling or critical phasing relation between segments or limbs. For example, human locomotion involves the cooperative activity of hundreds of muscles and joints. Identifying collective variables enables one to move beyond describing the details of these individual components and to uncover a key to the overall pattern that reflects the cooperation of the component parts. In studies of bipedal locomotion equations that predict the relation between velocity and displacement of limb segments throughout the step cycle and the relative timing of the oscillations of paired limbs during step cycles have been used as collective variables.

One form of a low-dimensional descriptor of a limb in motion is a phase portrait. This consists of a plot of displacement *vs* velocity at successive points throughout the movement. It thus represents the state (at each point) and dynamics (relation among successive points) of the system. When the system behaves in a stable manner, the trajectory of the phase portrait has a high probability of converging on a particular 'shape' and region of the state space. State space may be thought of as 'work space', or the boundaries within which movement trajectories are possible. The resulting shape of the attractor pattern can belong to one of four known classes: point, limit cycle, quasi-periodic, and chaotic (Crutchfield *et al.* 1986).

Defining the collective variables of motor behaviors by the type and shape of their attractor patterns or the phasing relations between segments provides an entry into investigating pattern stability and transitions between different coordinative modes. The utility of these techniques has been demonstrated at multiple levels. For example, medical scientists have modeled normal heart rhythms as single periodic attractors, reflecting a single pattern of the timing of muscle contractions and relaxations over consecutive cycles of heart activity. Phase shifts to period doubling (switching between two rhythmic patterns) and ultimately chaos (complex and seemingly random shifts among rhythms) reflect abnormal, yet patterned, behaviors induced by scaling up on control parameters, such as stress or drugs (Winfree 1983, Fruchter and Ben-Haim 1991, Weiss *et al.* 1994). By describing the dynamics of cardiac behavior the goal is to predict when transitions (instabilities) begin and ultimately to intervene before abnormal rhythms occur.

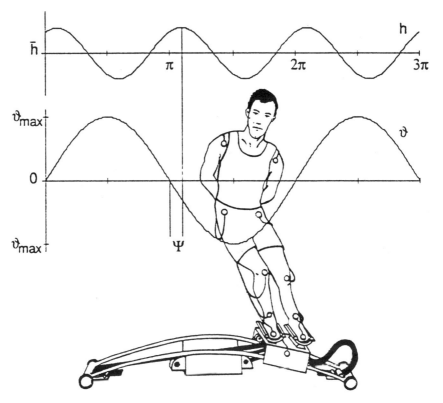

Fig. 15.5. Sketch of a performer on a ski-simulator apparatus. h = vertical displacement over time of the performer's center of mass; ϑ = angular displacement (to right and left) of the platform, a value of zero occurring when the platform reaches its highest point possible. Ψ = lag between when performer's center of mass and the platform reversed directions of movement around the highest point in their respective movement cycles. (Adaptted by permission from Vereijken 1991 and Vereijken *et al.* 1992.)

In their attempt to understand the effects of directed practice on learning, Vereijken *et al.* (1992) used two forms of collective variables (equations of motion and critical phasing relations) to reveal clues to the processes underlying change in performance. They proposed that the first question one must ask when studying learning is *what* must be learned and the second is *how* it is learned. To illustrate their points they analyzed the movements of adults learning to perform on a slalom ski-simulator. The apparatus consisted of two bowed, parallel rails over which a platform rolled (Fig. 15.5). The subjects' task as they stood on the platform was to move it from side to side with maximal amplitude and frequency. To address what must be learned, the researchers derived an equation of motion that described the subject–apparatus system. From this equation they identified the phase lag between oscillations of the height of the subject's center of mass and those of the platform ('Ψ' in Fig. 15.5) as the critical part of the equation, the essence of what must be learned. The lag between the platform reversal from moving upward to downward and when the body's center of mass reversed as well, reflected the timing of the forcing function, that is, when subjects gave a 'push' to keep the platform moving.

In the second part of their study Vereijken *et al.* (1992) addressed how the task was learned by examining the movement patterns of adults as they practiced the task. They found that global improvement in performance over time was reflected in successive changes in the timing of the phase lag, from pushing before the platform reached its peak (wasted energy) to pushing after the platform had reversed directions (when passive forces could be maximally exploited). Therefore, by describing the dynamics of the task, they were able to identify the critical component in the subject–apparatus system that defined the essence of the task and study changes in the behavior over time. Thus, collective variables served as tools for studying the process of motor skill learning.

By characterizing the behavior of a complex system as a phase portrait we can observe the dynamics of the behavior, its stability, and qualitative change over repeated cycles at any point in time as well as over longer periods of time. Those adopting the dynamic systems viewpoint suggest that from the topology of phase portraits it is possible to infer the underlying causal processes (Abraham and Shaw 1981, Garfinkel 1983). For example, a phase portrait (plot of velocity *vs* displacement) of a frictionless pendulum or spring would look smooth and round. Cooke (1979) utilized the shape of phase portraits generated during reaching to suggest that arm movements are controlled by a 'damped mass-spring' system. That is, people utilize the spring-like properties of their muscle–tendon units to control their movements. (For a useful tutorial on interpreting shapes of phase portraits, see Winstein and Garfinkel 1989.)

Fig. 15.6 illustrates phase portraits of the thigh segment of an infant with DS as he produced alternating steps on a treadmill at 16 and 18 months. At both ages, the thigh segment moved like a limit cycle attractor, repeating movement through the same region of state space over cycles. However, significant differences are readily apparent. The multiple shapes of successive trajectories indicate that behavior at 16 months was not very stable and control strategies varied with each cycle. Multiple cusps and loops reflect interruptions in movement, and shifts in location within the work space of successive cycles also occurred. By 18 months stability had improved; the shapes of the trajectories were similar across cycles, and greater overlap of successive cycles was evident. The smoothly rounded segments of the trajectory in the swing phase suggest that position dependent forces opposing motion occurred. This in turn suggests that the infant was taking advantage of the spring-like qualities of the muscles to produce thigh movement. Cusps occurring in a fairly consistent location early in the stance phase suggest active modulation of forces as the infant supported his weight after touchdown. Follow-up investigations using torque analysis or electromyography would help to verify or refute this interpretation. In this example, phase portraits of the infant's attractor pattern revealed clues to the underlying control characteristics and suggested an increase in the stability of the behavior over time.

Modeling the attractor dynamics
Traditional approaches to dynamics emphasize mathematically derived equations of motion that describe the patterned behavior. Terms in the equations include the components of the

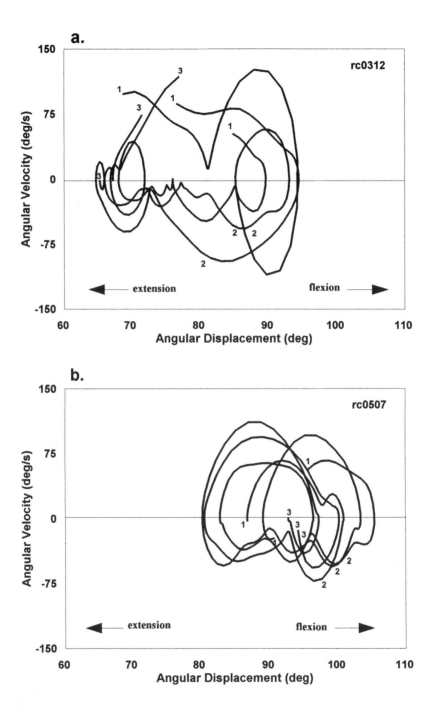

Fig. 15.6. Phase portrait of three cycles of the thigh segment movement of an infant with Down syndrome stepping on a treadmill at ages 16 months *(a)* and 18 months *(b)*. 1 = toe-off, 2 = touchdown, 3 = end of stance. (Phase portrait trajectories progress clockwise by definition.)

action system, representing, for example, the body's mechanical and material properties, the impact of gravity, and their interrelations. For the movement scientist the goal is "to place motor behavior in the context of natural physical law" (Goldfield *et al.* 1993). Few people concerned with development have pursued this specific goal to date.

One clever example of this type of analysis and its relevance is provided by the work of Goldfield *et al.* (1993). They observed infants longitudinally while the infants were supported in an upright position by a harness attached to a spring. This is sometimes known as a 'jolly jumper' apparatus. The task, learning to bounce in the harness, is clearly novel. Commands to generate this behavior could hardly be in the genetic code, yet it is a skill that infants readily acquire. The researchers predicted that infants would use visual and proprioceptive feedback from their own explorations to assemble appropriate moves to drive the spring and 'tune' it (that is, find the appropriate timing and energy) to find the stable pattern, or attractor.

Goldfield *et al.* modeled the action system (infant plus apparatus) as a forced mass-spring system. The measurable damping and stiffness characteristics could be used to parameterize the equation; the infant, of course, provided the source for the forcing function. Their model predicted a specific resonant frequency at which maximal efficiency occurs (maximum bounce for minimum energy). Thus frequency should act as an attractor, the 'location' in work space where the baby–jumper system should prefer to be. During early trials, infants' behaviors were quite varied as they explored the properties of their systems. But when infants settled into parallel leg kicks and adjusted the timing and energy to optimize the match between their system characteristics and those of the apparatus, sustained bouncing occurred. Goldfield *et al.* found a close fit between the resonant frequency that was predicted from the equation for each baby and their individual periodicity. Their data suggest that infants are able not only to assemble and tune their systems to acquire new tasks, but also to optimize the naturally occurring constraints on the system.

The compatibility of dynamic systems theory with a theory of brain organization
Dynamic systems theory proposes that structure and patterned behavior arise from self-organization at all levels, not only the overt behavior of an organism but subsystems levels as well. Therefore one could propose that out of the many components that interact within the brain (the circulating hormones, pressure gradients, efferent and afferent activity that link it to the periphery and context), the self-organization of neural structures can occur. For two reasons, however, it seems relevant to address in this chapter more directed efforts to develop a comprehensive understanding of the development of organization within the brain. First is the need for any theory of skill development to be compatible with contemporary data concerning relevant subsystems. Second, by understanding how the brain becomes organized, given its multimodal areas and peripheral connectivity, we may understand better one way in which multiple subsystems are linked and share in the process of generating the neural contribution to motor behavior.

Gerald Edelman's theory of neuronal group selection (Edelman 1987, Sporns and Edelman 1993) is compatible with dynamic systems theory and derives specifically from data reflecting what is known about neural development. Edelman integrated contemporary data from neuroembryology, neuroanatomy and developmental psychology to propose that through a process of exploration, interaction and selection, organization emerges in the brain. Briefly, during early brain development anatomical form and patterns of synaptic connectivity are elaborated through a series of mechanisms: cell proliferation, cell adhesion and movement, differentiated growth, cell death and the formation of vast numbers of connections (Cowan 1978, Edelman 1987). Because of their dynamic properties these mechanisms introduce individual variance, even in genetically cloned animals, into what Edelman refers to as the primary repertoire, or neuronal network. Over time, as the organism interacts with its environment, selection among diverse preexisting groups of cells is accomplished by differential modification of synaptic strengths. This process shapes the behavioral repertoire of the organism according to what is of adaptive value to it in its eco-niche.

More explicitly, Edelman suggests that an infant's own cycles of action and perception drive the organization of her nervous system (Sporns and Edelman 1993). As an infant moves in her environment a repertoire of groups of related neurons, associated with categories of action, is organized. The information resulting from the efferent neural activations that produce movements within a particular category (*e.g.* kicks, reaches) and the afferent information or sensory consequences of these movements are continuously and temporally correlated within and between local neuronal groups. Through this constant and multimodal flow of information between the CNS and the periphery, neuronal groups are selectively carved out. By this process global and hierarchical mapping also occurs. That is, neurons in local networks develop functional connections and strengthen their interconnections with related networks in other areas, such as visual and somatosensory areas. The sources of information, and subsequently the organization, depend as much on the morphology of non-neural structures and movement contexts as on the CNS.

Edelman and his colleagues have generated a series of computer simulations and, more recently, automata with which they have demonstrated that categories of recognition and action can be learned without preexisting instructions for behavior or error detection devices (Reeke and Sporns 1990; Reeke *et al.* 1990a,b). One robot in their series, Darwin III, was designed with a complex, multilevel 'brain', an arm and an eye. Areas in the brain included a 'cerebral cortex' that generated a primary repertoire of unstructured movements, and a 'cerebellum' that correlated feedback from the arm and eye with signals arising from random arm movements initiated by the motor cortex. The simple 'value', or preference, that was specified was a bias toward strengthening neural connections which were activated when the arm moved near a target within its perceptual–motor space. Without initial cortical representations for reaching, local and global groups of neural connections strengthened, and coordinated reaches improved, as a function of exploration coupled with sensory consequences (Reeke and Sporns 1990).

Simulations can verify models but more important is how well the model matches what it is supposed to reflect, the acquisition of human skill. When Thelen and her colleagues (Thelen *et al.* 1993, Thelen 1995) compared the 'output' of infants, whose real-world acquisition of reaching they had been studying longitudinally, with Darwin III's 'output' they observed amazing similarities. They compared the trajectories of their infants' arm movements in space to Darwin III's arm movements across periods of prereaching, unsuccessful attempts, and stable reaching. Both showed initially rather jerky and random pathways and displayed a large set of possible solutions for moving the arm to the target, as might be expected from a complex but unspecified neuromotor system. Over successive repetitions, the limb trajectories of both systems became less varied and more direct as they settled into stable attractor patterns that matched their intrinsic dynamics to the task.

While change in Darwin III's simulated brain could be observed, clearly change in the organization of the infants' neurons could not. Moreover, similar outcomes do not prove similar underlying processes. The growing evidence for brain plasticity in adults, as well as early in life, indicates the importance of experience and exploration in neural organization (Merzenich *et al.* 1990, Kaas 1991).

Recent technological advances in neuroscience have enabled the monitoring of neural properties as a function of the dynamics of the organism. The electrophysiological mapping of cortical areas in monkeys has changed the notion that neural order and functional relations are predetermined and fixed (Merzenich and Kaas 1980, Jenkins *et al.* 1990, Kaas 1991). By variously altering the afferent feedback or neural input to areas that supported a particular sensory or motor function, these authors have demonstrated that neural mappings and activity, even in adult animals, are dynamic. For example, when Jenkins *et al.* (1990) amputated one or two digits in owl monkeys the cortical representations of the adjacent digits and palm expanded to include areas formerly reflecting activity in the amputated segments. And when the monkeys practised a food retrieval task, the specific areas in the somatosensory cortex that represented the digits making tactile contact increased their area of representation. When practice stopped, area boundaries shifted again.

Therefore, fundamental to both dynamic systems theory and contemporary ideas on brain development is the concept of self-organization. Overt motor behavior and brain organization are quite flexible, influenced by multiple inputs, and not precoded. Recent advances in neuroscience provide the instantiation of the processes by which categories of skills may be learned.

The 'principled' story

In summary, there are several reasons to conclude that motor skill development is an emergent process. First, the results of many experiments, some of which I have described in this chapter, suggest that the organization of and changes in motor patterns of infants and children obey the principles of pattern generation common in dynamic systems. Second, while development may look inevitable, rule driven, or predesigned, this is no longer a plausible explanation. Genetic codes and neural maturation theories cannot explain the origin of commands for behavior or the emergence of novelty, individuality and adaptability inherent in complex human movements. Cognitive approaches also embed behavior in plans existing in advance of the action and are limited to CNS mechanisms. Most important, cognitive approaches ignore the dynamics of the movement pattern itself and the multiple and varied forces that exert effects on behavior.

Dynamic systems theory proposes instead that there are no rules of development. There is complexity and there are relations among subsystems in open, thermodynamic and active systems. There is real-time heterarchical cooperation among the organism's intrinsic dynamics (history of experience, cognition, and biomechanical, neural and physiological properties), the goal and the context. Solutions arise from the constraints inherent in the context and the task, given the many solutions available to complex human organisms. From the continuous process of multimodal and multilevel perception and action, infants and children discover the fit between their capabilities and their goals and acquire stable and functional motor behaviors.

REFERENCES

Abraham, R., Shaw, C. (1981) *Dynamics: the Geometry of Behavior.* Santa Cruz: Aerial Press.
Barclay, C.R., Newell, K.M. (1980) 'Children's processing of information in motor skill acquisition.' *Journal of Experimental Child Psychology*, **30**, 98–108.
Bayley, N. (1935) 'The development of motor abilities during the first three years.' *Society for Research in Child Development Monographs*, **1**, (1), 1–26.
Beilin, H. (1989) 'Piagetian theory.' *In:* Vasta, R. (Ed.) *Six Theories of Child Development: Revised Formulations and Current Issues.* Greenwich, CT: JAI Press, pp. 85–131.
Benson, J.B. (1993) 'Season of birth and onset of locomotion: theoretical and methodological implications.' *Infant Behavior and Development*, **16**, 69–81.
Bernstein, N. (1967) *The Co-ordination and Regulation of Movements.* Oxford: Pergamon Press.
Bosma, J.F. (1972) 'Form and function in the infant's mouth and pharynx.' *In:* Bosma, J.F. (Ed.) *Third Symposium on Oral Sensation and Perception. The Mouth of the Infant.* Springfield, IL: C.C. Thomas, pp. 3–27.
Clark, J.E. (1982) 'Developmental differences in response processing.' *Journal of Motor Behavior*, **14**, 247–254.
—— Whitall, J., Phillips, S.J. (1988) 'Human interlimb coordination: the first 6 months of independent walking.' *Developmental Psychobiology*, **21**, 445–456.
Connolly, K.J. (1970) 'Skill development: problems and plans.' *In:* Connolly, K.J. (Ed.) *Mechanisms of Motor Skill Development.* London: Academic Press, pp. 3–21.
Cooke, J.D. (1979) 'Dependence of human arm movements on limb mechanical properties.' *Brain Research*, **165**, 366–369.
Cowan, W.M. (1978) 'Aspects of neural development.' *International Review of Physiology*, **17**, 150–191.
Crutchfield, J.P., Farmer, J.D., Packard, N.H., Shaw, R.S. (1986) 'Chaos.' *Scientific American*, **254**, 46–57.
Cunningham, C. (1988) *Down's Syndrome: an Introduction for Parents.* Cambridge, MA: Brookline Books.
Dyer, S., Gunn, P., Rauh, H., Berry, P. (1990) 'Motor development in Down syndrome children: an analysis of the Motor Scale of the Bayley Scales of Infant Development.' *In:* Vermeer, A. (Ed.) *Motor Development, Adapted Physical Activity and Mental Retardation. Medicine and Sport Science, Vol. 30.* Basel: Karger, pp. 7–20.
Edelman, G.M. (1987) *Neural Darwinism.* New York: Basic Books.
Fletcher, S.G. (1973) 'Maturation of the speech mechanism.' *Folia Phoniatrica*, **25**, 161–172.
Forssberg, H. (1985) 'Ontogeny of human locomotor control. I. Infant stepping, supported locomotion and transition to independent locomotion.' *Experimental Brain Research*, **57**, 480–493.
Fruchter, G., Ben-Haim, S. (1991) 'Stability analysis of one-dimensional dynamical systems applied to an isolated beating heart.' *Journal of Theoretical Biology*, **148**, 175–192.
Gallagher, J.D., Thomas, J.R. (1984) 'Rehearsal strategy effects on developmental differences for recall of a movement series.' *Research Quarterly for Exercise and Sport*, **55**, 123–128.
Garfinkel, A. (1983) 'A mathematics for physiology.' *American Journal of Physiology*, **245**, R455–R466.
Gesell, A. (1928) *Infancy and Human Growth.* New York: Macmillan.
Glass, L., Mackey, M.C. (1988) *From Clocks to Chaos: the Rhythms of Life.* Princeton, NJ: Princeton University Press.
Goldfield, E.C. (1989) 'Transition from rocking to crawling: postural constraints on infant movement.' *Developmental Psychology*, **25**, 913–919.
—— Kay, B.A., Warren, W.H. (1993) 'Infant bouncing: the assembly and tuning of action systems.' *Child Development*, **64**, 1128–1142.
Haken, H. (1983) *Synergetics, an Introduction: Non-Equilibrium Phase Transitions and Self-Organization in Physics, Chemistry and Biology. 3rd Edn.* Berlin: Springer.

342

Halverson, H.M. (1931) 'An experimental study of prehension in infants by means of systematic cinema records.' *Genetic Psychology Monographs*, **10**, 107–286.

—— (1937) 'Studies of grasping responses of early infancy: I, II, III.' *Journal of Genetic Psychology*, **51**, 371–449.

Hellebrandt, F.A., Rarick. G.L., Glassow, R., Carns, M.L. (1961) 'Physiological analysis of basic motor skills. I. Growth and development of jumping.' *American Journal of Physical Medicine*, **40**, 14–25.

Jeannerod, M. (1988) *The Neural and Behavioural Organization of Goal-Directed Movements*. Oxford: Clarendon Press.

Jeka, J., Kelso, J.A.S. (1989) 'The dynamic pattern approach to coordinated behavior: a tutorial review.' *In:* Wallace, S.A. (Ed.) *Perspectives on the Coordination of Movement*. Amsterdam: Elsevier, pp. 3–45.

Jenkins, W.M., Merzenich, M.M., Recanzone, G. (1990) 'Neocortical representational dynamics in adult primates: implications for neuropsychology.' *Neuropsychologia*, **28**, 573–584.

Kaas, J.H. (1991) 'Plasticity of sensory and motor maps in adult mammals.' *Annual Review of Neuroscience*, **14**, 137–167.

Kelso, J.A.S., Holt, K.G., Kugler, P.N., Turvey, M.T. (1980) 'On the concept of coordinative structures in dissipative structures: II. Empirical lines of convergence.' *In:* Stelmach, G.E., Requin, J. (Eds.) *Tutorials in Motor Behavior*. New York: North-Holland, pp. 49–70.

Konner, M. (1991) 'Universals of behavioral development in relation to brain myelination.' *In:* Gibson, K.R., Petersen, A.C. (Eds.) *Brain Maturation and Cognitive Development: Comparative and Cross-cultural Perspectives*. New York: Aldine de Gruyter, pp. 181–223.

Kugler, P.N., Kelso, J.A.S., Turvey, M.T. (1980) 'On the concept of coordinative structures as dissipative structures: I. Theoretical lines of convergence.' *In:* Stelmach, G.E., Requin, J. (Eds.) *Tutorials in Motor Behavior*. New York: North-Holland, pp. 3–47.

Langendorfer, S. (1987) 'Prelongitudinal screening of overarm striking development performed under two environmental conditions.' *In:* Clark, J.E., Humphrey, J.H. (Eds.) *Advances in Motor Development Research*. New York: AMS Press, pp. 17–47.

Lerner, R.M. (1978) 'Nature, nurture, and dynamic interactionism.' *Human Development*, **21**, 1–20.

Lewis, V.A., Bryant, P.E. (1982) 'Touch and vision in normal and Down's syndrome babies.' *Perception*, **11**, 691–701.

Lydic, J.S., Steele, C. (1979) 'Assessment of the quality of sitting and gait patterns in children with Down's syndrome.' *Physical Therapy*, **59**, 1489–1494.

McGraw, M.B. (1932) 'From reflex to muscular control in the assumption of an erect posture and ambulation in the human infant.' *Child Development*, **3**, 291–297.

—— (1943) *The Neuromuscular Maturation of the Human Infant*. (Reprinted 1990 as *Classics in Developmental Medicine No. 4*. London: Mac Keith Press.)

Merzenich, M.M., Kaas, J.H. (1980) 'Principles of organization of sensory-perceptual systems in mammals.' *Progress in Psychobiology and Physiological Psychology*, **9**, 1–42.

—— Allard, T.T., Jenkins, W.M. (1990) 'Neural ontogeny of higher brain function: implications of some recent neurophysiological findings.' *In:* Franzn, O., Westman, P. (Eds.) *Information Processing in the Somatosensory System*. London: Macmillan, pp. 293–311.

Mounoud, P., Vinter, A. (1981) 'Representation and sensorimotor development.' *In:* Butterworth, G. (Ed.) *Infancy and Epistemology; an Evaluation of Piaget's Theory*. Brighton, Sussex: Harvester Press, pp. 200–235.

Newell, K.M., Scully, D.M., McDonald, P.V., Baillargeon, R. (1989a) 'Task constraints and infant grip configurations.' *Developmental Psychobiology*, **22**, 817–831.

—— —— Tenenbaum, F., Hardiman, S. (1989b) 'Body scale and the development of prehension.' *Developmental Psychobiology*, **22**, 1–13.

Oller, D.K. (1980) 'The emergence of the sounds of speech in infancy.' *In:* Yeni-Komshian, G., Kavanagh, J., Ferguson, C. (Eds.) *Child Phonology: Vol.1, Production*. New York: Academic Press, pp. 93–112.

—— (1986) 'Metaphonology and infant vocalizations.' *In:* Lindblom, B., Zetterstrom, R. (Eds.) *Precursors of Early Speech*. New York: Stockton Press, pp. 21–36.

Peiper, A. (1963) *Cerebral Function in Infancy and Childhood*. New York: Consultants Bureau.

Piaget, J. (1952) *The Origins of Intelligence in Children*. New York: International Universities Press.

Raibert, M.H. (1986) *Legged Robots That Balance*. Cambridge, MA: MIT Press.

Reeke, G.N., Sporns, O. (1990) 'Selectionist models of perceptual and motor systems and implications for functionalist theories of brain function.' *Physica D*, **42**, 347–364.

—— Finkel, L.H., Sporns, O., Edelman, G.M. (1990a) 'Synthetic neural modelling: a multi-level approach to brain complexity.' *In:* Edelman, G.M., Gall, W.E., Cowan, W.M. (Eds.) *Signal and Sense: Local and Global Order in Perceptual Maps*. New York: Wiley, pp. 607–707.

343

—— Sporns, O., Edelman, G.M. (1990b) 'Synthetic neural modeling: the 'Darwin' series of recognition automata.' *Proceedings of the IEEE*, **78**, 1498–1530.

Roberton, M.A. (1977) 'Stability of stage categorizations across trials: implications for the 'stage theory' of overarm throw development.' *Journal of Human Movement Studies*, **3**, 49–59.

—— (1978) 'Longitudinal evidence for developmental stages in the forceful overarm throw.' *Journal of Human Movement Studies*, **4**, 167–175.

Schmidt, R.A. (1975) 'A schema theory of discrete motor skill learning.' *Psychological Review*, **82**, 225–260.

Schöner, G., Kelso, J.A.S. (1988) 'Dynamic pattern generation in behavioral and neural systems.' *Science*, **239**, 1513–1520.

Seefeldt, V., Haubenstricker, J. (1982) 'Patterns, phases, or stages: an analytical model for the study of developmental movement.' *In:* Kelso, J.A.S., Clark, J.E. (Eds.) *The Development of Movement Control and Co-Ordination.* New York: John Wiley & Sons, pp. 309–318.

Shirley, M.M. (1931) *The First Two Years: a Study of 25 Babies. Postural and Locomotor Development, Vol 1.* Minneapolis: University of Minnesota Press.

Sporns, O., Edelman, G.M. (1993) 'Solving Bernstein's problem: a proposal for the development of coordinated movement by selection.' *Child Development*, **64**, 960–981.

Stark, R. (1980) 'Stages of development in the first year of life.' *In:* Yeni-Komshian, G., Kavanagh, J., Ferguson, C. (Eds.) Child Phonology. Vol.1, Productions. New York: Academic Press, pp. 73–92.

Sutherland, D.H., Olshen, R., Cooper, L., Woo, S.L-Y. (1980) 'The development of mature gait.' *Journal of Bone and Joint Surgery*, **62A**, 336–353.

Thelen, E. (1986) 'Treadmill-elicited stepping in seven-month-old infants.' *Child Development*, **57**, 1498–1506.

—— (1995) 'Motor development: a new synthesis.' *American Psychologist*, **50**, 79–95.

—— (1996) 'The improvising infant: learning about learning to move. *In:* Merrens, M.R., Brannigan, G.G. (Eds.) *The Developmental Psychologists: Research Adventures Across the Life Span.* New York: McGraw Hill, pp. 21–35.

—— Cooke, D.W. (1987) 'The relationship between newborn stepping and later locomotion: a new interpretation.' *Developmental Medicine and Child Neurology*, **29**, 380–393.

—— Ulrich, B.D. (1991) 'Hidden skills: a dynamic systems analysis of treadmill stepping during the first year.' *Society for Research in Child Development Monographs*, **56**, (1), 1–98.

—— Fisher, D.M., Ridley-Johnson, R. (1984) 'The relationship between physical growth and a newborn reflex.' *Infant Behavior and Development*, **7**, 479–493.

—— Skala, K., Kelso, J.A.S. (1987a) 'The dynamic nature of early coordination: evidence from bilateral leg movements in young infants.' *Developmental Psychobiology*, **23**, 179–186.

—— Ulrich, B.D., Niles, D. (1987b) 'Bilateral coordination in human infants: stepping on a split-belt treadmill.' *Journal of Experimental Psychology: Human Perception and Performance*, **13**, 405–410.

—— Bril, B., Brenière, Y. (1992) 'The emergence of heel strike in newly walking infants: a dynamic interpretation.' *In:* Woollacott, M., Horak, F. (Eds.) *Posture and Gait Control Mechanisms.* Eugene, OR: University of Oregon Books, pp. 334–337.

—— Corbetta, D., Kamm, K., Spencer, J.P., Schneider, K., Zernicke, R.F. (1993) 'The transition to reaching: mapping intention and intrinsic dynamics.' *Child Development*, **64**, 1058–1098.

Ulrich, B.D., Ulrich, D.A., Collier, D.H., Cole, E. (1992) 'Topology of supported stepping patterns in infants with Down syndrome.' *In: Proceedings of the Conference of the North American Society for the Psychology of Sport and Physical Activity, Pittsburgh, 1992. (Abstract.)*

—— —— Collier, D.H., Cole, E.L. (1995b) 'Developmental shifts in the ability of infants with Down syndrome to produce treadmill steps.' *Physical Therapy*, **75**, 14–23.

—— —— Angulo-Kinzler, R., Chapman, D.D. (in press) 'Sensitivity of infants with and without Down syndrome to intrinsic dynamics.' *Research Quarterly for Exercise and Sport.*

Vereijken, B. (1991) *The Dynamics of Skill Acquisition.* Meppel, Amsterdam: Krips Repro.

—— Whiting, H.T.A., Beek, W.J. (1992) 'A dynamical systems approach to skill acquisition.' *Quarterly Journal of Experimental Psychology*, **45A**, 323–344.

von Bertalanffy, L. (1968) *General Systems Theory.* New York: George Braziller.

von Hofsten, C. (1984) 'Developmental changes in the organization of prereaching movements.' *Developmental Psychology*, **20**, 378–388.

—— (1989) 'Motor development as the development of systems: comments on the special section.' *Developmental Psychology*, **25**, 950–953.

Waddington, C.H. (1966) *Principles of Development and Differentiation.* New York: MacMillan.

344

Waldrop, M.M. (1992) *Complexity.* New York: Simon & Schuster.

Weiss, J.N., Garfinkel, A., Spano, M.L., Ditto, W.L. (1994) 'Chaos and chaos control in biology.' *Journal of Clinical Investigation*, **93**, 1355–1360.

Whiting, H.T.A. (Ed.) (1984) *Human Motor Actions: Bernstein Reassessed.* Amsterdam: North-Holland.

Wild, M. (1938) 'The behavior pattern of throwing and some observations concerning its course of development in children.' *Research Quarterly*, **9**, 20–24.

Williams, K. (1980) 'The developmental characteristics of a forward roll.' *Research Quarterly for Exercise and Sport*, **51**, 703–713.

Winfree, A. (1983) 'Sudden cardiac death: a problem in topology.' *Scientific American*, **248** (5), 144–160.

Winstein, C.J., Garfinkel, A. (1989) 'Qualitative dynamics of disordered human locomotion: a preliminary investigation.' *Journal of Motor Behavior*, **21**, 373–391.

Zanone, P.G., Kelso, J.A.S., Jeka, J.J. (1993) 'Concepts and methods for a dynamical approach to behavioral coordination and change.' *In:* Savelsbergh, G.J.P. (Ed.) *The Development of Coordination in Infancy.* Amsterdam: Elsevier Science, pp. 89–135.

Zimmerman, H.M. (1956) 'Characteristic likenesses and differences between skilled and non-skilled performance of the standing broad jump.' *Research Quarterly*, **27**, 352.

16
ADAPTIVE MODEL THEORY: CENTRAL PROCESSING IN ACQUISITION OF SKILL

P.D. Neilson, M.D. Neilson and N.J. O'Dwyer

Important as it is to reduce spasm and spasticity in cerebral palsy (CP) to prevent development of muscle contractures and joint deformities (Neilson and McCaughey 1982; Nash *et al.* 1989; O'Dwyer *et al.* 1989, 1994; Neilson 1993a), spasm and spasticity are not the primary causes of functional disability in CP (Neilson and O'Dwyer 1981, O'Dwyer and Neilson 1988, Vaughan *et al.* 1988). We are drawn to this conclusion after many years of investigating the processing of purposive movement in both normal and CP subjects by means of visual tracking experiments. Even in a one-dimensional tracking task using isometric electromyography to control response cursor position on a display screen, the tracking behaviour of CP subjects is grossly abnormal (Neilson *et al.* 1990). While able to contract muscles through the full range at normal speeds or faster, CP subjects generate tracking responses which are abnormal in amplitude and timing, and there is excessive inappropriate activity unrelated to the task. Normal subjects quickly adapt their tracking behaviour to compensate for the dynamics of the tracking system (McRuer and Krendel 1974; McRuer 1980; Neilson *et al.* 1985, 1992, 1995) but CP subjects have difficulty doing so. Apart from reduction in the amount of inappropriate activity, their tracking does not improve with practice (Neilson *et al.* 1990). Because abnormal tracking behaviour in muscles without tonic stretch reflexes (such as lip muscles) is the same as the abnormal behaviour measured in muscles with tonic stretch reflexes, such as jaw closing and elbow flexion muscles (Vaughan *et al.* 1988), we have shown that abnormal tonic stretch reflex mechanisms responsible for spasticity are not primarily responsible for the disruption of muscle control in tracking tasks.

Variability of tracking behaviour across subjects does not correlate with the level of spasticity, whereas it does correlate with functional ability (Neilson and O'Dwyer 1981, Neilson *et al.* 1990). At a cognitive level, CP subjects can appreciate the tracking task and can provide an accurate verbal description of it. We have observed informally that, when given a video game requiring only a verbal response, CP subjects perform as well as normal ones. Thus, while people with CP can appreciate the perceptual goals of purposive movement, their damaged central nervous system (CNS) is unable to generate the appropriate motor commands to achieve those goals.

Visual tracking provides a valuable experimental tool with which to investigate both normal and pathophysiological mechanisms underlying perceptual–motor performance and skill acquisition. To provide the necessary bridge between behavioural observation and neural processing of sensory–motor signals we have developed Adaptive Model Theory (AMT). This is a computational theory based on recent advances in the fields of adaptive signal processing (Widrow and Stearns 1985, Haykin 1986) and adaptive control of dynamic systems (Goodwin and Sin 1984, Åström and Wittenmark 1989, Isermann *et al.* 1992). We have constructed a computer model of these self-tuning processes (Neilson *et al.* 1992, 1995) and are currently comparing its behaviour with that of human subjects acquiring tracking skills under different conditions, *e.g.* with changing levels of predictability of target motion, with changing dynamics of the tracking system, and when learning new movement synergies to perform two-dimensional and dual tracking tasks (Alafaci 1992, Neilson *et al.* 1993, Oytam 1993, Foo 1994, Gow 1994, Ho 1994).

In what follows we present a didactic description of AMT. In the latter part of the chapter we use AMT as a framework to discuss the development of movement in the neonate and the disruption of motor development in CP.

Overview of adaptive model theory
AMT represents the CNS as an adaptive optimal controller which transforms an intermittently planned response trajectory into a set of motor commands by means of an inverse internal model of the system lying between those motor commands and the desired response.

Adaptive control
A system with constant characteristics can be made to generate any desired output simply by transforming a representation of that output through an exact inverse model of the system, then using that signal as the system's input. For a system with changing characteristics the same principle applies but the inverse model must now be continuously updated if the output is to remain correct. This is known as adaptive control. Adaptive control uses both feedback and feedforward processes. The feedforward pathway consists of adaptive filters which transform the desired output through a model of the inverse of the system's current characteristics to generate the required input. The feedback pathway incorporates the modelling process, consisting of adaptive filters which repeatedly adjust their parameters to match the input–output characteristics of the controlled system. The controller then uses these parameters to implement the correct inverse model.

Three parallel processing systems
In AMT, feedforward is incorporated in what we term the response execution (RE) system (Fig. 16.1). This contains the controlled system consisting of muscle, biomechanical and external systems, and a controller consisting of adaptive neural filters which implement an inverse model of the system currently being controlled. The controller transforms a desired response trajectory R^*, preplanned by the response planning (RP) system in terms of desired reafference, into an appropriate set of motor commands to drive the controlled system and generate exactly the desired response trajectory R^*.

The feedback pathway responsible for maintaining the accuracy of the inverse model is incorporated in the sensory analysis (SA) system. The SA system uses networks of adaptive neural filters to condense incoming information and to model the interrelationships within

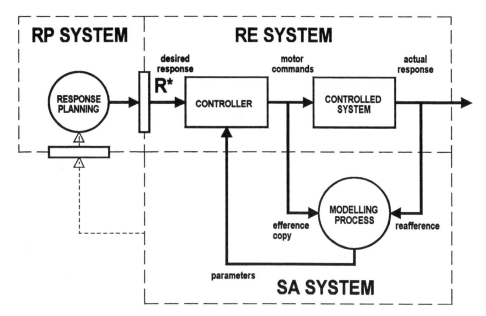

Fig. 16.1. Schematic diagram illustrating the three processing systems SA, RP and RE which are hypothesized to operate independently and in parallel. The rectangular blocks on the border of the RP system represent working memory buffers. Only modelling of the controlled system and adaptive tuning of the controller are illustrated. Other sensory inputs to the RP system are represented by the dashed line and open arrow.

and between these signals. Most importantly, this process includes information about the outgoing motor commands. Known as efference copy, this feedback and its relationship to the corresponding reafference from peripheral receptors provides the key for adaptive control. Within the circle labelled 'modelling process' in Figure 16.1, efference copy is transformed through an adaptive filter model of the controlled system to obtain the expected reafference. The adaptive filter circuitry automatically tunes its parameters to minimize the variance of the error between expected and actual reafference and hence matches the characteristics of the controlled system. These parameters are then used to tune the controller (inverse model) in the RE system.

As described previously (Neilson *et al.* 1992, 1995), the SA and RE systems operate continuously and in real-time in parallel with a third process, the RP system. This represents the lowest level of a hierarchy that potentially encompasses all cognitive processing (see Neilson *et al.* 1992). Diverse as this is, in the context of purposive movement the task of response planning ultimately reduces to the generation of a desired response trajectory. The three systems operate independently and in parallel with sequential transfer of information achieved by memory buffering (narrow rectangular blocks in Figure 16.1). The SA system writes information into working memory to be read independently by the RP system. Similarly, the RP system writes information into working memory to be read independently by the RE system.

348

The idea of sequential processing stages operating in parallel is by no means new in models of perceptual–motor performance (*e.g.* McLeod 1977, Requin 1980, Miller 1993). The conceptualization is underpinned by a wealth of evidence accumulated from the earliest reaction time experiments onwards that, while selecting an appropriate motor response, a subject is able simultaneously to execute a response to a previous stimulus and detect and register in memory a subsequent stimulus which may appear and disappear during the current reaction time (see Welford 1980). Likewise, the idea of memory buffering has strong support from neurophysiological experimentation. In delayed response tasks involving monkeys, for example, certain neurons in the prefrontal cortex possess 'memory fields'. When a visual target disappears from view, individual prefrontal neurons switch into an active state producing electrical activity at more than twice the baseline rate. They remain active until the end of the delay period (3–6 seconds) when the monkey delivers its response (Goldman-Rakic 1987, 1992).

We now review the processing underlying each of the three systems (for greater computational detail, see Neilson *et al.* 1992, 1995). Using results of computer simulations we show that processing within SA, RP and RE systems can be accomplished by biologically feasible neural networks which bear strong similarity from system to system. But whereas the networks of SA and RE systems function as adaptive filters operating continuously in real-time, the RP system requires a finite time to complete its processing and thereby introduces intermittency into movement control (Neilson *et al.* 1995). We begin with this system.

The response planning system
Studies of the 'psychological refractory period' in double stimulation reaction time experiments (Craik 1947; Welford 1952, 1980; Smith 1967; Pashler 1984, 1992; Pashler and Johnston 1989) provide convincing evidence for the existence of a central processing bottleneck associated with selection of a response. Accordingly, in AMT it is the RP system which limits and paces the flow of information from the occurrence of a perceptual event to the implementation of an appropriate motor response.

Elsewhere (Neilson *et al.* 1995) we describe a neural circuit called an optimum trajectory generator (OTG) which forms the basis of the RP system in our tracking simulations. The OTG plans an optimal S-shaped trajectory to move the response cursor from its current position into alignment with the predicted target motion. It employs a basic computational module similar to the adaptive filter circuit repeated throughout the SA and RE systems. Consequently, we are able to simulate the entire movement control system, comprised of SA, RP and RE, by a single basic circuit repeated many times in parallel. Simulation studies in our laboratory (Gow 1994, Ho 1994) demonstrate that the OTG generates responses with the same S-shaped temporal waveforms as actual error correction responses measured during visual tracking and reaching experiments. The OTG is designed such that the fastest desired response trajectory (R*) corresponds to a fast ballistic movement. Increasing the duration of R* alters the compromise between tracking accuracy (measured by mean square tracking error) and the mean square acceleration (the simulated equivalent of the input muscular energy required to accelerate an inertial system). The slower the movement the less muscular energy required but the greater the mean square tracking error. We have described the trajectories generated by the OTG mathematically (Neilson *et al.* 1995) and have shown that they match the speed–accuracy tradeoff inherent in Fitts' law and are consistent with trajectories based on minimization of mean square acceleration or jerk in reaching models (Nagasaki 1983; Hogan 1984, 1988; Flash and Hogan 1985; Hasan 1986; Meyer *et al.* 1988; Agarwal *et al.* 1993).

An important feature of the OTG is the finite interval of time (minimum 100ms) allocated for it to read sensory information from memory, generate an appropriate S-shaped R* and write this into memory ready for execution. The OTG plans only one R* at a time and does not commence planning a second until it has completed planning the first. This embodies our proposal in AMT that the RP system operates iteratively, generating a concatenated sequence of submovements, each preplanned on the basis of information available from the SA system and executed open-loop by the RE system. While one submovement is being executed by the RE system the next is being planned in parallel by the RP system, while the SA system processes external and internal information on which yet another submovement will be based. Although each system relies on the processing of another, it is the RP system that determines the duration of submovements and thereby paces the information transfer around the perceptual–motor loop.

Pashler (1992) showed that in reaction time tasks the response selection mechanism responsible for the central bottleneck is able to generate assemblages of motor behaviour as a single response without repeatedly employing the bottleneck mechanism. This is consistent with our findings comparing tracking performance across one- and two-dimensional visual tasks (Alafaci 1992, Oytam 1993, Chuin 1994, Foo 1994). Using a variety of experimental configurations, this work shows that subjects can control two degrees of freedom with no greater a central time delay (as measured by phase lag) than required to perform a one degree of freedom task, in agreement with a similar study by Navon *et al.* (1984). We incorporate this feature of response planning into AMT via what we term 'the N degrees of freedom controller hypothesis'. According to this hypothesis the RP system includes a finite number N of OTGs operating independently and in parallel. In the time required to plan a single R*, the RP system can plan a multidimensional desired response trajectory $R^* = [R_1^*, R_2^*, \ldots, R_N^*]$ and store it in memory ready for execution.

The value of N remains to be determined experimentally, but intuitively it is rather higher than the value of two demonstrated in the tracking studies. Consider, for example, the sprinter who jumps from the starting blocks using almost every muscle in the body with no greater reaction time than observed in lifting a single finger. The AMT solution to the degrees of freedom problem (Bernstein 1967) is discussed in the section on the RE system. Fundamental to that solution is the process of condensing highly redundant reafferent input into a smaller set of orthogonal feature signals, as described in the next section. Essentially, the SA system extracts feature signals which form the basis for a number of orthogonal coordinate systems. The dimension of the vector spaces defined by these coordinate systems has a maximum value N corresponding to the number of OTGs provided in RP. It is within the vector space of multimodal reafference that the RP system plans the desired response trajectory R*.

The sensory analysis system

The SA system continuously processes all exafferent and reafferent signals, in which there is massive redundancy. Its first task is to remove this redundancy, which we show is a necessary step before proceeding to the modelling of sensory and motor interrelationships that define the structure of the perceptual–motor world in general and which control perceptual–motor performance in particular. Because our focus here is on the control of purposive movement, we concentrate on the processing of reafferent information, but the same principles apply to exafference. As discussed elsewhere (Neilson *et al.* 1992), it is the ability of the SA system to form accurate sensory–motor models that allows exafference to be distinguished from reafference.

In Figure 16.1 we encapsulated the essential principle of SA as a modelling process using efference copy together with the corresponding reafference to establish the current controlled system characteristics. Figure 16.2 provides a more detailed picture. Efference consists of a multitude of motor command signals labelled **m** in vector notation. These form the input to a sequence of subsystems which together are equivalent to the controlled system in the original figure. Thus the motor commands **m** are transformed through the muscle control system **MCS** resulting in a set of muscle tension signals **t**, which operate on the biomechanical system **BM** to produce a set of signals θ representing the resulting movements of the body.*

When body movements are used to control an external system **E**, this generates a further set of multimodal reafferent signals **r**, such as the movements of the response cursor while tracking, or the visual, auditory and kinaesthetic consequences of accelerating a car around a corner. To provide adaptive feedforward control of the system consisting of **MCS**, **BM** and **E**, the dynamic relationships between the various sets of reafferent signals **m**, **t**, θ and **r** must be determined. To do this it is necessary first to remove the redundancy within each highly intercorrelated set of input signals. This is accomplished by the process of orthogonalization. As shown in Figure 16.2, each set of signals passes through an orthogonalizing network labelled *O* which extracts from each a smaller number of independently varying feature signals **M**, **T**, Θ and **R**. The number of independent feature signals in each set (*i.e.* the dimensions of the vectors **M**, **T**, Θ and **R**) corresponds to the number of degrees of freedom inherent in each of the original sets of redundant signals **m**, **t**, θ and **r** in the current task. We justify orthogonalization as an essential aspect of AMT on two counts. First, orthogonalization is the most efficient and numerically sound method for encoding the information in a large set of intercorrelated signals (see Neilson 1993b). Second, it is a mathematical necessity that intercorrelation within sets of variables be accounted for before the relationship between sets can be determined. Thus orthogonalization is an essential precursor to modelling the interrelationships in sensory input.**

*In some circumstances, muscle tension signals **t** will generate, in addition to or instead of body movements, changes in the force/pressure between body parts or against external objects. We used the signals θ to represent all such changes but for brevity refer to them generically as 'body movements'.

**For those more familiar with multivariate statistics than control theory, orthogonalization of input signals can be seen as a type of dynamic principal components analysis, while the separation of within-set and between-set relationships is essentially what occurs in canonical correlation, of which multiple regression and multivariate analysis of variance are special cases.

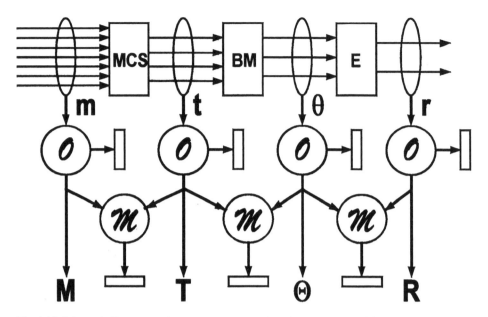

Fig. 16.2. Schematic illustration of sensory processing of reafferent signals. **MCS** = muscle control system, **BM** = biomechanical system, **E** = external system, **m** = feedback of motor commands, **t** = feedback of muscle tensions, θ = feedback of body movements, **r** = multimodal reafference, $\mathcal{O}$ = orthogonalizing network, $\mathcal{M}$ = modelling network, **M** = orthogonalized motor command feature signals, **T** = orthogonalized tension feature signals, Θ = orthogonalized body movement feature signals, **R** = orthogonalized multimodal reafferent feature signals. Small rectangular boxes represent working memory buffers. Arrows into small rectangular boxes represent parameter signals. Terms defined in text.

In Figure 16.2 we locate modelling networks $\mathcal{M}$ between the sequential sets of orthogonal feature signals **M** and **T**, **T** and Θ, and Θ and **R**. These networks identify the current characteristics of the controlled system comprising **MCS**, **BM** and **E** and, as discussed explicitly in the section on the response execution system below, provide the basis of feedforward control. While not depicted in the figures, we also construe there to be modelling between non-sequential sets of feature signals, such as **M** and **R**, **M** and Θ, **T** and **R**. Thus a nervous system deprived of kinaesthetic feedback of muscle tensions **T** and body movements Θ can still establish models of relationships between **M** and **R** and thereby retain control of the overall system. Such control in the absence of kinaesthetic feedback has been demonstrated experimentally (Taub and Berman 1968) and clinically (Rothwell *et al.* 1982). On the other hand, a system deprived of efference copy **M** is unable to transform any desired sensory response **T**, Θ or **R** into appropriate motor commands **M** to achieve it, and consequently movement control is severely impaired. As discussed later, disruption of the central processing of efference copy is the pathophysiological mechanism we believe underlies functional disability in CP.

The process of orthogonalization and the process of modelling, represented in Figure 16.2 by $\mathcal{O}$ and $\mathcal{M}$ respectively, can each be accomplished in computer simulations by networks of self-tuning adaptive filters (Neilson *et al.* 1992, 1995; Neilson 1993b). We now examine ways in which adaptive filtering might be implemented in the CNS. We find evidence for two types of adaptive neural circuitry. The first utilizes 'hard-wired' synaptic mechanisms which evolve slowly, the second employs modulatory signals to produce rapid changes in neural transmission.

Neural basis of slow adaptation

Sensory connections between the thalamus and sensory cortex have been shown to be organized into multiple but closely related sensory maps (Kaas *et al.* 1979). These sensory maps are not static anatomical constructs but are functional entities depending on the patterns of correlations between input signals (Merzenich and Jenkins 1993). Studies of neonatal synaptic plasticity in the visual cortex of kittens and monkeys (Hubel and Wiesel 1962, Wiesel and Hubel 1965, LeVay *et al.* 1978, Stryker and Harris 1986, Reiter and Stryker 1988) have shown that during a developmental time window of approximately three months in the cat (Frégnac and Imbert 1984), self-organizing synaptic mechanisms in the cortex strengthen synaptic inputs which fire synchronously and weaken those which fire asynchronously. The cortex segregates into columns of cells which respond to correlated inputs from the thalamus but with each column responding to a different and independently varying pattern of input. This leads to the formation of ocular dominance columns, orientation columns, colour blobs and other features. Stryker and Harris (1986) showed that the synaptic connections involved in the formation of ocular dominance columns can be strengthened or weakened depending on the correlation between electrical stimulation applied via implanted electrodes to the optic nerves in the kitten.

Experiments by Merzenich and colleagues have shown substantial reorganization of the topographic maps of skin surfaces within somatosensory cortical fields of adult rats, raccoons, cats and monkeys following various interventions (for reviews, see Clark *et al.* 1988, Jenkins *et al.* 1990, Merzenich and Jenkins 1993). In discussing the mechanisms of these self-organizing processes, Merzenich and colleagues have emphasized that, from the perspective of afferent inputs, input coincidence underlies the selection of effective inputs. They stress that cortical representations map probabilities of coincident or nearly coincident responses

The above gives ample evidence of the existence of self-tuning processes within the sensory system with the parameters of the filters being effectively 'wired-in' as the strength of synaptic connections. Such parameters describing relationships between sensory and motor signals computed on the basis of long-term correlations over days, weeks or months represent knowledge about the invariant (or only slowly changing) order in the perceived environment. These 'wired-in' networks form a type of 'world observer' from which noisy or partially sensed inputs can lead to a reconstruction (or estimation) of the most probable state of the perceived environment or, in other words, a most probable model of the world.

Piecemeal tuning of adaptive filters

Relationships between sensory signals, generally speaking, are more complex than those represented by the most probable model of the world. They are equivocal and vary momentarily depending on the task and conditions. A most probable model, derived long-term, cannot reflect the strong but fleeting relationships revealed by short-term correlations. To illustrate this, consider the problem of computing the relationship between two sine waves of identical frequency which for the first half of the analysis interval are in phase and for the second half are 180° out of phase. The correlation computed over the analysis interval is zero and the sine waves are said to be unrelated despite the fact that for half the time they are perfectly related with a correlation coefficient of one and for the remaining half they are perfectly related with a correlation coefficient of minus one.

The CNS is confronted with a similar problem in acquiring internal models of motor synergies and of sensory–motor relationships. During a particular reaching movement, for example, certain rotations at the shoulder and elbow will be highly correlated, but these correlations are fleeting and exist only for the duration of the movement, which may be as short as 0.5 seconds. If correlations were computed over intervals even as short as a few seconds during which different movements were executed, the rotations would appear to be uncorrelated and the CNS would be unable to identify the reduced degrees of freedom and the simplified sensory–motor relationships associated with the reaching synergy. Observations of baby movements during the first few months after birth reveal them to be highly variable, changing from one pattern of correlations between joint angles to another, often in rapid succession (Cooke and Thelen 1987). If the CNS is to learn about coordination by experiencing dynamic interactions with the outside world, it must possess mechanisms able to model fleeting, short-term relationships between sensory and motor signals.

We propose that the CNS is able to establish a repertoire of movement synergies and sensory–motor relationships in a 'piecemeal' fashion. That is, it is able to identify relationships between sensory and motor signals generated by a succession of changing motor behaviours. Each synergy and pattern of sensory–motor relationships appears for only a short interval of time and is then replaced by another pattern, but each behaviour is repeated on multiple occasions. For the CNS to compute relationships on a piecemeal basis it must be able to store sets of parameters in memory and retrieve them in association with the appropriate behaviour. The parameters can then be updated recursively during execution of the behaviour and returned to memory awaiting the next repetition. We now examine how such processes might be implemented.

Neural basis of rapid adaptation
To tune an adaptive filter to mimic the dynamic relationship between two signals it is necessary to pass one of the signals through the filter and then compare the output with the other signal. Self-tuning circuitry automatically tunes the parameters of the filter to minimize the discrepancy. We propose that in the CNS fast adapting neural filters are implemented by subcortical pathways through parts of the basal ganglia and cerebellum.

BASAL GANGLIA PATHWAYS
The basal ganglia are known to collect information from all over the neocortex and connect back into the supplementary motor area (SMA) and premotor regions of the cortex. The caudate nucleus and putamen receive topographically organized input from the full extent

of the neocortex (Côté and Crutcher 1991), and there is evidence for 'output channels' from the basal ganglia (Strick *et al.* 1993). Major outputs from the basal ganglia arise from the internal segments of the globus pallidus and from the pars reticulata of the substantia nigra and project to the ventrolateral, ventroanterior and mediodorsal nuclei of the thalamus. These in turn project to the prefrontal cortex, the premotor cortex, the SMA and the motor cortex, but the projections are predominantly to the more anterior regions (Graybiel 1990, DeLong 1993). Recordings of motor related cells in the basal ganglia (DeLong and Georgopoulos 1981, DeLong *et al.* 1983b) indicate that their discharge is not related to motor commands and muscle forces *per se*, but rather to the direction and extent of movements and to the perceptual goals of those movements (Crutcher and Alexander 1993).

The notion that transformation of neural signals through the basal ganglia is adaptive and modulated by central influences is not new. Inputs to the striatum from the thalamus and cortex end in modules analogous to the columns of the cortex (Graybiel 1984, Selemon *et al.* 1994). The smaller of these neurochemically specialized compartments are called 'striasomes' while the larger compartments are called 'the matrix'. The majority of cortical projections to the striatum terminate in the matrix compartments. The striasomes, on the other hand, receive cortical input from the limbic system and project to the dopaminergic neurons of the substantia nigra pars compacta. This is consistent with these inputs being derived ultimately from long-term memory via the limbic system. The striasomes appear to modulate the dopaminergic pathways. Dopamine-containing axon terminals are known to converge with corticostriatal axon terminals on individual dendritic spines of striatal neurons (Freund *et al.* 1984) and could determine the postsynaptic sensitivity of striatal cells to corticostriatal input. A leading hypothesis is that dopaminergic striatal terminals modulate the through traffic of the matrix compartment (Graybiel 1990), and this is supported by the observations (DeLong *et al.* 1983a, Grace and Bunney 1985) that neurons in the substantia nigra pars compacta fire at very low frequencies and are not tightly coupled to details of ongoing movements but are involved in the acquisition of learned movement (Kimura *et al.* 1993) and respond to rewards such as food and drink (Schultz *et al.* 1993). Physiological and anatomical findings imply that distinct input–output subsystems in the striatum are modulated by different sets of dopaminergic neurons and participate in neural processing related to movement control. Clinical and laboratory evidence suggests that the modulatory loops are crucial in controlling the motor functions of the basal ganglia (Graybiel 1990).

CEREBELLAR PATHWAYS

We have argued previously that adaptive neural pathways through parts of the cerebellum are involved (i) in the adaptive formation of models of motor synergies, muscle control systems and biomechanical systems by the SA system, and (ii) in feedforward control of movement in the RE system (Neilson *et al.* 1985, 1988, 1992). We have also provided detailed descriptions of corticocerebellar circuitry (Neilson *et al.* 1992) and shown that the arrangement of microzone circuits in parasagittal strips lying across the folia receiving synaptic inputs from parallel fibres running along the folia is consistent with the structure required to form adaptive neural filter models of multiple-input–multiple-output nonlinear dynamic relationships between neural signals. We argue that the sensitivity of Purkinje cell synapses to their parallel fibre inputs can be modulated by inferior olive climbing fibre inputs. The corticonuclear microcomplex (the functional module of the cerebellum—see Ito 1984, 1990) resembles the circuitry of an adaptive linear combiner described in adaptive signal processing literature (Widrow and Stearns 1985, Haykin 1986). We will not discuss mathematical details of the circuit here, but our computer simulation of it (Neilson *et al.* 1992) shows that it can automatically tune itself within a few seconds to form a model of a nonlinear dynamic relationship between input and output signals (Wu 1992). As pointed out by Ito (1990), based on the synaptic plasticity between parallel fibres and Purkinje cells, the functional module which occurs repeatedly in sagittal slices of the cerebellum can function as an adaptive controller and can be inserted in reflex arcs, command systems of voluntary motor control, and probably even in cortical systems performing mental activities. In AMT it is hypothesized that, similar to the modulatory role of the dopaminergic cells in the substantia nigra, the low frequency discharges of inferior olive cells modulate the transmission of information through the microzone circuits of the cerebellum by way of climbing fibre inputs.

Two types of central sensory signals

In summary, we see the SA system as establishing a repertoire of sensory–sensory and sensory–motor relationships. Sensory information is initially processed through adaptive filters with 'wired-in' parameters which reflect long-term most probable relationships. Thereafter processing is carried out by the adaptive filter circuits of the basal ganglia and cerebellum, the parameters of which are sustained by electrical activity which may change rapidly. This latter filtering process effectively provides two types of electrical signals representing sensory information. The first type corresponds to the orthogonal feature signals extracted by the self-tuning orthogonalizing networks. These provide task-dependent orthogonal coordinate systems which encode all the information presented redundantly by the receptor input signals. The second type of signal represents the parameters describing the relationships between neural signals and these provide perceptual knowledge about the structure of the world. For example, in stretching an elastic band, forces and movements are detected by sensory receptors but we have no difficulty perceiving the 'stiffness' of the band which is a parameter of the relationship between force and movement.

In the terminology used by Barlow (1994) when discussing the role of the neocortex, the two types of electrical signals mentioned above can be referred to as 'information' and 'knowledge', respectively. The orthogonal feature signals encode information about the particular environment, while the parameters represent knowledge about the structure of the environment and of the body in interaction with the environment. For example, when driving a car in the country as compared to the city, the visual feature signals encoding the scene are completely different but the rules of visual perspective represented by the relationships between visual signals (and hence by the parameter signals) remain unchanged.

The response execution system

In Figure 16.1 we depicted the RE system as a controller and a controlled system, its task being to transform the desired response trajectory $\mathbf{R}^*$ into an appropriate set of motor commands to produce a response $\mathbf{R}$ matching the desired $\mathbf{R}^*$. In Figure 16.2 we showed the

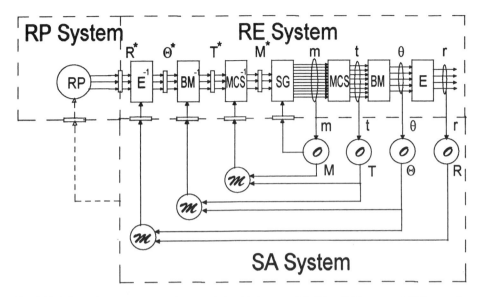

Fig. 16.3. Schematic diagram illustrating the relationship between SA, RP and RE systems. **MCS** = muscle control system; **BM** = biomechanical system; **E** = external system; **E**⁻¹ = internal model of inverse dynamics of **E**; **BM**⁻¹ = internal model of inverse dynamics of **BM**; **MCS**⁻¹ = internal model of inverse dynamics of **MCS**; 𝓜 = modelling networks; 𝒪 = orthogonalizing networks that transform efference copy **m**, muscle tensions **t**, body movements θ and multimodal reafference **r** into a reduced number of orthogonal feature signals **M**, **T**, Θ and **R**, respectively.

controlled system as a sequence of three subsystems, the muscle control system **MCS**, the biomechanical system **BM** and the external system **E**, and discussed how the sensory analysis processes of orthogonalization and modelling provide parameters defining the current characteristics of each subsystem. In Figure 16.3 we now show that these parameters serve to implement the inverse models of **E**, **BM** and **MCS**. These inverse models, denoted respectively by **E**⁻¹, **BM**⁻¹ and **MCS**⁻¹, together with a synergy generator **SG** (discussed below), are implemented as adaptive neural filters and form the feedforward controller within the RE system. Our initial discussion of RE concerns these feedforward processes. We subsequently show how the RE system also incorporates feedback processes in the form of reflexes which correct for unexpected disturbance forces and for inaccuracies in the feedforward models **BM**⁻¹ and **MCS**⁻¹.

Adaptive inverse models
Figure 16.3 shows the RE system operating in concert with the SA and RP systems in the context of an ongoing task such as pursuit tracking in which the requirement is to manipulate a control in such a way that a response cursor follows the path of the tracking target as accurately as possible. SA processes continuously orthogonalize the signals **m**, **t**, θ and **r** and model the relationships between the reduced sets of feature signals **M**, **T**, Θ and **R** to give the prevailing characteristics of subsystems **MCS**, **BM** and **E**. Any change in the

characteristics of a subsystem is transmitted in terms of new parameter signals which adapt the weights of the neural filters representing the equivalent inverse model. If the characteristics of the tracking equipment change, as happens if there is a change of gain between the subject's control and the response cursor, this is detected by SA as a change in the external system **E**, leading to a corresponding change in $\mathbf{E}^{-1}$ to restore correct feedforward control. Likewise, if a weight is attached to the subject's controlling arm, a change in the biomechanical system **BM** is detected and $\mathbf{BM}^{-1}$ altered accordingly. Effects such as fatigue, which alter the characteristics of the muscle control system **MCS**, will likewise bring about the appropriate change in $\mathbf{MCS}^{-1}$ via the continuous modelling processes of the SA system.

Provided the models $\mathbf{E}^{-1}$, $\mathbf{BM}^{-1}$ and $\mathbf{MCS}^{-1}$ remain accurate inverses of their counterparts **E**, **BM** and **MCS**, the RE system will generate the correct set of motor commands **M*** to move the tracking response cursor appropriately with a trajectory signalled visually by reafference **R** = **R***. Our computer simulations verify this performance. Yet to be discussed, however, is the generation of the set of highly redundant descending motor commands **m** from the smaller centrally derived set of orthogonalized motor commands **M***. We refer to this as synergy generation, accomplished by the process **SG** in Figure 16.3.

Synergy generation

A major theme in discussions of motor control is the issue of redundancy, or the so-called degrees of freedom problem described by Bernstein (1967), in which it is recognized that there are many different patterns of muscle activation which can be used to achieve a given perceptual goal. In terms of SA processes, we can restate the problem as there being many more descending motor pathways carrying signals **m** than there are independent reafferent responses **R**. In AMT the key step in solving this disparity is the process of orthogonalizing **m** to produce **M**, accompanied by the inverse process of using **M*** to produce **m** (Neilson 1993b). As shown in Figure 16.3, the orthogonalization of the redundant set of motor command signals **m** into the reduced set of independent feature signals **M** produces parameter signals which set the weights of the adaptive filter circuits of the synergy generator **SG**. In this way the small set of independently varying central command signals **M*** is transformed via divergent adaptive neural filter pathways into a large number of highly intercorrelated motor command signals **m** at the periphery. The generation of effective synergies thus depends on the effectiveness of the SA process of orthogonalization of redundant motor commands **m**, or rather, of their efference copy. As discussed later, we are of the opinion that disruption of these self-tuning processes involved in sensory analysis of efference copy is the primary cause of functional disability in cerebral palsy.

Task dependence

If purposive movement is generated by transforming a trajectory of desired reafference **R*** through a controller consisting of inverse models $\mathbf{E}^{-1}$, $\mathbf{BM}^{-1}$, $\mathbf{MCS}^{-1}$ and a synergy generator **SG**, it is clear that these controller elements will need to vary according to the particular task. Take the example of tracking discussed above. We have already indicated how the models $\mathbf{E}^{-1}$, $\mathbf{BM}^{-1}$ and $\mathbf{MCS}^{-1}$ can be tuned on-line and, if the task is unidimensional, requiring only a one degree of freedom movement of a manual control, the synergy generator **SG** will likewise be tuned throughout the task performance. Thus, while the models may alter, and alter dramatically as would occur with a large change in the gain of the tracking system **E**, they do so in a generic way, tied to the multimodal task-dependent coordinate space in which the desired response **R*** is planned. Such variation is distinct from the alteration in the models which must occur when the task itself is altered.

To continue with the tracking example, suppose the task is changed such that the manual control which previously moved vertically now moves horizontally. This requires a new synergy, not just an adjustment of the old one, with corresponding changes in the operative muscles and biomechanical characteristics **MCS** and **BM**, as well as a new relationship **E** between movement of the body and the corresponding movement of the response cursor. If the task is further changed to involve two-dimensional tracking movements, all of the models **MCS**, **BM** and **E** as well as the synergy generator **SG** will change again.

In general we see purposive movement as encompassing a repertoire of models which differ according to the task and which determine the N-dimensional coordinate system in which the RP system plans the desired trajectory of the multimodal reafference **R***. Such models are implemented by adaptive neural filters, and, thus far, we have shown the parameters from these filters as being supplied on-line by the SA system's processing of reafference during an ongoing task. In AMT we also see this 'short-term' modelling as informing a 'long-term' central store of modelled relationships. Once stored, parameters can be retrieved from long-term memory and used to tune the appropriate adaptive neural filters in the SA and RE systems to suit the task. Thus, based on previous experience, the CNS can adapt rapidly from one task to another by selecting appropriate parameters from memory to tune the adaptive neural filters throughout the SA and RE systems. During execution of the new task, sensory analysis of response feedback can fine-tune the retrieved models. In highly skilled movements, we see central influences as capable of modulating the characteristics of adaptive filters as rapidly as from one submovement to the next, although this is an extreme example. Thus the adaptability and flexibility of the skilled performer can be attributed in large measure to the ability of the CNS to select from a variety of previously learned synergies and sensory–motor models and to transfer smoothly from one to another in rapid succession. Sophisticated motor skills, such as speech or playing a musical instrument, not only involve learning the many synergies and sensory–motor relationships involved but also require learning the transitions from one synergy to the next in the correct sequence and with the right melody.

While changing models from task to task may seem a complication, it also brings the simplification that much of the planning and sequencing of movement can remain independent of the precise means by which it will be effected, a view not without support (*e.g.* Garcia-Colera and Semjen 1988, Glencross *et al.* 1995). Consider the planning and sequencing involved in steering a car or writing with a pen. In these examples the desired reafferent signal **R*** is planned principally in terms of how the equipment is to respond, rather than in terms of the exact body movement that generates the response. Thus we plan our steering in terms of the translation of the visual field as the car turns the corner, and our writing in terms of the visual feedback of the characters traced out on the page. While these visual

359

consequences are condensed by SA orthogonalization with other correlated sensory information such as kinaesthetic, labyrinthine and cutaneous input, the primacy of the visual planning allows us readily to transfer our steering skill to a bus or our writing skill to a blackboard simply by invoking the appropriate synergies and inverse models.

When we change from car to bus or from pen on paper to chalk on board, we are clearly dealing with a changed relationship between multimodal reafference $\mathbf{R}$ and kinaesthetic feedback Θ as a result of changing the external system $\mathbf{E}$. Many learned skills such as riding a bicycle, sailing a boat or flying a plane obviously require the acquisition of a repertoire of appropriate inverse models $\mathbf{E}^{-1}$. Not so obvious is the fact that much of human performance that does not involve external equipment nevertheless still requires the acquisition of inverse models $\mathbf{E}^{-1}$. Take a reaching movement for example. Here the relationships between the multimodal feedback of hand position and kinaesthetic feedback of joint angles and muscle lengths provides an internal model of the inverse kinematics of the arm (Hollerbach 1982; Hogan 1984, 1985). Likewise in speech, the relationships between auditory and kinaesthetic feedback provide a model of the inverse dynamics of the acoustic characteristics of the vocal tract. The blind and the deaf are unable to form these external models and, if made to see or hear, are unable to perform appropriately despite their new sensory input until an adequate $\mathbf{E}^{-1}$ is acquired.

There is another reason for describing the relationships between multimodal reafference and kinaesthetic feedback as an inverse model of an external system. As we show below, the model $\mathbf{E}^{-1}$ differs from the other models $\mathbf{BM}^{-1}$, $\mathbf{MCS}^{-1}$ and $\mathbf{SG}$ involved in feedforward control of movement by the way in which it is integrated with reflex feedback systems. In a sense, the inverse model $\mathbf{E}^{-1}$ is external to the reflex feedback systems while the other models are not. Errors in the inverse models $\mathbf{BM}^{-1}$ and $\mathbf{MCS}^{-1}$ bring reflex feedback systems into play while errors in $\mathbf{E}^{-1}$ do not. Errors in $\mathbf{E}^{-1}$ can only be corrected intermittently at reaction time rates via feedback through the perceptual–motor loop which, in general, involves the external world.

Feedforward and feedback control within RE

As well as feedforward via the inverse models $\mathbf{E}^{-1}$, $\mathbf{BM}^{-1}$ and $\mathbf{MCS}^{-1}$ as discussed above, the RE system also includes reflex (feedback) systems which lessen the effects of model errors and disturbances and which regulate the effective shock absorber characteristics (stiffness and viscosity) of the joints. Figure 16.4 shows this interplay between feedforward and feedback control within the RE system.

The rectangular block at top left in Figure 16.4 represents working memory holding the multimodal desired response trajectories, $\mathbf{R}^* = [R_1^*, R_2^*, \ldots, R_N^*]$, preplanned by the RP system. Similarly to Figure 16.3, $\mathbf{R}^*$ is transformed by $\mathbf{E}^{-1}$ into a vector of desired body movements Θ^*. As previously, $\mathbf{E}^{-1}$ functions as an adaptive model of the inverse dynamics of the external system. It is assumed that the internal model $\mathbf{E}^{-1}$ has sufficient parallel pathways to implement an N-input to N-output transformation, where N corresponds to the number of OTGs in the RP system, equivalent to the maximum number of degrees of freedom that can be controlled simultaneously. The relationships between $\mathbf{R}^*$ and Θ^* depend on the motor synergy involved and vary from task to task. Consequently, the internal model $\mathbf{E}^{-1}$

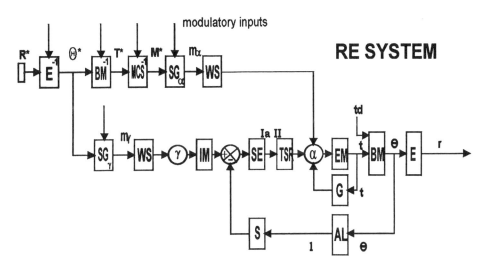

modulatory inputs

RE SYSTEM

Fig. 16.4. Block diagram illustrating the flow of information hypothesized in AMT to be involved in feedback and feedforward control of movement within the response execution (RE) system. E^{-1} = inverse model of external system; BM^{-1} = inverse model of biomechanical system; MCS^{-1} = inverse model of muscle control system; SG_α = synergy generator for alpha-motoneurons; SG_γ = synergy generator for gamma-motoneurons; WS = wired-in synergies; α = alpha-motoneurons; γ = gamma-motoneurons; IM = intrafusal muscles; SE = primary and secondary spindle endings; TSR = tonic stretch reflex pathways; EM = extrafusal muscles; G = Golgi tendon organ feedback; BM = biomechanical system; E = external system; AL = transformation of joint angles into muscle lengths; S = viscoelastic coupling of spindle endings to extrafusal muscle lengths; R^* = high level desired response trajectory; Θ^* = high level desired body movement trajectory; T^* = high level desired tension trajectory; M^* = high level desired motor command trajectory; m_α = motor commands to alpha-motoneurons; m_γ = motor commands to gamma-motoneurons; Ia and II = afferent activity from primary and secondary spindle endings; t = tensions developed by skeletal muscles; td = disturbance tensions; θ = body movements; r = multimodal sensory response; l = length of extrafusal muscles.

must be able to change from one submovement to the next to suit the task. Descending modulation of E^{-1} is indicated by the modulatory input arrow at the top of the E^{-1} block in Figure 16.4.

The desired kinaesthetic response trajectory Θ^* provides a source of excitation for both closed-loop control via gamma-motoneurons and open-loop control via alpha-motoneurons. Let us follow the flow of information along the top of Figure 16.4 for pathways involved in open-loop feedforward control of alpha-motoneurons. Similarly to Figure 16.3, BM^{-1} transforms the desired body movements Θ^* into required muscle tensions T^*, and MCS^{-1} transforms T^* into appropriate motor commands M^*.

Figure 16.4 shows a synergy generator in both the alpha and gamma pathways. The adaptive synergy generator SG_α contains slave copies of adaptive models of the dynamic relationships between the m_α signals formed by orthogonalizing circuits within the SA system. Central modulatory control of the adaptive neural filter circuits in SG_α is indicated by the input arrow at the top of the block in Figure 16.4. Similarly, the block labelled SG_γ in

Figure 16.4 functions as an adaptive self-tuning synergy generator for gamma motor commands $\mathbf{m}_\gamma$, and the central modulatory control is indicated by the input arrow at the top of that block.

Thus the blocks $\mathbf{BM^{-1}}$, $\mathbf{MCS^{-1}}$ and $\mathbf{SG}_\alpha$ along the top of Figure 16.4 represent self-tuning pathways modulated by central influences to provide open-loop adaptive feedforward control of muscles via alpha-motoneurons. In line with proposals by Ito (1984, 1990), Miyamoto *et al.* (1988), Kawato (1992, 1993), Kawato and Gomi (1992) and Shidara *et al.* (1993), we locate these adaptive transformations in the cerebellum (Neilson *et al.* 1985, 1992). The suggestion in AMT that the outputs of feedforward adaptive neural pathways through the cerebellum provide inputs to brainstem and motor cortex centres which, in turn, drive descending pathways (both directly and indirectly via interneurons and wired-in synergies) to alpha-motoneurons, is supported by the observation that local stimulation of regions of the cerebellar nuclei providing thalamocortical projections in alert baboons causes muscle contractions with a fine somatotopic organization of either simple or synergistic movements depending on the site of stimulation (Rispal-Padel *et al.* 1983).

Alpha–gamma coupling

The desired movement signals Θ^* at the output of $\mathbf{E^{-1}}$ provide an appropriate drive to gamma-motoneurons via the adaptive synergy generator $\mathbf{SG}_\gamma$. Since the descending drives to alpha- and gamma-motoneurons derive from a common set of central signals Θ^*, it follows that they are dynamically related, hence the appropriateness of the term 'alpha–gamma coupling'. However, relationships between alpha and gamma are variable and can change between submovements depending on changes in the adaptive models $\mathbf{BM^{-1}}$, $\mathbf{MCS^{-1}}$, $\mathbf{SG}_\alpha$ and $\mathbf{SG}_\gamma$. Descending drives to alpha- and gamma-motoneurons can be transformed by circuitry within the cortex, brainstem or spinal cord. We label such circuitry 'wired-in synergies' (WS) in Figure 16.4. Brainstem circuits for controlling conjugate, vergence and accommodation movements of the eyes provide an excellent example of such wired-in synergies.

If the adaptive models $\mathbf{BM^{-1}}$ and $\mathbf{MCS^{-1}}$ in the feedforward pathways are accurately tuned, the open-loop drive $\mathbf{m}_\alpha$ to the alpha-motoneurons α will cause the extrafusal muscle fibres $\mathbf{EM}$ to develop exactly the tensions $\mathbf{t}$ required to pull on the prevailing biomechanical loads $\mathbf{BM}$ to produce the desired body movements θ and changes in muscle lengths $\mathbf{l}$. When coupled to muscle spindle endings by viscoelastic elements $\mathbf{S}$, these muscle length changes unload mechanical deformations of spindle endings by exactly the amounts required to offset deformations caused by contractions of the intrafusal muscle fibres $\mathbf{IM}$ driven by descending motor commands $\mathbf{m}_\gamma$. Consequently, as demonstrated by Vallbo (1981), the spindle endings maintain a steady discharge rate throughout the movement despite the length change of the muscle, and there is no changing stretch reflex contribution to the movement. On the other hand, if the movement deviates from the desired change in muscle lengths Θ^* either because of unexpected disturbance forces $\mathbf{td}$, internally generated perturbations, or inaccuracies in the feedforward models $\mathbf{BM^{-1}}$ or $\mathbf{MCS^{-1}}$, then the unloading of spindle endings will not exactly compensate for deformation caused by fusimotor drive, and the stretch reflex will be brought into play. As learning progresses and the internal models become more accurate, one might expect a gradual transfer from feedback control via gamma-motoneurons and the stretch reflex loop, to open-loop feedforward control via more direct descending pathways to alpha-motoneurons. This is in keeping with Matthew's (1972) servo assist theory of muscle control, but it extends the theory by providing insights as to how the appropriate alpha–gamma coupling might be formed within the CNS.

Sensory–motor modelling in motor development

Ultrasound studies have revealed that as early as eight to ten weeks after conception, the human fetus already has a repertoire of movements (J.I.P. DeVries *et al.* 1985) produced by a coordinated pattern of activity involving many muscles. At this time the brain is early in development. Proliferation of neurons within the ventricular zone occurs from approximately two to four months after conception, and the peak time period for the migration of neurons from their sites of origin in ventricular and subventricular zones to sites where they will reside for life awaits the third to fifth month of gestation (Volpe 1987). The coordination of muscles involved in fetal movements is unlikely to be attributable to processes similar to those of the mature CNS. More likely, they are produced by 'pattern generators' within the evolving spinal cord, brainstem and cortical circuitry.

This is probably true not only for fetal movements but also for many neonatal responses which persist for the first few months. Cioni and Prechtl (1988) demonstrated a progression of spontaneous movements from fetus to neonate with no delineation evident between fetus and newborn infant. Likewise, Thelen and colleagues (Thelen and Fisher 1982, 1983; Thelen *et al.* 1984; Thelen 1985) showed that stepping and kicking movements of infants during the first few months exhibit the same temporal patterning and rates as those of newborn babies. From comparison of locomotor patterns of spinal cats with walking in the human neonate (elicitable within minutes of birth) Trevarthen (1984) argued that the human pattern is produced in rudimentary form by autonomous activity of the spinal 'locomotor generator' and that effective walking is 'learned' as supraspinal control circuits mature and establish influence over spinal circuits. These views are consistent with the conclusions of Thelen (1985, 1990) that the process assembles under some higher level task goal and that the emergence of walking is the expression of a self-organizing system, the outcome of which depends on factors including pattern generation, tone, articulator differentiation, muscle strength, postural control, visual flow sensitivity, body constraints and motivation.

The spurt of motor development that occurs at about two months after birth probably coincides with developmental processes within the CNS, such as myelination of the cerebellar peduncles and striatum (Yakovlev and Lecours 1967). According to AMT, these maturational processes bring into play cortico-basal ganglia and cortico-cerebellar mechanisms associated with the self-tuning modelling circuitry of the SA system described earlier. Initially, the signals driving the modelling circuitry correspond to the activity produced by the pattern generators underlying fetal and neonatal responses. Driven by the correlations between these sensory and motor signals, the modelling circuits automatically tune themselves, piecemeal, to extract feature signals and to form internal models (albeit inaccurate ones) of the interrelationships. Once established, even in rudimentary form, the models provide the infant with the necessary neural pathways to transform desired perceptual outcomes (for example, the smell of the breast, the taste of the milk) into appropriate motor commands to generate them. Initially, the goal-directed movements roughly mimic the neonatal responses, but, with time, amplitude and timing of desired response trajectories and the correlations between them can be altered. Feedback from these novel responses drives the modelling circuitry leading to the formation and storage of an expanding repertoire of new synergies and sensory–motor models. According to this view, the pattern generators function as a 'bootstrap' to initiate motor development.

Our computer simulations of this process are revealing interesting phenomena. Starting with responses from pattern generators, it is a simple matter for the adaptive filter circuits within the simulator to tune themselves to extract orthogonal feature signals and form models of the synergies and sensory–motor relationships involved. Using the coordinate system of these feature signals, a simulated RP system then generates desired response trajectories which are transformed into appropriate motor commands by the previously formed sensory–motor models and synergy generators. Once the simulator has acquired sensory–motor models and synergy generators for performing, for example, a two degrees of freedom tracking task, it can be forced to learn new synergies with either one or two degrees of freedom by introducing new dynamic relationships between the target waveforms. Initially, tracking errors introduced by the now incorrect 'start-up' synergy are detected and corrected by feedback through the perceptual–motor loop. These corrections alter the correlations between outgoing motor commands and response feedback and this, in turn, retunes the adaptive filters in the orthogonalizing and modelling networks. As the parameters of the synergy generator tune towards their correct values, feedback correction via the perceptual–motor loop diminishes. Thus we have a method by which the simulator, starting from pattern generator responses, develops a repertoire of new synergies.

Much is yet to be learned from these simulations. We have observed already, however, that the number of degrees of freedom in the new synergy is always equal to or less than the number of degrees of freedom in the 'seed' synergy. In other words, we cannot achieve formation of a new synergy with a large number of degrees of freedom by having the simulator practise a task with a smaller number. This is not to deny that reducing the degrees of freedom is a simplifying strategy adopted in learning new skills (Bernstein 1967, Vereijken et al. 1992). It does, however, question the mechanisms for acquiring synergies with increased degrees of freedom and suggests a role for the random high degrees of freedom movements produced by the newborn infant.

Disruption of motor development in cerebral palsy

In several major studies of the neuropathology of CP (e.g. Towbin 1960, Christensen and Melchior 1967), the cerebral cortex, hemispheric white matter, basal ganglia and cerebellum were all found to be affected in varying combinations. Although their occurrence was recognized, lesions of the cerebral white matter received little emphasis despite the realization that white matter is particularly vulnerable to insult in the immature brain (e.g. DeReuck et al. 1972, Gilles 1977, Rorke 1982). In perinatal autopsies, white matter damage has been reported to be far more frequent than signs of neuronal necrosis. The importance of infarcts in the white matter surrounding the lateral ventricles (periventricular leukomalacia or PVL) in CP was emphasized by Banker and Larroche (1962) and has been verified subsequently by others (DeReuck *et al.* 1972, Armstrong and Norman 1974, Pape and Wigglesworth 1979). The most frequent location of structural abnormalities observed during computer tomographic studies in children and adolescents with CP is the cerebral white matter, especially in the periventricular region, and there are similar findings from brain scan studies of preterm infants and asphyxiated term infants who subsequently developed CP (Adsett *et al.* 1985; L.S. DeVries *et al.* 1985, 1987; Volpe *et al.* 1985; Weindling *et al.* 1985; Wilson and Steiner 1986). Indeed, PVL revealed by routine ultrasound brain scans in preterm infants is proving a valuable early predictor of CP. But why should such relatively small infarcts in the deep white matter lead to the familiar syndrome of motor disabilities in CP?

According to AMT, there are critically important cortico-basal ganglia and cortico-cerebellar pathways involved in self-tuning adaptive neural filter circuits. These circuits are essential both for acquisition of motor synergies and for formation of sensory–motor models for transforming perceptual goals into appropriate motor commands. We propose that the periventricular lesions associated with CP are critically located to disrupt the self-tuning circuits involved in processing efference copy. Consequently, during the period of motor development, ability of the damaged CNS to model motor synergies and compute relationships between motor commands and sensory consequences is impaired on the motor side. Normal motor development cannot occur. The damaged CNS is unable to transform an appreciation of the desired perceptual goals of a movement into appropriate motor commands. Inappropriate motor commands are generated instead. With the damaged CNS unable to form accurate internal models of its own muscle control systems, interaction between feedback and feedforward mechanisms provides an explanation of why reflex activity is abnormal in CP. However, there are other factors involving faulty descending modulation of reflex transmission which must be taken into account when discussing CP spasticity (Neilson 1993a). Moreover, since the damaged CNS is unable to relate feedback from inappropriate movements with the motor commands that generated them, such movements are experienced as involuntary, as if caused by unknown external disturbances rather than by internally generated motor commands. With the CNS unable to distinguish between external disturbances and internal model errors, inaccurate models lead to illusions of movement (Lackner and Graybiel 1981, 1984). Increased levels of cocontraction and increased stretch reflex sensitivities may, in part, represent the body's normal stiffening reaction to protect against perceived external disturbances. Thus spasticity and inappropriate movement may be aspects of CP secondary to the primary cause of functional disability. Lesions in the periventricular white matter around the time of birth may disrupt sensory–motor modelling on the motor side, and consequently, although able to model the external world and the body biomechanics, the CNS is unable to form accurate sensory–motor models required to transform perceptual goals of movements into appropriate synergies of motor commands to achieve them. Normal motor development would be impaired, and the syndrome of motor control known as CP would follow. The crucial question is, how can lesions in the periventricular white matter be bypassed so that normal functioning of cortico-basal ganglia and cortico-cerebellar neuronal circuitry is restored from as early an age as possible?

REFERENCES

Adsett, D.B., Fitz, C.R., Hill, A. (1985) 'Hypoxic–ischaemic cerebral injury in the term newborn: correlation of CT findings with neurological outcome.' *Developmental Medicine and Child Neurology*, **27**, 155–160.

Agarwal, G.C., Logsdon, J.B., Corcos, D.M., Gottlieb, G.L. (1993) 'Speed–accuracy trade-off in human movements: an optimal control viewpoint.' *In:* Newell K.M., Corcos, D.M. (Eds.) *Variability and Motor Control.* Champaign, IL: Human Kinetics Publishers, pp. 117–155.

Alafaci, M. (1992) 'Identification of the human operator functioning as an adaptive self-tuning regulator.' (Thesis, School of Electrical Engineering, University of New South Wales.)

Armstrong, D., Norman, M.G. (1974) 'Periventricular leucomalacia in neonates. Complications and sequelae.' *Archives of Disease in Childhood*, **49**, 367–375.

Åström, K.J., Wittenmark, B. (1989) *Adaptive Control.* Reading, Berkshire: Addison–Wesley.

Banker, B.Q., Larroche, J-C. (1962) 'Periventricular leukomalacia of infancy. A form of neonatal anoxic encephalopathy.' *Archives of Neurology*, **7**, 386–410.

Barlow, H. (1994) 'What is the computational goal of the neocortex?' *In:* Koch, C., Davis, J.L. (Eds.) *Large-Scale Neuronal Theories of the Brain.* Cambridge, MA: MIT Press, pp. 1–22.

Bernstein, N. (1967) *The Co-ordination and Regulation of Movements.* London: Pergamon Press.

Christensen, E., Melchior, J.C. (1967) *Cerebral Palsy—a Clinical and Neuropathological Study. Clinics in Developmental Medicine No. 25.* London: Spastics Society Medical Education and Information Unit.

Chuin, K.Y. (1994) 'Studies of human eye–hand coordination. One dimension vs two dimension tracking.' (Thesis, School of Electrical Engineering, University of New South Wales.)

Cioni, G., Prechtl, H.F.R. (1988) 'Development of posture and motility in preterm infants.' *In:* von Euler, C., Forssberg, H., Lagercrantz, H. (Eds.) *Neurobiology of Early Infant Behaviour.* Stockholm: Stockton Press, pp. 69–77.

Clark, S.A., Allard, T., Jenkins, W.M., Merzenich, M.M. (1988) 'Receptive fields in the body-surface map in adult cortex defined by temporally correlated inputs.' *Nature*, **332**, 444–445.

Cooke, D.W., Thelen, E. (1987) 'Newborn stepping: a review of puzzling infant co-ordination.' *Developmental Medicine and Child Neurology*, **29**, 399–404.

Côté, L., Crutcher, M.D. (1991) 'The basal ganglia.' *In:* Kandel, E.R., Schwartz, J.H., Jessell, T.M. (Eds.) *Principles of Neural Science, 3rd Edn.* New York: Elsevier, pp. 647–659.

Craik, K.J.W. (1947) 'Theory of the human operator in control systems. I. The operator as an engineering system.' *British Journal of Psychology*, **38**, 56–61.

Crutcher, M.D., Alexander, G.E. (1993) 'Neuronal correlates of a sensorimotor transformation in monkey putamen.' *In:* Mano, N., Hamada, I., DeLong, M.R. (Eds.) *Role of the Cerebellum and Basal Ganglia in Voluntary Movement.* Amsterdam: Excerpta Medica, pp. 71–81.

DeLong, M.R. (1993) 'Overview of basal ganglia function.' *In:* Mano, N., Hamada, I., DeLong, M.R. (Eds.) *Role of the Cerebellum and Basal Ganglia in Voluntary Movement.* Amsterdam: Excerpta Medica, pp. 65–70.

—— Georgopoulos, A.P. (1981) 'Motor functions of the basal ganglia.' *In:* Brooks, V.B. (Ed.) *Handbook of Physiology. Section I. The Nervous System. Vol. II. Motor Control, Part 2.* Bethesda, MD: American Physiological Society, pp. 1017–1061.

—— Crutcher, M.D., Georgopoulos, A.P. (1983a) 'Relations between movement and single cell discharge in the substantia nigra of the behaving monkey.' *Journal of Neuroscience*, **3**, 1599–1606.

—— Georgopoulos, A.P., Crutcher, M.D. (1983b) 'Cortico-basal ganglia relations and coding of motor performance.' *In:* Massion, J., Paillard, J., Schultz, W., Wiesendanger, M. (Eds.) *Neural Coding of Motor Performance (Experimental Brain Research*, Suppl. 7), Berlin: Springer-Verlag, pp. 30–40.

DeReuck, J., Chattha, A.S., Richardson, E.P. (1972) 'Pathogenesis and evolution of periventricular leukomalacia in infancy.' *Archives of Neurology*, **27**, 229–236.

DeVries, J.I.P., Visser, G.H.A., Prechtl, H.F.R. (1985) 'The emergence of fetal behaviour. II. Quantitative aspects.' *Early Human Development*, **12**, 99–120.

DeVries, L.S., Dubowitz, L.M.S., Dubowitz, V., Kaiser, A., Lary, S., Silverman, M., Whitelaw, A., Wigglesworth, J.S. (1985) 'Predictive value of cranial ultrasound in the newborn baby: a reappraisal.' *Lancet*, **2**, 137–140.

—— Connell, J.A., Dubowitz, L.M.S., Oozeer, R.C., Dubowitz, V., Pennock, J. (1987) 'Neurological, electrophysiological and MRI abnormalities in infants with extensive cystic leukomalacia.' *Neuropediatrics*, **18**, 61–66.

Flash, T., Hogan, N. (1985) 'The coordination of arm movements: an experimentally confirmed mathematical model.' *Journal of Neuroscience*, **5**, 1688–1703.

366

Foo, H.C. (1994) 'Studies of human eye–hand co-ordination: one-dimension compatible and incompatible versus two-dimension incompatible tracking.' (Thesis, School of Electrical Engineering, University of New South Wales.)

Frégnac, Y., Imbert, M. (1984) 'Development of neuronal selectivity in primary visual cortex of cat.' *Physiological Reviews*, **64**, 325–434.

Freund, T.F., Powell, J.F., Smith, A.D. (1984) 'Tyrosine hydroxylase-immunoreactive boutons in synaptic contact with identified striatonigral neurons, with particular reference to dendritic spines.' *Neuroscience*, **13**, 1189–1215.

Garcia-Colera, A., Semjen, A. (1988) 'Distributed planning of movement sequences.' *Journal of Motor Behavior*, **20**, 341–367.

Gilles, F.H. (1977) 'Lesions attributed to perinatal asphyxia in the human.' *In:* Gluck, L. (Ed.) *Intrauterine Asphyxia and the Developing Fetal Brain.* Chicago: Year Book, pp. 99–107.

Glencross, D.J., Piek, J.P., Barrett, N.C. (1995) 'The coordination of bimanual synchronous and alternating tapping sequences.' *Journal of Motor Behavior*, **27**, 3–15.

Goldman-Rakic, P.S. (1987) 'Circuitry of primate prefrontal cortex and the regulation of behavior by representational memory.' *In:* Plum, F. (Ed.) *Handbook of Physiology: Section 1. The Nervous System. Vol. V. Higher Functions of the Brain, Part 1.* Bethesda, MD: American Physiological Society, pp. 373–417.

—— (1992) 'Working memory and the mind.' *Scientific American*, **267**, 110–117.

Goodwin, G.C., Sin, K.S. (1984) *Adaptive Filtering Prediction and Control.* Englewood Cliffs, NJ: Prentice–Hall.

Gow, S.M. (1994) 'Computer analysis of hand-writing movements.' (Thesis, School of Electrical Engineering, University of New South Wales.)

Grace, A.A., Bunney, B.S. (1985) 'Opposing effects of striatonigral feedback pathways on midbrain dopamine cell activity.' *Brain Research*, **333**, 271–284.

Graybiel, A.M. (1984) 'Neurochemically specified subsystems in the basal ganglia.' *In:* Evered, D., O'Connor, M. (Eds.) *Functions of the Basal Ganglia. Ciba Foundation Symposium 107.* London: Pitman, pp. 114–143.

—— (1990) 'The basal ganglia and the initiation of movement.' *Revue Neurologique*, **146**, 570–574.

Hasan, Z. (1986) 'Optimized movement trajectories and joint stiffness in unperturbed, inertially loaded movements.' *Biological Cybernetics*, **53**, 373–382.

Haykin, S. (1986) *Adaptive Filter Theory.* Englewood Cliffs, NJ: Prentice–Hall.

Ho, K.T. (1994) 'Studies of human eye–hand coordination optimal control of hand movement.' (Thesis, School of Electrical Engineering, University of New South Wales.)

Hogan, N, (1984) 'An organizing principle for a class of voluntary movements.' *Journal of Neuroscience*, **4**, 2745–2754.

—— (1985) 'Impedance control: an approach to manipulation. Part I: Theory.' *Journal of Dynamic Systems, Measurement, and Control*, **107**, 1–7.

—— (1988) 'Planning and execution of multijoint movements.' *Canadian Journal of Physiology and Pharmacology*, **66**, 508–517.

Hollerbach, J.M. (1982) 'Computers, brains and the control of movement.' *Trends in Neuroscience*, **5**, 189–192.

Hubel, D.H., Wiesel, T.N. (1962) 'Receptive fields, binocular interaction and functional architecture in the cat's visual cortex.' *Journal of Physiology*, **160**, 106–154.

Isermann, R., Lachmann, K.-H., Matko, D. (1992) *Adaptive Control Systems* New York: Prentice–Hall.

Ito, M. (1984) *The Cerebellum and Neural Control.* New York: Raven Press.

—— (1990) 'A new physiological concept on cerebellum.' *Revue Neurologique*, **146**, 564–569.

Jenkins, W.M., Merzenich, M.M., Recanzone, G. (1990) 'Neocortical representational dynamics in adult primates: implications for neuropsychology.' *Neuropsychologica*, **28**, 573–584.

Kaas, J.H., Nelson, R.J., Sur, M., Lin, C-S., Merzenich, M.M. (1979) 'Multiple representations of the body within the primary somatosensory cortex of primates.' *Science*, **204**, 521–523.

Kawato, M. (1992) 'Optimization and learning in neural networks for formation and control of coordinated movement.' *In:* Meyer, D.E., Kornblum, S. (Eds.) *Attention and Performance XIV: Synergies in Experimental Psychology, Artificial Intelligence, and Cognitive Neuroscience.* Cambridge, MA: MIT Press, pp. 821–849.

—— (1993) 'Inverse dynamics model in the cerebellum.' *In: Proceedings of 1993 International Joint Conference on Neural Networks, Nagoya, Japan.* Piscataway, NJ: Institute of Electrical and Electronic Engineers, pp. 1329–1335.

—— Gomi, H. (1992) 'A computational model of four regions of the cerebellum based on feedback-error learning.' *Biological Cybernetics*, **68**, 95–103.

Kimura, M., Aosaki, T., Graybiel, A. (1993) 'Role of basal ganglia in the acquisition and initiation of learned movement.' *In:* Mano, N., Hamada, I., DeLong, M.R. (Eds.) *Role of the Cerebellum and Basal Ganglia in Voluntary Movement.* Amsterdam: Excerpta Medica, pp. 83–87.

Lackner, J.R., Graybiel, A. (1981) 'Illusions of postural, visual, and aircraft motion elicited by deep knee bends in the increased gravitoinertial force phase of parabolic flight. Evidence for dynamic sensory-motor calibration to earth gravity force levels.' *Experimental Brain Research*, **44**, 312–316.

———— (1984) 'Perception of body weight and body mass at twice earth-gravity acceleration levels.' *Brain*, **107**, 133–144.

LeVay, S., Stryker, M.P., Shatz, C.J. (1978) 'Ocular dominance columns and their development in layer IV of the cat's visual cortex: a quantitative study.' *Journal of Comparative Neurology*, **179**, 223–244.

Matthews, P.B.C. (1972) *Mammalian Muscle Receptors and Their Central Actions.* London: Arnold.

McLeod, P. (1977) 'Parallel processing and the psychological refractory period.' *Acta Psychologica*, **41**, 381–396.

McRuer, D.T. (1980) 'Human dynamics in man–machine systems.' *Automatica*, **16**, 237–253.

—— Krendel, E.S. (1974) *Mathematical Models of Human Pilot Behavior. AGARDograph No. 188.* Neuilly-sur-Seine, France: Advisory Group for Aerospace Research and Development/NATO Aerospace Medical Panel.

Merzenich, M.M., Jenkins, W.M. (1993) 'Reorganization of cortical representations of the hand following alterations of skin inputs induced by nerve injury, skin island transfers, and experience.' *Journal of Hand Therapy*, **6**, 89–104.

Meyer, D.E., Abrams, R.A., Kornblum, S, Wright, C.E., Smith, J.E.K. (1988) 'Optimality in human motor performance: ideal control of rapid aimed movements.' *Psychological Review*, **95**, 340–370.

Miller, J. (1993) ' A queue-series model for reaction time, with discrete-stage and continuous-flow models as special cases.' *Psychological Review*, **100**, 702–715.

Miyamoto, H., Kawato, M., Setoyama, T., Suzuki, R. (1988) 'Feedback-error-learning neural network for trajectory control of a robotic manipulator.' *Neural Networks*, **1**, 251–256.

Nash, J., Neilson, P.D., O'Dwyer, N.J. (1989) 'Reducing spasticity to control muscle contracture of children with cerebral palsy.' *Developmental Medicine and Child Neurology*, **31**, 471–480.

Navon, D., Gopher, D., Chillag, N., Spitz, G. (1984) 'On separability of and interference between tracking dimensions in dual-axis tracking.' *Journal of Motor Behavior*, **16**, 364–391.

Neilson, P.D. (1993a) 'Tonic stretch reflex in normal subjects and in cerebral palsy.' *In:* Gandevia, S.C., Burke, D., Anthony, M. (Eds.) *Science and Practice in Clinical Neurology.* Cambridge: Cambridge University Press, pp. 169–190.

—— (1993b) 'The problem of redundancy in movement control: the adaptive model theory approach.' *Psychological Research*, **55**, 99–106.

—— McCaughey, J. (1982) 'Self-regulation of spasm and spasticity in cerebral palsy.' *Journal of Neurology, Neurosurgery and Psychiatry*, **45**, 320–330.

—— O'Dwyer, N.J. (1981) 'Pathophysiology of dysarthria in cerebral palsy.' *Journal of Neurology, Neurosurgery and Psychiatry*, **44**, 1013–1019.

—— Neilson, M.D., O'Dwyer, N.J. (1985) 'Acquisition of motor skill in tracking tasks: learning internal models.' *In:* Russell, D.G., Abernethy, B. (Eds.) *Motor Memory and Control.* Dunedin, New Zealand: Human Performance Associates, pp. 25–36.

———— (1988) 'Internal models and intermittency: a theoretical account of human tracking behavior.' *Biological Cybernetics*, **58**, 101–112.

—— O'Dwyer, N.J., Nash, J. (1990) 'Control of isometric muscle activity in cerebral palsy.' *Developmental Medicine and Child Neurology*, **32**, 778–788.

—— Neilson, M.D., O'Dwyer, N.J. (1992) 'Adaptive model theory: Application to disorders of motor control.' *In:* Summers, J.J. (Ed.) *Approaches to the Study of Motor Control and Learning.* Amsterdam: Elsevier, pp. 495–548.

————— (1993) 'What limits high speed tracking performance?' *Human Movement Science*, **12**, 85–109.

————— (1995) 'Adaptive optimal control of human tracking.' *In:* Glencross, D., Piek, J. (Eds.) *Motor Control and Sensory-Motor Integration: Issues and Directions. Advances in Psychology Series No. 111.* Amsterdam: Elsevier, pp. 97–140.

Nagasaki, H. (1983) 'Asymmetric velocity and acceleration profiles of human arm movements.' *Experimental Brain Research*, **74**, 319–326.

O'Dwyer, N.J., Neilson, P.D. (1988) 'Voluntary muscle control in normal and athetoid dysarthric speakers.' *Brain*, **111**, 877–899.

—— —— Nash, J. (1989) 'Mechanisms of muscle growth related to muscle contracture in cerebral palsy.' *Developmental Medicine and Child Neurology*, **31**, 543–547.

—— —— —— (1994) 'Reduction of spasticity in cerebral palsy using feedback of the tonic stretch reflex: a controlled study.' *Developmental Medicine and Child Neurology*, **36**, 770–786.

Oytam, Y. (1993) 'Human eye–hand coordination (etch-a-sketch mode).' (Thesis, School of Electrical Engineering, University of New South Wales.)

Pape, K.E., Wigglesworth, J.S. (1979) *Haemorrhage, Ischaemia and the Perinatal Brain. Clinics in Developmental Medicine No. 69/70.* London: Spastics International Medical Publications.

Pashler, H. (1984) 'Processing stages in overlapping tasks: evidence for a central bottleneck.' *Journal of Experimental Psychology: Human Perception and Performance*, **10**, 358–377.

Pashler, H. (1992) 'Dual-task interference and elementary mental mechanisms.' *In:* Meyer, D.E., Kornblum, S. (Eds.) *Attention and Performance XIV: Synergies in Experimental Psychology, Artificial Intelligence, and Cognitive Neuroscience.* Cambridge, MA: MIT Press, pp. 245–264.

—— Johnston, J.C. (1989) 'Chronometric evidence for central postponement in temporally overlapping tasks.' *Quarterly Journal of Experimental Psychology*, **41A**, 19–45.

Reiter, H.O., Stryker, M.P. (1988) 'Neural plasticity without postsynaptic action potentials: less-active inputs become dominant when kitten visual cortical cells are pharmacologically inhibited.' *Proceedings of the National Academy of Sciences of the USA*, **85**, 3623–3627.

Requin, J. (1980) 'Toward a psychobiology of preparation for action.' *In:* Stelmach, G.E., Requin, J. (Eds.) *Tutorials in Motor Behavior.* Amsterdam: North Holland, pp. 373–398.

Rispal-Padel, L., Cicirata, F., Pons, J-C. (1983) 'Neocerebellar synergies.' *In:* Massion, J., Paillard, J., Schultz, W., Wiesendanger, M. (Eds.) *Neural Coding of Motor Performance. (Experimental Brain Research Suppl. 7.)* Berlin: Springer-Verlag, pp. 213–223.

Rorke, L.B. (1982) *Pathology of Perinatal Brain Injury.* New York: Raven Press.

Rothwell, J.C., Traub, M.M., Day, B.L., Obeso, J.A., Thomas, P.K., Marsden, C.D. (1982) 'Manual motor performance in a deafferented man.' *Brain*, **105**, 515–542.

Schultz, W., Ljungberg, T., Apicella, P., Romo, R., Mirenowicz, J., Hollerman, J.R. (1993) 'Primate dopamine neurons: From movement to motivation and back.' *In:* Mano, N., Hamada, I., DeLong, M.R. (Eds.) *Role of the Cerebellum and Basal Ganglia in Voluntary Movement.* Amsterdam: Excerpta Medica, pp. 89–97.

Selemon, L.D., Gottlieb, J.P., Goldman-Rakic, P.S. (1994) 'Islands and striosomes in the neostriatum of the rhesus monkey: non-equivalent compartments.' *Neuroscience*, **58**, 183–192.

Shidara, M., Kawano, K., Gomi, H., Kawato, M. (1993) 'Inverse-dynamics model eye movement control by Purkinje cells in the cerebellum.' *Nature*, **365** (2), 50–52.

Smith, M.C. (1967) 'Theories of the psychological refractory period.' *Psychological Bulletin*, **67**, 202–213.

Strick, P.L., Hoover, J.E., Mushiake, H. (1993) 'Evidence for "output channels" in the basal ganglia and cerebellum.' *In:* Mano, N., Hamada, I., DeLong, M.R. (Eds.) *Role of the Cerebellum and Basal Ganglia in Voluntary Movement.* Amsterdam: Excerpta Medica, pp. 171–180.

Stryker, M.P., Harris, W.A. (1986) 'Binocular impulse blockade prevents the formation of ocular dominance columns in cat visual cortex.' *Journal of Neuroscience*, **6**, 2117–2133.

Taub, E., Berman, A.J. (1968) 'Movement and learning in the absence of sensory feedback.' *In:* Freedman, S.J. (Ed.) *The Neuropsychology of Spatially Oriented Behavior.* Homewood, IL: Dorsey, pp. 173–192.

Thelen, E. (1985) 'Developmental origins of motor coordination: leg movements in human infants.' *Developmental Psychobiology*, **18**, 1–18.

—— (1990) 'Coupling perception and action in the development of skill: a dynamic approach.' *In:* Bloch, H., Bertenthal, B. (Eds.) *Sensory-motor Organization and Development in Infancy and Early Childhood.* Dordrecht: Kluwer, pp. 273–283.

—— Fisher, D.M. (1982) 'Newborn stepping: an explanation for a 'disappearing' reflex.' *Developmental Psychology*, **18**, 760–775.

—— —— (1983) 'From spontaneous to instrumental behavior: kinematic analysis of movement changes during very early learning.' *Child Development*, **54**, 129–140.

—— —— Ridley-Johnson, R. (1984) 'The relationship between physical growth and a newborn reflex.' *Infant Behavior and Development*, **7**, 479–493.

Towbin, A. (1960) *The Pathology of Cerebral Palsy. The Causes and Underlying Nature of the Disorder.* Springfield, IL: Charles C. Thomas.

Trevarthen, C. (1984) 'How control of movement develops.' *In:* Whiting, H.T.A. (Ed.) *Human Motor Actions – Bernstein Reassessed.* Amsterdam: Elsevier, pp. 223–262.

369

Vallbo, Å. (1981) 'Basic patterns of muscle spindle discharge in man.' *In:* Taylor, A., Prochazka, A. (Eds.) *Muscle Receptors and Movement.* London: Macmillan, pp. 263–275.

Vaughan, C.W., Neilson, P.D., O'Dwyer, N.J. (1988) 'Motor control deficits of orofacial muscles in cerebral palsy.' *Journal of Neurology, Neurosurgery and Psychiatry,* **51**, 534–539.

Vereijken, B., van Emmerik, R.E.A., Whiting, H.T.A., Newell, K.M. (1992) 'Free(z)ing degrees of freedom in skill acquisition.' *Journal of Motor Behavior,* **24**, 133–142.

Volpe, J.J. (1987) *Neurology of the Newborn. 2nd Edn.* Philadelphia: W.B. Saunders.

—— Herscovitch, P., Perlman, J.M., Kreusser, K.L., Raichle, M.E. (1985) 'Positron emission tomography in the asphyxiated term newborn: parasagittal impairment of cerebral blood flow.' *Annals of Neurology,* **17**, 287–296.

Weindling, A.M., Rochefort, M.J., Calvert, S.A., Fok, T-F., Wilkinson, A. (1985) 'Development of cerebral palsy after ultrasonographic detection of periventricular cysts in the newborn.' *Developmental Medicine and Child Neurology,* **27**, 800–806.

Welford, A.T. (1952) 'The "psychological refractory period" and the timing of high-speed performance—a review and a theory.' *British Journal of Psychology,* **43**, 2–19.

—— (1980) 'The single channel hypothesis.' *In:* Welford, A.T. (Ed.) *Reaction Times.* London: Academic Press, pp. 215–252.

Widrow, B., Stearns, S.D. (1985) *Adaptive Signal Processing.* Englewood Cliffs, NJ: Prentice–Hall.

Wiesel, T.N., Hubel, D.H. (1965) 'Comparison of the effects of unilateral and bilateral eye closure on cortical unit responses in kittens.' *Journal of Neurophysiology,* **28**, 1029–1040.

Wilson, D.A., Steiner, R.E. (1986) 'Periventricular leukomalacia: evaluation with MR imaging.' *Radiology,* **160**, 507–511.

Wu, J.Z. (1992) 'Real-time modelling of non-linear systems with non-white, non-Gaussian inputs.' (Thesis, School of Electrical Engineering, University of New South Wales.)

Yakovlev, P.I., Lecours, A-R. (1967) 'The myelogenetic cycles of regional maturation of the brain.' *In:* Minkowski, A. (Ed.) *Regional Development of the Brain in Early Life.* Oxford: Blackwell Scientific, pp. 3–70.

INDEX